Tissue Expansion in Reconstructive and Aesthetic Surgery

Gordon H. Sasaki, M.D., F.A.C.S.
Diplomat of the American Board of Plastic Surgery
Plastic and Reconstructive Surgery
Pasadena, California
Provisional Courtesy Staff
Loma Linda University
Loma Linda, California

with 859 illustrations

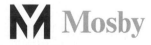

St. Louis Baltimore Boston Carlsbad Chicago Naples New York Philadelphia Portland
London Madrid Mexico City Singapore Sydney Tokyo Toronto Wiesbaden

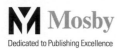

Dedicated to Publishing Excellence

A Times Mirror
Company

Senior Editor: Laurel Craven
Developmental Editor: Wendy Buckwalter
Project Manager: Peggy Fagen
Production Editor: Marian S. Hall
Designer: Dave Zielinski
Manufacturing Manager: William A. Winneberger, Jr.

Printed in Canada
Composition by Graphic World, Inc.
Lithography/color film by Graphic World, Inc.
Printing/binding by Friesens Printing Company

Mosby, Inc.
11830 Westline Industrial Drive
St. Louis, Missouri 63146

Library of Congress Cataloging-in-Publication Data

Sasaki, Gordon H.
    Tissue expansion in reconstructive and aesthetic surgery / Gordon
  H. Sasaki.
      p. cm.
    Includes bibliographical references and index.
    ISBN 0-8016-4320-1
    1. Tissue expansion.   I. Title.
    [DNLM: 1. Tissue Expansion—methods.   WO 600 S252t 1998]
  RD119.5.T57S27   1998
  617.9′5—dc21
  DNLM/DLC
  for Library of Congress   98-9639
                                                                  CIP

98 99 00 01 02 / 9 8 7 6 5 4 3 2 1

Foreword

This observation by Emerson introduced the foreword to the first edition of Grabb and Smith's classic textbook, *Plastic Surgery,* in 1968. The authors of those few introductory pages, Drs. Herbert Conway and Reed Dingman, were accurate in noting, "The need for replacement of tissues and organs presents the medical profession with one of its greatest challenges . . ." and prescient in their prediction, ". . . [T]he solution of replacement of parts of the human body" will come from a combination of clinical experience and new technology.

The process we have come to call tissue expansion certainly is not the only example of this evolution, but it illustrates a quantum leap in our ability to care for patients by manipulating normal biological processes in a beneficial way. In a single generation of surgeons, tissue expansion has progressed from its early days as a clinical oddity to its current status as one of the basic techniques taught to every plastic surgery resident. Although other specialties have incorporated some specific aspects or capabilities of tissue expansion, it is legitimate for plastic surgeons to claim its inception and development as their own. The author of this text, Dr. Gordon Sasaki, has provided us with a book for this age, and it is a fine one.

This book is a huge undertaking, encompassing the author's extensive and scholarly experience with the technique and the patients who have experienced it in his care. In its scope and style, it is reminiscent of Dr. Ralph Millard's *Cleft Craft,* and I use the analogy in the full knowledge that this sets an extremely high standard. I believe that readers expecting such quality and depth will find both in this book. It describes a large array of very specific and different clinical applications of tissue expansion, ranging from male-pattern baldness to expansion of radiated tissue, and does so from the perspective of a single author. The reader is afforded an extensive review of the world's literature pertaining to tissue expansion and, perhaps more importantly, the author's experience in operating rooms and laboratories throughout the world. As

an invited guest of leading medical centers, research institutes, and other facilities, the author has seen and discussed the successes and failures of other surgeons firsthand. We and our patients are the ultimate beneficiaries of those hundreds of thousands of miles he has traveled.

A certain symmetry exists in citing Bill Grabb's exhaustive and scholarly work, *Plastic Surgery,* in reference to this present volume. I first met Gordon Sasaki 20 years ago, when Dr. Grabb invited him to Ann Arbor, Michigan, for a mini-symposium centered on various hamartomas. A second component of the meeting, seemingly unrelated, was to present and discuss our rudimentary experience at Michigan with the new technique of tissue expansion. Gordon and I were both residents then, and it was clear that Dr. Grabb invited him to this meeting primarily to recruit him to our faculty after completion of his training. Bill viewed him as one of the brightest and most talented young plastic surgeons in the world, an appraisal only a few of us thought was not entirely compatible with his ultimate decision to stay in California. We knew of Dr. Sasaki's experience with hamartomas, the topic selected in his honor, but he amazed us all by taking an active part in discussions during the tissue expansion component of the program. As we soon learned, Gordon already was quite familiar with the work of another California plastic surgeon, Dr. Chedomir Radovan; he and Dr. Radovan had jointly treated several patients, and Gordon already was taking some of the basic questions of tissue expansion to the laboratory. I am not aware of any subsequent symposium on tissue expansion, national or international, that has not included Dr. Sasaki as a principal speaker. In fact, he has been the chairman of most of them.

It is an honor to write this foreword. My scientific objectivity here may be somewhat attenuated by my long friendship with Gordon Sasaki, but I believe that this is balanced by the many opportunities I have had to observe the skill, precision, and integrity of his work. As tissue expansion and other forms of tissue engineering find new and even more dramatic clinical applications in the next century, this book will be a foundation for new generations of surgeons and other conductors of the biological symphonies we are beginning to hear and understand. Many biological "dividends" can be gained by the judicious manipulation of living tissue at its many levels of organization, and tissue expansion is a prime example.

This book will prove valuable in current practice, but I believe that its second and third editions will be as different from it as later editions of Grabb and Smith's *Plastic Surgery* differed from their 1968 predecessor. This is clearly the best news of all: tissue expansion and other means of inducing desired biological responses will become more and more sophisticated, and new books will never contain them all.

Eric David Austad, M.D.
Ann Arbor, Michigan

Preface

The continual quest of the plastic and reconstructive surgeon is to provide ideal tissue replacement for defects. To achieve this goal, surgeons historically have developed means to transfer tissues that range from "simple" (skin grafts) to "complex" (composite free tissue transfer) procedures. Because all results must be judged by both functional and aesthetic considerations, it is the surgeon's responsibility to select a method that is reliable, safe, and efficacious, and that produces the least morbidity at the donor site.

Chronic, or long-term, tissue expansion represents a major innovation to plastic and reconstructive surgery and has evolved since 1976 from an experimental curiosity to a worldwide procedure in more than 75,000 cases. In some areas of the world, tissue expansion has been slow to develop because of unavailability of expanders due to problems of supply and distribution and to restrictive administrative regulations and because of inadequate current technical information for surgeons.

It has been stated that tissue expansion provides tissue with a near-perfect color match, texture, sensation, and special adnexal characteristics (hair, sweat and sebaceous glands). In most patients, donor tissue is expanded from adjacent areas. However, the use of regional and free tissue transfer of expanded flaps is testing the surgeon's ingenuity to solve selected distant soft tissue problems. Expansion of skin for harvesting large areas of skin grafts provides increased coverage material for specific defects. The hallmark of tissue expansion remains the creation of a hemispheric domed flap, which produces a minimal or no donor site scar after the transfer.

Chronic tissue expansion is a labor-intensive procedure. It requires that the surgeon understand the proper indications for expansion, master the technical aspects of the procedure, anticipate and convey to the patient the benefits and limitations of the procedure, and be able to manage complications. It is important to remember that not every defect should be managed surgically by long-term tissue expansion and that not all patients are candidates for this reconstructive procedure.

In contrast to the technique of chronic expansion, short-term or intraoperative expansion takes advantage of the intrinsic ability of skin to stretch. The increased amount of tissue generated by acute expansion can be used to cover smaller defects. Intraoperative expansion also may be used as a more effective means to accomplish serial reduction when long-term expansion is not an acceptable alternative for the reconstructive patient. The benefits and limitations of intraoperative expansion in aesthetic surgery still are being explored, especially in the areas of male-pattern baldness, cervicofacial rhytidoplasty, and augmentation mammoplasty. Correction of problems in aesthetic surgery using intraoperative expansion has been partially successful and requires further experience to determine its potential.

As with every new concept and technique, the "pendulum of theory and experience" is continually swinging back and forth. It presently is unclear where tissue expansion will ultimately find itself within the surgeon's armamentarium. Refinements in technique and use in areas of the body other than skin, such as nerve and vessel elongation and bladder and intestinal reconstruction, continue to evolve and challenge the surgeon to satisfy the requirements of reconstruction.

Acknowledgments

I undertook to write this book to record my personal 15-year experience in tissue expansion for residents in training and practitioners. This effort acknowledges the contributions from my plastic surgical colleagues who, through communications, meetings, and shared surgical endeavors, generously shared their experiences and philosophies with me. This book represents an amalgamation of all our ideas.

A partial list of tissue "expansionists" throughout the world includes the following colleagues: from Brazil, J. Anger and R. Gemperli; from Finland, R. Nordstrom; from France, J. Aubert, G. Magalon, and D. Marchac; from Germany, W. Audretsch, E. Biemer, K. Exner, and G. Lemperle; from Great Britain, O. Fenton and D. Sharpe; from Italy, A. Azzolini; from Japan, T. Ohura, T. Shirakabe, Y. Iwahira, T. Hirayama, and R. Tanino; from Korea, C. Park; from the Netherlands, P. van Damme and J. van Rappard; from Sweden, M. Olenius and J. Wieslander; and from the United States, L. Argenta, B. Bauer, H. Becker, J. Gibney, E. Manders, and A. Versaci.

Other individuals have had a profound influence on shaping my career in expansion work. William Grabb introduced me to the initial phases of tissue expansion and always supported my academic interests. Chedomir Radovan conveyed his enthusiasm and generously shared his clinical applications and patient results with me. Cho Pang listened patiently to my research aims and imposed the rigors of the scientific method on our experimental work. Thomas Krizek provided me with the academic environment to reach the limits of my abilities. Eric Austad exemplified the

ideal companion from whom to seek advice and rationality in this dynamic field.

I have appreciated the steadfastness of the manufacturers of expander devices in supporting basic research and clinical requirements, as well as the myriad teaching courses around the world. In particular, my profound gratitude is extended to Bruce Reuter, Gene Jackubczak, and Lois Duel for their continued friendship and professionalism.

I wish to thank Mosby, Inc. for their confidence and patience in the preparation of this book. Wendy Buckwalter, my Developmental Editor, endured my procrastinations but never wavered in her belief that I would complete this odyssey. The precise line drawings and artistic illustrations were created by my gifted medical illustrator, Cathy Reichel-Clark, who was never flustered by deadlines and revisions.

I am fortunate to have an outstanding office staff who unfailingly gave their all to care for our patients and to fulfill my requests. In particular, I wish to thank my private surgical nurse, Rita Muschenheim, who made me a better surgeon by providing the optimal surgical fields, handing me the needed instruments, and never keeping me waiting for suture cuttings.

Lastly, I am grateful to my wife, Joanne, and our children, Lindsey and Matthew, whose unconditional love and support permitted me to pursue my professional career at the expense of missing a few ball games.

It is to these individuals and our trusting patients that this text is dedicated.

Contents

PART One

FUNDAMENTALS

1

History and Evolution of Tissue Expansion

The ability of human tissue to expand and stretch has been observed and documented through history. In his "Invited Discussion" to Dr. Chedomir Radovan's first article,[1] Dr. William Grabb at the University of Michigan wrote in 1982, "Heaven only knows that the principle of skin expansion has been staring us in the face. The loose skin of the abdominal wall following pregnancy and body skin following massive weight loss have been there for all to see."[2] Therapeutic use of these mechanisms of natural tissue expansion with the aid of balloon expanders has evolved dramatically in the last two decades.

Human tissue readily adapts to physiologic expansion without thinning of the overlying skin. If adaption did not occur, significant functional and aesthetic deformities would result during the individual's growth phases. Although human skin is often described as an "anisotropic elastic membrane," living integumentary tissue in vivo responds to gradual stress stimuli by increasing mitotic activity to maintain its thickness and protective integrity. In a true anisotropic state the material becomes thinner as stretching proceeds, much as a rubber band reduces its diameter as it elongates. In contrast, the enlarging fetal brain stretches the calvaria at suture lines to accommodate the rapid growth of the cerebral hemispheres. During puberty, breast tissue responds to hormonal stimuli by slowly enlarging the overlying skin to produce the ptotic breast mound (Figure 1-1). In pregnancy the enlarging fetus and uterus stretch the abdominal and pelvic structures over 9 months to accommodate fetal growth and facilitate parturition (Figure 1-2). All these tissues increase or maintain their thickness with growth.

In a similar response to tension, the tissues overlying the growth of benign subcutaneous tumors such as ganglia or lipomas (Figure 1-3) and malignant tumors such as sarcomas (Figure 1-4) maintain their integrity.

Artificially induced expansion continues to be an integral part of the aesthetic and ethnographic characteristics of certain cultures. Anthropologists have recorded progressive lip expansion with substitution of enlarging plates by Chadian women in Africa[3] (Figure 1-5) and gradual elongation of neck length with metal rings by the Paduang women of Burma.[4]

EARLY DEVELOPMENTS

Clinically controlled femoral limb elongation using bone traction rather than expander balloon was first reported in 1905 by Codvilla.[5] Paul Magnuson[6] at the University of Pennsylvania in 1908 confirmed that soft tissue structures of the leg could be safely stretched by an external traction device with surgical lengthening of shortened bones. Victorio Putti[7] at the University of Bologna emphasized in 1921 that internal lengthening of bone by 3 to 4 inches (7.5 to 10 cm) could be achieved by constant tension for 30 days. Putti focused on concomitant stretching of muscles, nerves, and vessels and reported one neurologic complication involving the crural and sciatic nerves.

Dr. Charles Neumann of New York City is credited with the first clinical report of a latex balloon to reconstruct an ear (Figure 1-6). Neumann presented his findings to the American Society of Plastic and Reconstructive Surgeons (ASPRS) in October 1956 and published "The Expansion of an Area of Skin by Progressive Distention of a Subcutaneous Balloon"[8] in 1957. He inserted a "collapsed rubber balloon . . . introduced beneath the skin of the side of the head in the region of the missing portion of the ear. A flexible polyethylene tube, . . . through which the balloon could be inflated, was allowed to pass from the balloon via a subcutaneous tunnel." The tubing was exteriorized behind the ear, connected to a stopcock, and filled incrementally with air for 2 months. After expansion, measurements indicated a 50% increase in the skin's surface area. At the second stage a cartilaginous graft was inserted and covered with the expanded bipedicle flap for a successful reconstruction. Neumann's original work created little enthusiasm because no further publications or presentations appeared until 20 years later. Unfortunately, Neumann died in 1972[9] before witnessing the pioneering works of Radovan and Austad.

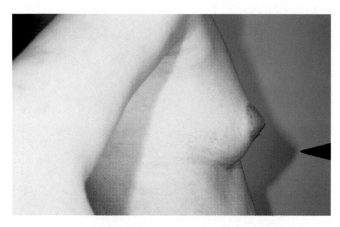

Figure 1-1 Adolescent breast buds begin to develop in response to hormonal changes during puberty. As the breast mounds become larger, the overlying skin stretches to accommodate their increased size and shape.

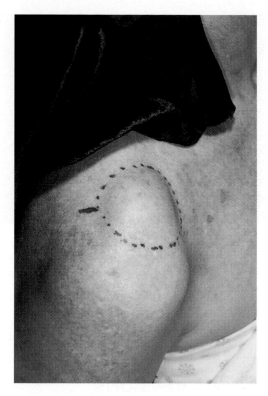

Figure 1-3 A 5 × 5 cm lipoma has grown slowly on the anterior shoulder of this 55-year-old patient. The overlying soft tissue has stretched to accommodate the fatty tumor.

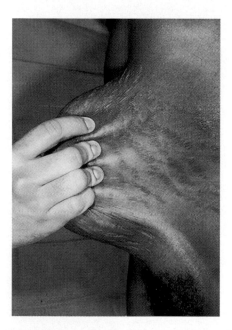

Figure 1-2 During pregnancy the developing fetus and uterus slowly force the confining pelvis to stretch. At parturition the overlying abdominal tissue has been expanded, with striae formation on the skin. The resulting pannus is removed by an abdominoplasty, with repair of the separated rectus abdominis muscles.

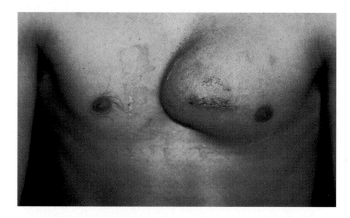

Figure 1-4 Chondrosarcoma occupies the parasternum of this 16-year-old male. This malignant tumor developed over 3 years, stretching the overlying skin.

As a plastic surgical resident at Georgetown University, Dr. Chedomir Radovan (Figure 1-7) conceived of inserting a silicone balloon and two separate valve systems under skin as a closed system.[10] One valve was for filling saline, and the second valve withdrew fluid. Radovan brought his idea to Rudi Schulte at Heyer-Schulte Corporation, who made a prototype expander for clinical use. Radovan inserted his first expander in January 1976 at Georgetown University to resurface a 7 × 11 cm (17½ × 27½–inch) defect on a patient's arm. This flap was expanded for only 3 weeks. A second patient had surgery 2 months later to cover an exposed fractured tibia.

Before these initial clinical trials by Radovan, Dr. Eric Austad[11] (Figure 1-8) was proceeding with his concepts of tissue expansion, unaware of Neumann's and Radovan's previous publications. Austad sought the advice of Drs. Reed Dingman and William Grabb about the potential applications for a self-inflating tissue expander. He then consulted with the research and development staff at Dow-Corning Medical Products in Midland, Mich., on Jan. 13, 1976. A few weeks

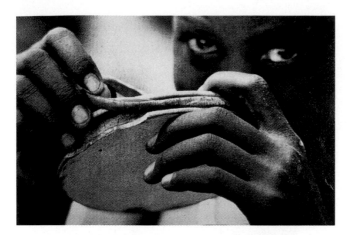

Figure 1-5 Chadian women beautify themselves by slowly expanding their lips with different-sized plates. They begin by inserting small disks into slits in their lips, then replace them with larger plates over time.

later, Radovan performed his first clinical case at Georgetown University.

SCIENTIFIC SESSIONS

Radovan presented his early experience with expansion technique at the ASPRS meeting in Boston in 1976.[12] This presentation was met with skepticism partly because of the success achieved by the concept's simplicity and the developer's overenthusiasm. Radovan displayed a poster (Figure 1-9) titled "Development of the Adjacent Rotation Flaps and of the Breast after Mastectomy Using the 'Radovan Expander'" the following year in 1977 at the annual meeting in San Francisco.[13] From 1977 to 1978 Radovan accumulated a variety of cases and presented his clinical experience at the scientific session at Toronto in 1979.

At the same Toronto meeting, Dr. Eric Austad also presented his limited clinical experience with an osmotically driven, self-inflating expander at the University of Michigan and the first evaluation of laboratory histomorphologic changes during expansion. For this work, Austad received first prize in the clinical category competition sponsored by the ASPRS.[14] Austad and his co-workers performed their first clinical cases in 1977 and published both their experience with the self-inflating expander[15] and their animal study[16] in 1982.

The author (Dr. Gordon Sasaki) first met Radovan at his poster display at the 1977 meeting. Through Radovan's encouragement and advice, the author's first experience with this new technique was in 1979 with the insertion of an expander in the upper arm of a 13-year-old patient. The goal was to resurface a large skin graft on thin tissue covering a metal plate

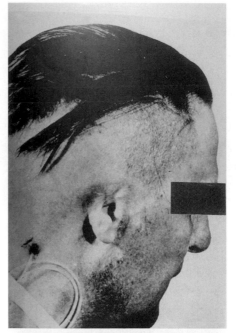

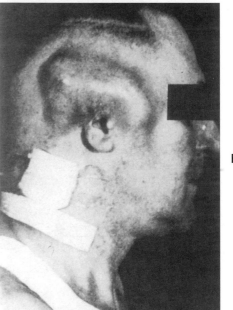

Figure 1-6 A, Dr. Neumann's patient, a 52-year-old male, sustained a traumatic amputation of the upper two thirds of his right ear. A delayed reconstruction was begun by inserting a 5-inch (12.5 cm) rubber balloon just above the ear remnant. A $\frac{1}{8}$-inch-diameter flexible polyethylene tubing from the balloon exits through a stab wound in the neck. **B,** The patient's balloon has been inflated gradually over 6 weeks. Measurements 2 months after the first surgery revealed about a 50% increase of the skin above the expander from its original area of 12 square inches (30 cm²). This additional skin was considered sufficient to provide anterior and posterior coverage for a cartilaginous graft. At the second surgery the expanded skin was advanced as a double-pedicled tube flap over the cartilaginous framework. A third procedure of multiple Z-plasties was required to blend in the seam lines.

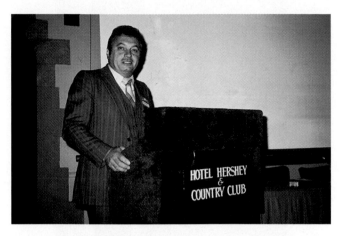

Figure 1-7 Dr. Chedomir Radovan delivered one of his first lectures on tissue expansion at a meeting hosted by Dr. Ernest Manders in Hershey, Pennsylvania.

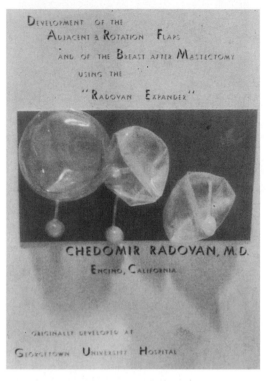

Figure 1-9 At the 1977 meeting of the American Society of Plastic and Reconstructive Surgeons in San Francisco, Radovan displayed his concept of breast reconstruction with a tissue expansion technique performed within a subcutaneous pocket.

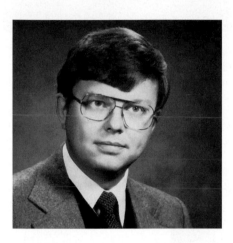

Figure 1-8 Dr. Eric Austad developed his concepts of tissue expansion at the University of Michigan (Ann Arbor). His early experimental studies and clinical experience coincided with Radovan's efforts.

on her humerus (Figure 1-10). A single, round 300 cc expander was inserted adjacent to the skin graft through a 10 cm (4-inch) paralesional incision (Figure 1-11). Expansion proceeded without complications for 10 weeks. The skin graft was replaced with her stable expanded skin flap, leaving a depression on the anteromedial aspect of the upper arm (Figure 1-12). The plate was removed safely 1 year later after bone union had occurred.

The presentations at the 1979 Toronto meeting generated significant interest in tissue expansion as an innovative concept and technique throughout the United States, especially at academic centers. At this early developmental stage the few clinicians with sufficient experience emphasized the importance of proper indications and attention to technique. Because of the high incidence of "major and minor complications," however, especially in pediatric patients, in certain anatomic

areas (e.g., lower extremities), and in compromised tissue (e.g., resulting from radiation, infection, or diabetes), many questioned the value of this reconstructive procedure and expressed concern about the expansion process inducing irreversible ischemic changes.

Despite these setbacks, continued research and improved results led to the first informal gathering to discuss tissue expansion at the University of Michigan in 1981, under the guidance of Grabb and chaired by Austad (Figure 1-13). With their cumulative experience of probably less than 200 cases, the attendants included Chedomir Radovan, Louis Argenta, Ernest Manders, and the author, who would continue their pioneering efforts.

In 1982 the First National Tissue Expansion Symposium, cosponsored by the Plastic Surgical Educational Foundation (PSEF) and the University of Michigan, convened at Ann Arbor and invited Drs. Armand Versaci and John Gibney to join the faculty. In the next decade more than 100,000 tissue expansion surgeries were documented worldwide. Variations and improvements of technique were presented every 2 years at five subsequent National Tissue Expansion Symposia (Figures 1-14 and 1-15) and four International Tissue Expansion Symposia. Audiences' increasing sophistication indicated the level to which tissue expan-

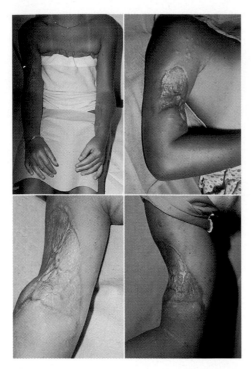

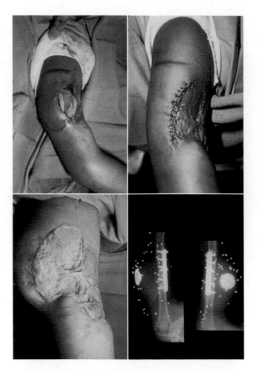

Figure 1-10 Tissue trauma from accidental shotgun blast to right upper extremity of this 13-year-old female. She sustained damage to her biceps and triceps muscles, a mid-shaft humeral fracture, and associated nerve injuries. A split-thickness skin graft provided temporary coverage over the defect.

Figure 1-11 Patient in Figure 1-10, first surgery 6 months later. Round, 300 cc tissue expander was inserted under the adjacent normal skin through a 10 cm (4-inch) paralesional incision. Serial expansion, averaging 20 to 30 cc (ml) per fill, was performed each week for 10 filling sessions. The radiograph shows the expander with its incorporated valve stretching tissue within a field of metallic fragments.

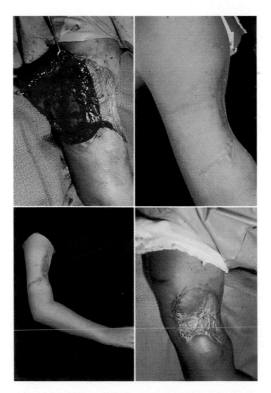

Figure 1-12 Patient in Figures 1-10 and 1-11, second surgery. The expanded tissue was advanced to replace the skin graft. Expansion reduced the amount of subcutaneous fat by compression ischemia, leaving a depression within the reconstructive field. The final vertical scar measured about 12 cm (5 inches) in length. *Lower right,* Preoperative reference photograph of defect.

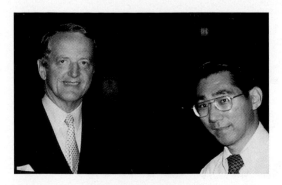

Figure 1-13 Dr. William Grabb *(left)* and the author at the first informal meeting on tissue expansion at the University of Michigan in 1981.

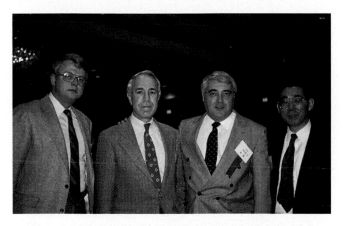

Figure 1-14 The First National Tissue Expansion Symposium convened at the Huntington-Sheraton Hotel in Pasadena, Calif., in October 1984. *Left to right,* Drs. Eric Austad, Armand Versaci, John Gibney, and the author.

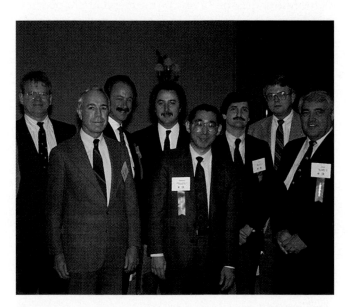

Figure 1-15 The 5th National Tissue Expansion Symposium, under the auspices of the Plastic Surgery Educational Foundation, was held at the Century Plaza Hotel in Century City, Calif., in 1989. *Left to right,* Drs. Ernest Manders, Armand Versaci, Alan Gold, Hilton Becker, the author, Jacic Fisher, Eric Austad, and John Gibney.

sion had evolved in different countries, with major complication rates reduced currently to 3% to 5%.

The future of tissue expansion depends on the creativity of plastic and reconstructive surgeons and those in related specialties as they apply its principles to solve tissue problems. Their efforts will ensure that tissue expansion remains an established and dynamic procedure.

REFERENCES

1. Radovan C: Reconstruction of the breast after radical mastectomy using a temporary expander, *Plast Reconstr Surg* 69:195, 1982.
2. Grabb WC: Discussion: breast reconstruction using the temporary expander, *Plast Reconstr Surg* 69:207, 1982.
3. Weeks GS: Into the heart of Africa, *National Geographic* 110:257, 1956.
4. Burnett W: Yank meets native, *National Geographic* 88:124, 1945.
5. Codvilla A: On the means of lengthening in the lower limbs, the muscle and tissues which are shortened through deformity, *Am J Orthop Surg* 2:353, 1905.
6. Magnuson PS: Lengthening shortened bones of the leg by operation, *Univ Penn Med Bull,* 1908, p 103.
7. Putti V: The operative lengthening of the femur, *JAMA* 77:934, 1921.
8. Neumann CG: The expansion of an area of skin by progressive distention of a subcutaneous balloon, *Plast Reconstr Surg* 19:124, 1957.
9. Obituary: Charles G. Neumann, *Plast Reconstr Surg* 52:690, 1973.
10. Radovan C: Personal communication, annual meeting of the American Society of Plastic and Reconstructive Surgeons, San Francisco, October 1977.
11. Austad ED: Evolution of the concept of tissue expansion, *Facial Plast Surg* 5:277, 1988.
12. Radovan C: Adjacent flap development using expandable Silastic implants. Paper presented at annual meeting of the American Society of Plastic and Reconstructive Surgeons, Boston, September 1976.
13. Radovan C: Development of the adjacent rotation flaps and of the breast after mastectomy using the "Radovan expander." Poster presented at annual meeting of the American Society of Plastic and Reconstructive Surgeons, San Francisco, October 1977.
14. Austad E: A self-inflating tissue expander. Paper presented at annual meeting of the American Society of Plastic and Reconstructive Surgeons, Toronto, October 1979.
15. Austad E, Rose GL: A self-inflating tissue expander, *Plast Reconstr Surg* 70:107, 1982.
16. Austad E et al: Histomorphologic evaluation of guinea pig skin and soft tissue after controlled tissue expansion, *Plast Reconstr Surg* 70:704, 1982.

2

Tissue Expanders and General Guidelines for Tissue Expansion Technique

TISSUE EXPANDER SYSTEMS

Composition

Tissue expander balloons are composed of silicone and filler ingredients. Silicone is a synthetic polymer produced by the heating (vulcanization) of oxygen, carbon, and silica. The final products exist in a solid, liquid, or gel state. Rigorous standards are required to qualify a silicone prosthesis as a medical-grade product for implantation within the human body.

Expander Balloon

The balloon is a preshaped prosthesis that is filled with saline fluid through an incorporated or a remote valve system. The envelope may possess either a smooth or textured surface. The thickness, durometer (stiffness) strength, and elasticity of the silicone envelope vary with the manufacturer's specifications.

Types of Balloons

Balloons can be divided into four categories: standard, differential, custom, and breast expanders.

Standard Expanders
Standard expanders are those commercially available from manufacturers that require no special features. These expander units may have a smooth or textured surface and an incorporated or remote valve system. Manufacturers have selected volumes and sizes based on most common uses by surgeons.

Round expanders, available in incremental volumes from 100 to 2000 cc, produce a hemispheric flap during expansion. Skin gain is about half the length of the dome's diameter. The larger the balloon's base diame-

ter, the more tissue is available for advancement. Round-shaped balloons are indicated for round lesions and are useful in head and neck expansions.

Rectangular expanders, available in volumes of 100 to 1000 cc, produce a sausage-shaped flap. The tissue gain is about half the dome's width. Rectangular expanders are useful in scalp, trunk, and extremity expansions.

Crescent expanders, available in volumes from 100 to 1000 cc, have greater expansion in the center than at the tips of the expander. This design matches the contour of a round-shaped defect, minimizing "dog-ear" deformities. Tissue gain from crescent-shaped expanders is usually less than that expected from round or rectangular expanders. Implantation is more challenging with the crescent configuration.

Differential Expanders
Differential expanders were designed to expand more in one site than another within the same implant. This effect was obtained by altering the durometer (stiffness) of the silicone envelope. Today's manufacturers have removed this type of nonbreast expander from the standard lines because of less interest and increased cost.

Custom Expanders
Custom expanders are specially ordered from the manufacturer based on the unit's design (volume, width, length, projection), thus increasing delivery time and cost. Most defects can be covered with standard expanders.

Anatomic Expanders for Breast Reconstruction
Anatomic breast expander units are designed to mimic breast proportions during the expansion phase. This ef-

fect produces varying degrees of success because surgically changing the shape of the expanded tissue affects the final breast profile more than the unit's shape. Nevertheless, some surgeons endorse expanders for breast reconstruction as a way to obtain better results.

A variation of the expander–permanent implant is available for breast reconstruction. This type of prosthesis serves both as an expander and an implant, thus eliminating the need for a second procedure. The device may consist of a single lumen that is filled with saline through a temporary remote valve and tubing. The tubing is curled within the prosthesis, and its removal by traction at the end of adjustment seals the opening. Another device (Becker system) consists of a double lumen with two separate chambers: an inner one filled with saline to achieve expansion and an outer chamber prefilled with gel to provide natural softness to the implant. The Becker system also has a temporary valve and tubing that are removed after adjustment. Permanent expander-implant systems usually do not provide significant expansion and are most effective when the skin envelopes are large enough but the implants require volume adjustment.

Filling Tubes

Filling tubes connect the valve to the expander unit through a reinforced patch at the tube-expander juncture. The tube may enter at (1) the lower third of the balloon, (2) the edge of its base, or (3) the center of its base. The third configuration permits greater versatility in placement of the system. The first design may produce tissue thinning or exposure by compressing the skin patch during expansion.

Connectors

Metal or plastic connectors are necessary to adjust tube length according to the position of the valve and expander. Some plastic connectors have a self-locking system that eliminates the need for suture fastening. A connector may become a site for leakage (detachment) or tissue ingrowth (capsule formation). Capsular containment at the connector site can make removing the system difficult, especially in an adjustable expander-implant system when the tubing and valve must be removed. Forceful dislodgement and separation of the connector will result in saline decompression of the balloon.

Valves

Valves permit saline injection into the expander without back-pressure leakage. Three types of valves are currently available: incorporated (self-contained), internal remote, and external.

Self-contained valves are incorporated into the expander's dome. The valve's bottom layer is made of an impregnable material (metal or substitute) to prevent perforation of the expander envelope. A self-sealing silicone material within the valve resists leakage at the multiple needle perforation sites. A raised silicone ring facilitates palpation to locate the valve. Some valves are located with a magnetic metal finder to pinpoint their epicenter. The self-contained valve eliminates the need for additional undermining to create a distant valve site, facilitates removal of the expander system, and removes the risks of valve migration or overturn, connector leakage, and tubing obstruction. Pressure on the overlying tissue from the valve at the expander's apex can lead to valve erosion or exposure. Risk of inadvertent puncture of the expander is increased because of the valve's proximity to the main expander unit.

Internal remote valves consist of a dome of silicone, self-sealant gel, and a metallic disk base to avoid perforation. The primary advantage of a remote valve system is to isolate the balloon from the valve, thereby eliminating inadvertent puncture of the silicone expander. Also, the valve can be more easily palpated because the surgeon can position it at a more superficial level under thin subcutaneous fat. A buried remote valve system, however, increases the risks of valve migration, leakage, overturn, and obstruction. Remote valves can also be a source of valve erosion and bacterial contamination of the entire system.

External valves are placed outside the skin to avoid valve overturn, migration, obstruction, leakage, and percutaneous needle-stick pain. The disadvantages include possible retrograde infection of the expander unit and chronic bacterial inflammation along the tube tract. A permanent alloplastic prosthesis or autogenous graft within the reconstructed site may be at greater risk for postoperative infection after using an external valve system.

Selection of Optimal System

Various systems are available for reconstructive needs. The surgeon can select a system that provides sufficient tissue with minimal risk by assessing the advantages and disadvantages of each type. The clinical setting determines the expander's shape and size. The outcome is influenced more by the surgical manipulation of available tissue than by the system's features. However, inappropriate selection and insertion of an expander system will nullify initial efforts to gain tissue.

GENERAL GUIDELINES

Tissue expansion is one of the reconstructive surgeon's alternatives in providing optimal tissue replacement when skin shortage is a major problem. To be useful, this technique must be simple, reliable, safe, effective, and cost competitive with other standard procedures. Successful reconstruction requires careful attention to optimal patient selection, preoperative planning, insertion of expander, the expansion process, and the delivery of tissue during the final procedure. The outcome depends on the size of the anticipated defect, extent and characteristics of the donor tissue site, degree of patient discomfort and distortion of body image, duration of expansion, and reduction of complications. Other factors include the patient's and surgeon's expectations and the surgeon's "artistry" during flap advancement.

PATIENT SELECTION

Tissue Stability

Tissue expansion requires a favorable environment to accommodate a temporary expander because it gradually stretches the overlying stable soft tissue over time (Figure 2-1). This implant is not only a foreign body, but also a dynamic structure that imposes forces of expansion on surrounding areas. The donor site should be free of bacterial contamination, infection, unstable scar tissue, and poorly vascularized tissue. For these reasons, this technique is primarily an elective surgical pro-

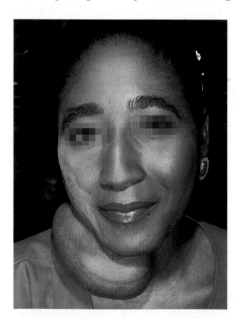

Figure 2-1 This 25-year-old patient sustained a full-thickness burn to her right midface that required a split-thickness graft for coverage. Because of hyperpigmentation and surface irregularities, the graft was camouflaged with makeup. A 300 cc rectangular tissue expander was inserted under the stable neck skin through a 3.5 cm incision behind the ear lobule. Serial expansion progressed for 10 weeks, after which the expanded neck skin was advanced up the midface, replacing the unsightly and asensory graft. Long-term expansion was successfully completed as an elective procedure in a favorable environment free of bacterial contamination.

cedure to provide coverage with the same type of tissue. Although expanders can be inserted at the time of trauma or adjacent to an open wound, the complication rate in these cases may be increased because of the potential for contaminated, ischemic, or devitalized tissue.

Patient Stability

The creation of a hemispheric mound (or mounds) adjacent to the reconstruction site is inherent in tissue expansion. Most patients accept the cosmetic or functional deformities associated with the buried expanders throughout the expansion period. Patients should be informed, however, that a hemispheric dome in certain areas of the body (scalp, face, neck, exposed areas of extremities) may produce aesthetic or functional problems during the early, middle, or late phases of expansion (Figure 2-2).

Temporary disfigurement or dysfunction of the lower lid, nasal alar, oral commissure, and lips and re-

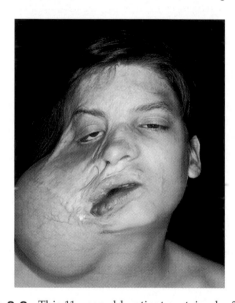

Figure 2-2 This 11-year-old patient sustained a 35% full-thickness burn to the forehead, nose, and right midface, trunk, and extremities after a gasoline explosion. The split-thickness skin graft to the midface was patient's primary concern because of its masklike appearance and lack of sensation. In the first expansion a 300 cc round expander was inserted through a 3.0 cm incision behind the ear lobule. The plane of dissection was performed above the superficial musculoaponeurotic system (SMAS) layer in neck below the mandible. After 7 weeks of expansion the expanded neck flap was advanced in a cephalad direction. Reexpansion of the midface portion of the neck skin was performed 1 year later with the same expander. During the second expansion phase, depicted in the photograph, temporary lower lid ectropion, lateral distortion of the nose and lips, and mild intrusion of the balloon into the oral cavity occurred after 5 weeks of expansion. The second reconstructive phase required release and suspension of the lower lid and oral commissure, further cephalomedial flap advancement, and creation of a more natural nasolabial fold.

striction of mastication and joint motion may result from tissue stretching and the physical and gravitational effects of saline within the enlarging expander. Patients may want to camouflage the deformity by wearing a ski cap, hat, or scarf at the workplace or in public (Figure 2-3). Occasionally, the only option for the patient is to remain at home during the final phases of expansion. Almost all aesthetic and dys-

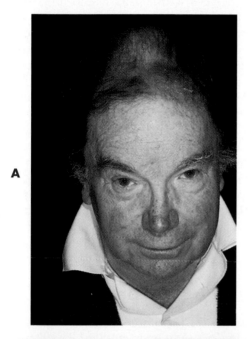

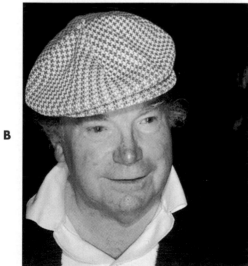

Figure 2-3 A, This 52-year-old patient had a malignant melanoma excised from his left forehead and scalp, which were resurfaced with a skin graft. One year later, a 300 cc round tissue expander was inserted under the galea aponeurotica of adjacent hair-bearing scalp through a 3.0 cm left postauricular incision. Serial expansion at 330 cc (ml) of saline produced a noticeable deformity. **B,** Patient began wearing a tam-o'-shanter cap to camouflage the bulge, which increased with further expansion to 500 cc of saline. Patient continued to work at his clothing store until his reconstruction was completed 3 months after initial insertion procedure.

functional side effects return to normal once the balloon is removed. Secondary remedial correction may be required, however, if significant complications or residual deformities persist. In general, children tolerate the process of expansion more readily than adolescents or adults. In selected cases, the expander may be deflated before an important occasion and reinflated later.

Development of an enlarging mound(s), as in breast reconstruction, may not always be a concern because symmetry and fullness are being achieved. If patients are unable to tolerate the inconveniences and side effects of the expansion process, alternative methods of reconstruction should be considered early in the formative phases of evaluation.

PREOPERATIVE PLANNING

During the initial consultation the surgeon and patient determine whether local tissue is both available and stable, whether expansion is a viable option to solve the problem, and whether the patient can accept the side effects and possible complications. To facilitate selection of an expander(s), the surgeon should have a centimeter tape measure, straight ruler, transparent wrap, and marking pens available during the examination (Figures 2-4 and 2-5). In special cases, unmarked radiographic film may be necessary to produce a template, which will then be designed into a custom-made expander to fit a specific donor site(s) for an irregularly shaped defect (Figures 2-6 and 2-7).

Implant Size, Shape, and Volume

Many clinicians[1-9] have proposed and evaluated methods to select the proper size, shape, and volume of

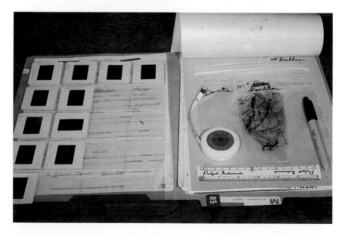

Figure 2-4 Patient's office chart should have complete and up-to-date information. Sequential slides or Polaroid prints should clearly document preoperative problems and surgical improvements. Accurate measurements of the defect and donor site(s) with a tape measure and straight ruler may be recorded on a transparency for future reference.

tissue expanders that will yield sufficient new tissue to complete the reconstruction. The calculated surface area over the expander is always overestimated when compared with the actual amount of tissue gain.[3,9] That is, the surgeon can always expect to have less usable tissue for the farthest reconstruction point after the expansion period than anticipated.

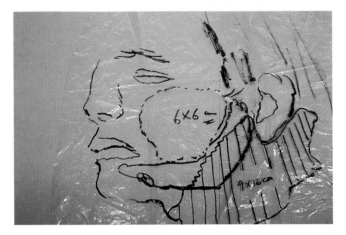

Figure 2-5 Transparent wrap is placed on the patient's neck and face for an accurate tracing of normal facial features and landmarks, including the defect and donor sites. This provides a permanent record to determine preoperatively the appropriate size and location of the expander unit.

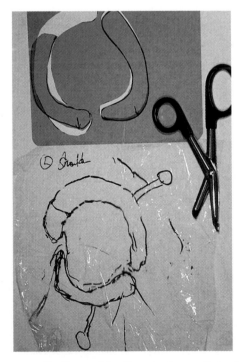

Figure 2-6 Radiographic film can be used to duplicate the defect's dimensions, and templates of the expander(s) can be taken from the transparency. The templates can be designed into custom expanders to fit the special requirements of the donor site for an irregular defect.

If the real skin gain equals the surface area gain over the expander, Radovan[6] and Morgan and Edgerton[10] suggest that the expander base should have the same size as the defect to be closed. Theoretically, a doubling of the dome surface would permit coverage of both the defect and the donor sites. On the other hand, Gibney[11] recommends that the expander base should be two and one-half to three times the defect's width. This would limit the use of commercial rectangular expanders, whose largest base width is about 8 to 10 cm, to small defects. Surgeons would predominantly use round expanders, whose base diameters are larger than those of rectangular expanders for equivalent volumes. Unfortunately, round-shaped expanders are difficult to fit into confined and narrow donor sites. In response, Manders and co-workers[12] recommend using as large an expander (rectangular or round) as possible in most reconstructions.

After addressing these concerns, the surgeon must select expanders based on (1) size of the defect, (2) size and location of the available donor site(s), and (3) expected advancement of a hemispheric domed flap that has been expanded to its safest limits of tissue tolerance and patient acceptance.

Size of Defect

The degree of difficulty in reconstructing a given defect depends not only on its greatest length and width dimensions, but also on the special characteristics that will be replaced. In general, the larger and more irregular the defect's shape, the more sophisticated are analytic assessment and tissue replacement. Therefore a first step is to measure the defect's maximum width and length and record its exact configuration on a transparent wrap.

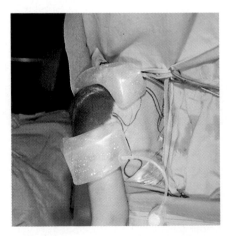

Figure 2-7 This 5-year-old patient demonstrates the custom-made expanders that will be inserted circumferentially around large congenital nevus on the left shoulder.

Size and Location of Donor Sites

The "clinically" available donor site is the total region of adjacent uninvolved tissue that can be used for expansion. The "practically" available donor site represents a partial region of the clinically available site or the entire site. This distinction is based on the respect for and preservation of the aesthetic and functional units within the donor region. For example, insertion of an expander under the nasolabial fold line or infraorbital skin may produce a distortion or obliteration of this medial cheek landmark or creation of lower lid ectropion. Therefore expansion should be limited to the practically available donor skin (i.e., lateral to the nasolabial and labiomandibular folds).

To determine the practically available donor skin, a template with the expander's exact base dimensions or the expander itself is outlined on the donor skin (Figure 2-8). Occasionally, more than one expander may be required for a "best fit" along one side of the donor tissue adjacent to the defect. At times, one expander on each side of the defect may be necessary to produce enough tissue for the reconstruction and to reduce the bulging deformity from a single implant. In

both these cases, the same principles apply regarding preservation of form and function within the available donor sites.

Expected Advancement of Expanded Flap

As previously mentioned, a discrepancy exists between the real tissue surface gain and the expander surface increase. Because of this limitation, expansion should proceed until sufficient tissue is stretched to complete the coverage. The surgeon should even overexpand and obtain more tissue than the estimated requirement. The extra skin may not be used, but enough will be available for the farthest and widest portion of the reconstruction.

The surgeon also must incorporate the phenomenon of tissue stretchback into this imprecise formula. *Tissue stretchback*[13] refers to the ability of chronically stretched skin (and/or muscle) either to contract immediately after tissue release or to shorten slowly over time. If this adverse effect is significant, immediate closure may be difficult, a wider scar may develop, or a secondary deformation of an adjacent mobile structure may occur postoperatively. The resulting degree of a hypertrophic scarring depends on the tension across the line of closure and factors such as scar direction, position across joints, and location on extremities.

The surgeon can estimate the amount of tissue advancement anticipated from expansion from the width of the hemispheric domed flap (Figure 2-9). As

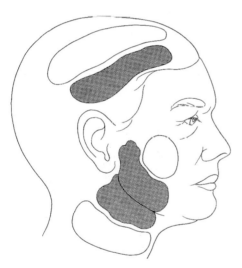

Figure 2-8 To resurface a right temporal-frontal scalp defect *(top shaded outline)*, the only "practically" available donor tissue (see text) is adjacent to the defect under normal hair-bearing scalp. The expander's exact base dimensions *(clear outline)* should be at least as long as the defect. Insertion of another expander on the opposite side of the defect (along the frontal-temporal hairline) would violate this important landmark and could influence the eventual position of the right brow. In contrast to this situation, reconstruction of a large, lower lateral midface defect that extends below the mandible's margin into the neck *(lower two shaded outlines)* is optimally approached by inserting two expanders on each side of the defect *(two clear outlines)*. Sufficient "practically" available donor tissues exists in the midface and neck that does not violate any functional or aesthetic units within these areas. The final scar location would be parallel and below the mandibular margin.

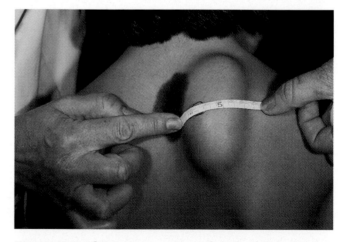

Figure 2-9 Surgeon can estimate length of flap advancement anticipated after each expansion by measuring width of the expanded flap. Amount of forward advancement on a flat surface is slightly less than half the width of the flap at that interval of expansion. By this method the surgeon can predict with some certainty when enough tissue has been stretched to proceed with the final stage of reconstruction. In general, 5 to 10 mm of additional tissue length is expected after each expansion session.

gradual expansion proceeds, the surgeon can measure in centimeters the width of the flap after each expansion period. The amount of advancement is then expected to be less than one-half the flap width at that interval of expansion. Thus, if the widest portion of the defect measures x cm, the surgeon should fill the expander until the width of the domed flap is 2.0 to 2.5 times x cm for a linear horizontal advancement over a planar defect. For reconstruction over curvatures (e.g., calvaria), joints, and dimensional structures of the ear, nose, and breast, more expansion is required to compensate for additional skin drape. Therefore the domed flap's width should be 2.5 to 3.0 times the defect's width.

The author's clinical experience in more than 1500 cases suggests that tissue gain depends more on size of the expander when filled to its stated or overinflated volume, the maximal safe limits to which tissues in a given region can be expanded, and the limits of patient tolerance. If the patient and tissue are used as the internal monitors for a successful expansion, the surgeon can accurately predict and advise the patient whether a single or second procedure is necessary.

Table 2-1 provides the typical expanded hemispheric domed flap width that can be expected for a given anatomic region.

Multiple expanders, positioned on each side of the defect, may be necessary for larger defects whose widths exceed the measurements in Table 2-1. Multiple expanders are used to (1) ensure enough tissue for coverage, (2) decrease the duration of expansion, and (3) reduce the overall bulge of the expanders because each contributes half the anticipated amount (with two expanders). The use of more than one expander

usually increases the incidence of implant complications and the cost. If the donor site cannot accommodate two or more expanders, the surgeon may consider reexpansion of the original site ("leapfrog" technique) 4 to 6 months later to complete the reconstruction (Figure 2-10).

Other factors that affect the expected advancement of the expanded flap are the patient's age, location on the body, and the expander's shape.

Age of Patient

Sugihara and associates[14] performed in vivo studies on 94 males from 3 months to 73 years of age by measuring skin extensibility with a Bio-skin Tensiometer. The skin of subjects younger than 2 years exhibited a higher degree of extensibility than skin in males 20 to 29 years of age. The skin at any site from all the other age groups by decades was not significantly different than the skin from the 20s group.

Despite Sugihara's objective findings, the author believes that the more pliable, softer, and thinner skin of prepubertal patients allows expansion to proceed more easily than with skin from postpubertal patients. However, skin from patients whose tissue elasticity is greatly diminished also exhibits rapid expansion, possibly because of the greater abundance, laxity, and actinic damage of skin in the older population.

■ **Table 2-1** Anticipated Advancement of Expanded Flaps*

Anatomic region	Expanded domed flap width (cm)	Expected flap advancement (cm)
Scalp	12-16	Up to 8
Forehead	8-14	Up to 7
Midface	10-14	Up to 7
Ear	4-8	Up to 4
Neck	12-16	Up to 8
Breast	Use linear and volumetric measurements (see Chapter 12)	
Trunk	14-24	Up to 12
Upper arm	12-18	Up to 9
Forearm	10-12	Up to 6
Thigh	12-20	Up to 10
Below knee	12-14	Up to 7

*For a given anatomic region, this table gives the flap advancement that can be expected from the expanded hemispheric domed flap on a planar reconstruction for that region.

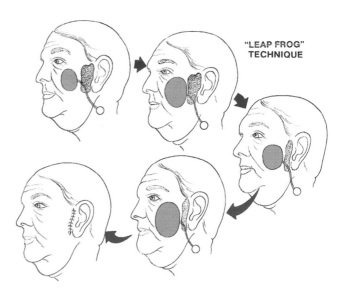

Figure 2-10 When a partial advancement of expanded skin is anticipated or realized at the second stage, reexpansion of the flap is possible after 4 to 6 months. This "leapfrog" technique enables surgeon to cover a complex or large defect completely. Although an expander may be left under an advanced flap to obviate the need for a second procedure, its presence can hinder healing at the suture line. This usually results in implant exposure and infection, which complicates subsequent stages of reconstruction.

Location on Body

Sugihara et al.,[14] Stark,[15] and Ohura, Sugihara, and Honda[16] observed variations in skin extensibility at different locations on the body. The thinner and more elastic skin of the face expands more rapidly than the thicker back skin. The skin's ability to accept expansion without complications is not directly related to its degree of extensibility. In evaluating tolerance to tissue expansion, van Rappard and colleagues[17] found that scalp, breast, trunk, and facial tissues were somewhat tolerant, while tissues on the back, upper leg, upper arm, forearm, and lower leg were the most intolerant. In the author's clinical experience, tissue from the upper or lower extremities can be expanded as easily as skin in other areas. The difficulty lies in the increased risk of implant exposure (i.e., intolerance) because of the relative thinness of distant extremity skin and the paucity of musculocutaneous perforators of skin over bone and tendons.

Shape of Expander

The three most frequently used expander shapes are round, rectangular, and crescent. The choice depends on the configuration and amount of practically available donor tissue. The expander's shape contributes to the overall efficiency of tissue gain. Van Rappard and associates[18] achieved the most effective surface area gain with rectangular expanders, calculating that 38% of the surface area increase was actually gained on the overlying skin. With crescent-shaped expanders the gain was 32%, and with round expanders only 25% of the calculated increase was achieved on the skin surface.

INSERTION OF EXPANDER

Skin Site for Expander Unit

The surgeon outlines the base dimensions of the selected expander, tubing, and valve on the patient's skin (Figure 2-11). The selection and location of the donor skin have been previously discussed. The site for the remote valve pocket should be in a "safe" position superior or lateral to the expander balloon. Valves positioned inferior and near the expander may be encroached on by the enlarging balloon above it. Inadvertent injury to the balloon from a needle stick may occur during filling of the encroached valve. To prevent this catastrophe, which requires surgical replacement with a new balloon, the valve must be inserted far enough away from the expander unit.

Skin Preparation and Local Anesthesia

After induction of general anesthesia (in children), the patient's skin at the operative site is painted with a bactericidal solution such as povidone iodine (Betadine). A local anesthetic agent (1% lidocaine [Xylocaine], 1:200,000 epinephrine) is diluted in a 1:1 ratio with saline if the calculated amount of *undiluted* Xylocaine or epinephrine would produce significant side effects or toxicity. For normal healthy adults the individual maximum recommended dose of Xylocaine with epinephrine should not exceed 7 mg/kg (3.5 mg/lb) of body weight, and the maximum total dose generally should not exceed 500 mg. For healthy children over 3 years of age who have normal lean body mass and body development, the maximum dose is determined by the child's age and weight; the total dose should not exceed 3 mg/kg (1.4 mg/lb). A generous amount of this solution is injected, as in dermatoclysis, into the operative site to aid in tissue dissection and to control bleeding. If the procedure is done under local anesthesia (in adults), the addition of a buffering agent (e.g., sodium bicarbonate) to the local anesthetic solution (in a 2:8 ratio) will reduce the burning sensation produced by the acidic mixture (pH 4.5).

Incision Sites

The most frequently used incisions are within the lesion, adjacent to the lesion, or remote from the defect.

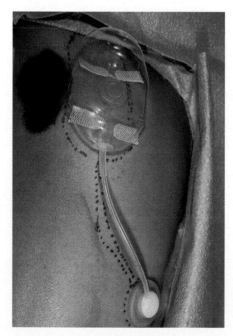

Figure 2-11 This 12-year-old patient has a congenital nevus measuring 4 × 8 cm on the interscapular region of the back. An exact outline of the expander unit is marked on the donor skin. Sketched locations of the expander balloon, tubing, and remote valve on the patient's skin enables the surgeon to determine the safest, most accessible incision to create the pockets to accommodate the unit. The surgeon also can estimate length of the tubing between the expander and its valve.

The incision choice is based on facilitating insertion of the balloon and valve system and reducing potential complications of expansion. Whenever possible, the direction of the incision should be radial (perpendicular) to the expander to oppose the forces of expansion and thus lessen the risk of wound dehiscence before and during expansion.

Intralesional Incision

An intralesional incision may be used when the lesion is large enough to accommodate incision length and stable enough to withstand dissection trauma and implant insertion (Figure 2-12). The major advantages with this approach are the incision's proximity to the anticipated area of expander pocket dissection, no additional visible incision scars, and relative safety of this incision, with reduced incidence of wound separation. However, if the defect (e.g., skin graft) is expected to become unstable after the trauma of dissection, ischemic changes and skin sloughing can lead to implant exposure and infection. Occasionally, tenting of the skin graft or unstable skin by the implant during expansion can cause delayed ischemia and blistering with cellulitis and possible exposure. These complications are preventable if the surgeon recognizes preoperatively that the skin, graft, or scar covering the lesion cannot withstand an intralesional approach.

Paralesional Incision

An incision at the defect–donor tissue interface may minimize incisional scars and facilitate dissection of the implant pocket (Figure 2-13). This surgical approach is most often used because it affords the easiest and most accessible exposure for flap elevation and implant insertion. Of all the incisions, however, the paralesional approach is most closely associated with implant exposure and infection. Because the incision is adjacent to the implant, it may be too weak to withstand the stresses of early expansion. The easiest surgical approach may not be the safest.

The ability to begin expansion with minimal concern for wound dehiscence is important to prevent formation of a thickened capsule, which can jeopardize effective expansion. A fibrotic capsule can develop from the inflammation of delayed wound healing (hematoma, seroma, bacterial contamination) and from the maturation of the surrounding capsule against the implant over time. Early expansion also helps to smooth out implant folds, which can erode through the overlying skin.

Remote Incision

Any incision made away from the defect reduces the incidence of wound healing problems, which can delay or abort the expansion process (Figure 2-14). A remote incision usually is made between the anticipated expander pocket (adjacent to the defect) and the remote valve pocket. This approach eliminates an incision near the expander balloon and defect, which could jeopardize early expansion. The incision should be made perpendicular (radial) to the implant and valve pockets to reduce the stresses of expansion forces. A disadvantage of a remote incision is creation of an additional scar; if possible, it is strategically hidden in a crease line, fold, or previous scar (Figure 2-15). Another disadvantage is the extended dissection of the pockets on each side of the incision.

Level of Dissection

The expander unit is usually inserted in the deep subcutaneous fat just above the muscle fascia (Fig-

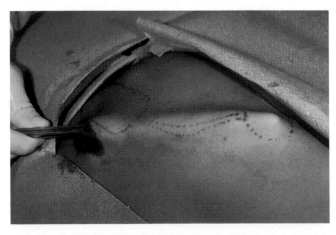

Figure 2-12   In this procedure an intralesional approach was a safe, effective means to dissect the pockets for the expander and its remote valve system. The lesion was stable enough to withstand the trauma of dissection and could accommodate the 3.5 cm incision.

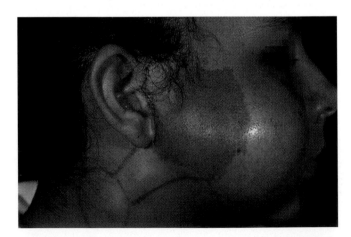

Figure 2-13   A 4.0 cm paralesional incision was made in the preauricular zone to gain access to the medial half of the midface. This approach is most frequently used because it permits the most accessible exposure for flap elevation and implant insertion. Of all incision choices, this selection places the most stress on the closure because of the expander's proximity.

ure 2-16). This surgical plane is relatively avascular and permits easier elevation of the overlying flap than with dissection in the middle subcutaneous fatty tissue. However, the surgeon must decide the safest, most efficient depth of dissection based on the clinical findings. If the overlying skin is scarred or unstable, the level should be deeper to ensure sufficient skin vascularity and integrity to contain the expander and withstand the expansion process. If the skin is thick and resistant to expansion, however, the balloon may be better inserted in the middle subcutaneous fat level to overcome these resistant layers. The pocket for the remote valve should be deep enough to prevent

skin erosion from the valve's firm dome but shallow enough to permit valve palpation.

Creation of the pockets can be accomplished easily in most cases by finger dissection or the spreading action of double-edged cutting scissors. Blunt dissection rather than cutting significantly reduces the incidence of hematomas or seromas.

Special instrumentation is useful to facilitate the creation of adequate pockets through a small (3.5 cm) incision. The author has developed a versatile tool, the "Helper"* dissector, for this purpose (Figure 2-17). The instrument is narrow (2.5 cm), long (25 cm), and malleable with a spoon-shaped dissecting blade on one end and a shoe-shaped receptacle to hold the valve on the opposite end. The Helper is inserted into the small incision, and the spoon-shaped end is pushed forward above the fascia and swept back and forth in an area 1 cm larger than the expander base outlined on the skin. This larger pocket ensures that the expander will be flat and not buckle with folds, which could lead to pressure necrosis and implant extrusion. The pocket for the valve is similarly made by passing the Helper away from the balloon pocket through the same incision. This malleable instrument also permits the surgeon to dissect around curved surfaces under the galea aponeurotica or subcutaneous plane, as on the scalp and joints.

Another instrument, the "Spreader,"† can also create a subcutaneous pocket by spreading apart the blades through the small incision (Figure 2-18). The use of both instruments enables the surgeon to complete the formation of the valve and balloon pockets safely and efficiently.

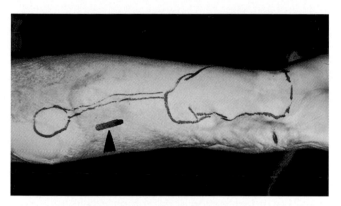

Figure 2-14 A remote incision is made away from the defect and expander. In general the incision is placed between the balloon and its valve. This approach reduces the risk of implant exposure but creates an additional scar.

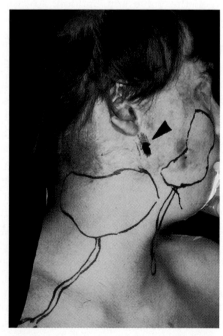

Figure 2-15 A 3.5 cm remote incision was made along a scar below the ear lobule in this 16-year-old patient with burn scars in the postauricular area and lateral midface. Pockets for two expander units were elevated from this access point, which was distant and perpendicular to the units.

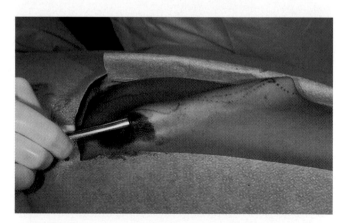

Figure 2-16 Expander pocket is usually located in the deep subcutaneous fatty plane above the muscle fascia. It is created safely by finger dissection or by the spreading action of an instrument, such as a long Metzenbaum scissors. The dissection is begun at the incision site (intralesional, paralesional, or remote), down to the appropriate subcutaneous plane, and then to the balloon site.

---

*Wells Johnson Co., Tucson, Arizona.
†Robbins Instruments, Chatham, New Jersey.

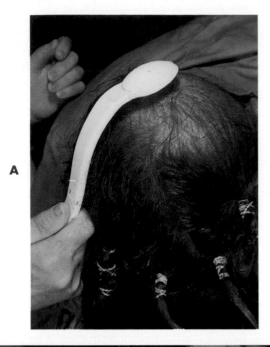

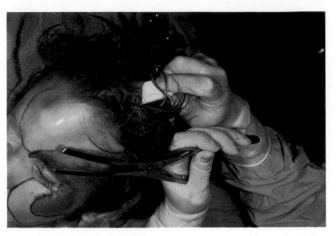

Figure 2-18 "Spreader" instrument rapidly creates a pocket or tract by inserting and gently spreading the long blades in the tissue. This initial dissection can be refined with the Helper instrument, which can more precisely develop the pockets for the expander and its valve.

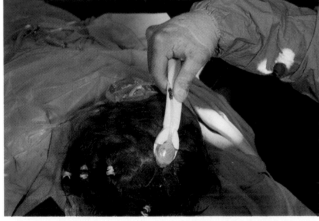

Figure 2-17 **A,** Malleable Teflon "Helper" instrument can facilitate the dissection of pockets around curved planes, such as the scalp. It can be autoclaved safely for repeated use. **B,** The Helper's opposite end houses the remote valve in a shoe-shaped receptacle, which is accurately positioned and left in the reservoir pocket as the instrument is removed.

Preparation of Dissected Pockets

An antibiotic solution (500,000 U bacitracin/500 ml saline) is used to irrigate the dissected pockets. The use of surgical drains depends on the amount of bleeding present or expected after the extensive undermining is completed. Surgical drainage is seldom necessary, however, because of the vasoconstrictive effect of epinephrine and the filling of the balloon to tissue capacity at surgery.

Preparation of Expander Unit

The surgeon removes the expander unit, consisting of the balloon, tubing, and valve, from its sterile package and inspects it for any imperfections that could lead to an eventual implant failure, especially herniations of the envelope, improper sealing at joints, and structural defects in the valve system. If the entire unit requires sterilization, insertion of a 23-gauge needle into the valve or transection of the tubing is required to decompress the expander and prevent overinflation or rupture during sterilization under vacuum pressure. A metal in-line connector is used to reassemble the transected tubing or to adjust the distance and tension between the valve and balloon. An appropriate tension across the tubing is imperative to prevent curling or kinking, which can cause skin erosion or flow obstruction.

The expander is partially filled with 10 to 20 ml of saline containing bacitracin by inserting a 23-gauge scalp vein needle perpendicularly into the soft spot on the remote valve. A drop of methylene blue dye may be added to the original saline solution as a marker. The integrity of the entire unit is examined by gently squeezing the balloon to determine any leakage from the balloon, tubing, and remote valve (Figure 2-19). If the full solution is too deeply colored, the implant may become discolored (precipitation of dye) and produce a cosmetic concern to the patient.

Insertion of Unit

The partially underfilled expander is carefully pushed through the 2.5 to 4.0 cm incision. The balloon is filled to tissue tolerance with the methylene blue saline solution through the remote valve (left temporarily outside the skin) with a 23-gauge scalp vein needle. The balloon is positioned by massaging the implant into its final location. Then the remote valve is inserted through the same incision into its separate snug pocket

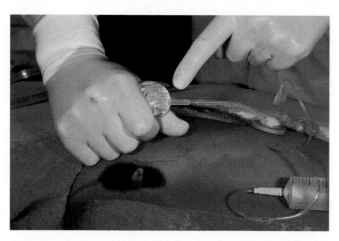

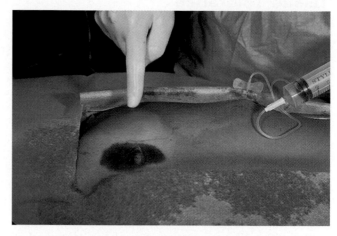

Figure 2-19 After expander unit is partially filled with saline or methylene blue–colored saline, the unit's integrity is determined by squeezing the balloon. The entire system must be checked for weak spots at joints and in the patch behind the expander. The soft spot on the reservoir must be able to seal repeated punctures by the 23-gauge needle.

Figure 2-20 Balloon is inserted and filled to tissue tolerance in its pocket, which is about 1 cm larger than the expander base. The balloon is expanded to smooth out wrinkles and folds. The valve is fitted snugly in its cavity to reduce the risk of overturning. The tubing is kept taut to prevent curling and kinking. Before leaving the operating room, the surgeon must ensure the expander unit is functioning perfectly by testing it for easy injection and withdrawal of saline through the remote valve system. Serial expansion is begun 1 to 2 weeks after surgery. Sterile technique is required to fill the expander by spreading Betadine paint and antibiotic ointment over the target zone on the valve. The amount of filling is determined by patient and tissue tolerance.

(Figure 2-20), which prevents overturning of the valve. The valve is placed deep but should be palpable under the tissue. Valve placement in a thin-skinned region is discouraged because of the increased chance for erosion. The length of tubing should be taut, not loose. If a curl or kink forms in the extended tubing, the valve pocket should be repositioned farther away or the tubing shortened at the in-line connector.

Exteriorization of the valve is an alternative to burying it, as is done in a closed system. An external reservoir eliminates the pain of percutaneous needle puncture and provides controlled drainage of a hematoma or seroma. The disadvantage of an external valve is possible contamination of the balloon and capsule, which may jeopardize the reconstruction, especially one using autogenous grafts or alloplastic implants. In addition, inflammation and contamination of the tract in which the tubing lies may result in an internal linear scar with skin hyperpigmentation. Pain from the percutaneous needle stick in a closed system can be reduced with the application of topical 2% Xylocaine jelly on the skin for 15 to 30 minutes.

Before skin closure (in a closed system), the valve should be tested in situ to ensure easy fluid withdrawal and injection. The expander should be filled with sterile isotonic saline containing bacitracin to (1) decrease the collection of seromas or hematomas by obliterating dead space in the pocket, (2) maintain the pocket size, (3) smooth out envelope folds and wrinkles, and (4) reduce the incidence of implant contamination.

Incision Closure

An absorbable suture(s) is placed at the balloon pocket–incision interface to prevent the expander from bulg-

ing into the dissection pathway. The tubing that crosses the access site is displaced into a separate tract by a few sutures to prevent its migration back into the incision line. The skin approximation is meticulously closed to ensure primary healing. The skin sutures are removed within 2 weeks to avoid suture tract infections.

SERIAL EXPANSION PROCESS

Expanders are inflated 1 to 2 weeks postoperatively before a firm capsule has formed and can inhibit the expansion process. The surgeon avoids increased tension on the suture line, fills the prosthesis under sterile conditions, and wipes the skin overlying the valve with an alcohol swab. After applying Betadine solution, the surgeon dabs Garamycin (gentamicin) ointment on the skin over the valve's soft spot. Wearing sterile gloves, the surgeon withdraws saline from a disposable 50 ml bottle using a 30 ml syringe. Small, one-time-use saline vials are preferred to larger containers to limit possible cross-contamination from multiple use. The prosthesis is expanded by introducing a 23-gauge butterfly (scalp vein) needle perpendicularly into the reservoir to minimize the risk of the needle tearing the valve. Trauma to the valve is more likely when a larger-gauge needle is attached directly to the syringe. Expanders are filled to tissue and patient tolerance.

Tissue Tolerance

Saline is injected until the skin feels firm to palpation. Inflation is stopped before capillary perfusion is compromised, as determined by the degree of pallor and blanching.

Patient Tolerance

The patient complains of discomfort or pain when tissue ischemia becomes significant from increased volume and pressure with overfill. If too much tension is produced, saline can be immediately withdrawn to reverse tissue ischemia and pain. No patient should experience significant pain after each serial expansion. Within 6 to 12 hours the tissues have stretched to accommodate the increased volume.

The interval between injections depends on the tissue's elasticity. Weekly intervals are generally convenient and provide enough time for the tissues to expand safely. Overly aggressive expansion causes not only patient discomfort but also tissue ischemia and necrosis. Inflation every 2 weeks is better tolerated by some patients and does not affect the final result. Some patients can respond to serial injections at 4-day intervals without major complications.

The primary criterion for adequate expansion is the generation of sufficient or slightly more tissue to reconstruct the defect successfully. The expansion process is complete when the measured width of the expanded hemispheric domed flap will provide the needed flap advancement to cover the defect, as previously described.

DELIVERY OF TISSUE

Preoperative preparation, surgical insertion, and serial expansion culminate in the final procedure of adequate flap coverage. At this point, another principle of soft tissue planning for flap advancement must be emphasized: produce the smallest but most functional and aesthetic scar. To achieve this goal, the surgeon must decide where the final scar should be located. After marking the skin with the final line of closure, which will be hidden as much as possible and directed in the lines of least skin resistance, the advancing flap can be best fitted to this pattern. The surgeon may stray from these markings once the flap is advanced.

Intraoperative Expansion

The surgeon may perform intraoperative expansion when additional tissue is required at the second surgery (Figure 2-21). After the patient or tissue is anesthetized, the expander can be filled to beyond tissue tolerance. Blanching, pallor, and increased firmness should be carefully monitored so that the ische-

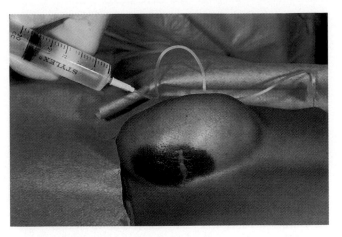

Figure 2-21   At second reconstructive stage, intraoperative expansion of the prosthesis can further stretch the overlying tissue to gain quickly 1 to 2 cm of skin. The surgeon fills the expander until skin blanching occurs for 5 to 10 minutes. A convenient approach is to perform intraoperative expansion immediately after the patient is anesthetized. By the time the surgeon has finished handwashing and the patient's skin is prepared and draped, the maximum amount of tissue stretch has occurred. Because of this small additional tissue gain at surgery, the surgeon is more confident that enough tissue is available to finish the reconstruction.

mic time does not exceed 10 to 15 minutes. In general, irreversible tissue ischemia does not occur within this brief period of increased volume and stretch and decreased perfusion pressure. The amount of saline added depends on the local conditions. Intraoperative expansion can sometimes gain 1 to 2 cm of additional tissue, allowing the surgeon to proceed with the reconstruction more confidently.

Flap Design for Advancement

The incision starts at the border between the lesion and the expander (Figure 2-22). Use of the cutting cautery allows dissection down to the capsule without injury to the expander. After the expander is removed from its pocket, the capsule surrounding the tubing is cut with the cautery and then split to free the encapsulated valve. Rarely, removal of the remote valve is so difficult that a separate incision over the reservoir is needed, resulting in an additional scar.

During the lesion's excision, the surgeon should attempt to preserve any uninvolved subcutaneous fat under the lesion (Figure 2-23). This tissue can provide added fill to the reconstruction.

A trial advancement of the hemispheric flap across the defect will indicate whether further releasing procedures are necessary (Figure 2-24, *A*). If the flap falls short of its intended forward position, an incision around the base of the capsule with further dissection into normal tissue will allow the flap to be moved forward more effectively. Extensive capsulectomy of the

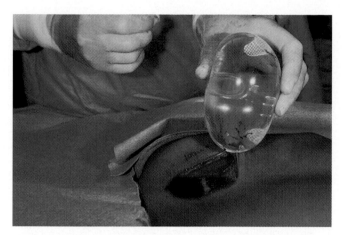

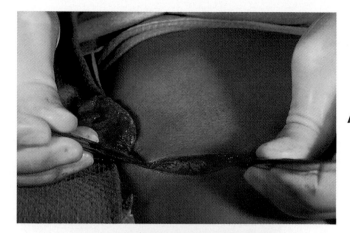

A

Figure 2-22 After expander unit is removed, the stretched flap will contract and appear insufficient for the intended coverage. The flap must be maximally reexpanded by releasing its base through a capsulotomy and, if needed, unfurling the domed flap by removing the capsule. This maneuver increases the area of usable tissue needed to cover the defined defect. Since the expansion process encourages the development of a highly vascular flap (delay phenomenon), capsulotomy and capsulectomy are not likely to compromise tissue perfusion.

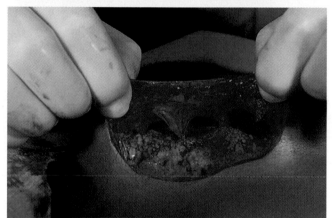

B

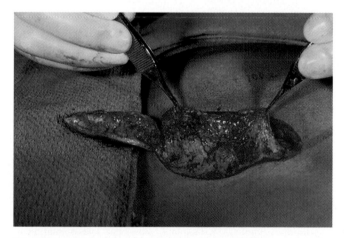

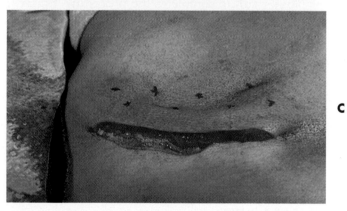

C

Figure 2-23 Whenever subcutaneous tissue under the defect can be safely preserved, it should be retained to provide more bulk to fill the compressed site. An additional incentive to utilize this tissue is the presence of sensory corpuscles and nerves.

Figure 2-24 **A,** The expanded flap is advanced to determine adequacy of coverage. Further surgical release may be required for further coverage. **B,** Expanded flap is gently pulled forward and stabilized in that position by dermal-advancing sutures (absorbable 3-0 or 4-0 material). These fixation sutures counter the stretchback phenomenon and lessen tension at the line of closure. **C,** These sutures are placed in a staggered triangular pattern so as not to compromise blood flow within the flap.

dome, especially at the leading edge of the expanded flap, may be necessary to unfurl and open the restricted flap. Double cutback, single backcut, or over-the-top advancement designs may be considered to maximize delivery of tissue, but additional scars may mar the final reconstruction.[19]

During flap advancement across the defect, absorbable tacking sutures from the capsule and dermis to stable underlying tissue will drag the flap forward and anchor it in a forward position (Figure 2-24, *B*). Such a maneuver may decrease the amount of flap retraction and the width of the inci-

sion scar. Positioning the anchor-advancing sutures in a triangulated distribution removes tension from the suture line closure (Figure 2-24, *C*). Any skin dimpling produced by these buried sutures disappears within 6 weeks. A two-layered skin closure

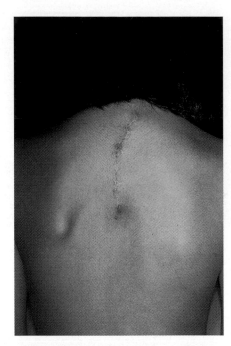

Figure 2-25 Final scar should be placed in the line of maximum skin relaxation, with minimal tension across the line of closure. The degree of scar hypertrophy is determined by several factors, including the patient's age and genetics and the scar site and its location on the body.

with an absorbable subdermal stitch and permanent outer suture completes the procedure. Surgical drains may be required to eliminate the dead space.

POSTOPERATIVE MANAGEMENT

Sutures are cleansed daily with hydrogen peroxide and lubricated with an antibiotic ointment. Sutures are usually removed in 2 to 3 weeks. The patient should use a sunscreen lotion for at least 6 weeks postoperatively to diminish discoloration of the flap or incision scar (Figure 2-25). If a hypertrophic scar develops, a pressure garment and silicone dressing may be beneficial.

SUMMARY

Meticulous attention to proper patient selection, preoperative planning, surgical technique, judicious tissue expansion, and delivery of tissue is essential to a successful outcome with ideal tissue replacement for patients who need reconstructive skin surgery. These general considerations apply to tissue reconstruction in all areas of the body. However, each region has special needs, which are explored later in the appropriate chapters.

REFERENCES

1. Austad ED, Thomas SB, Pasyk K: Tissue expansion: dividend or loan? *Plast Reconstr Surg* 78:63, 1986.
2. Brobmann GF, Huber J: Effects of different-shaped tissue expanders on transluminal pressure, oxygen tension, histopathologic changes, and skin expansion in pigs, *Plast Reconstr Surg* 76:731, 1985.
3. Duits EHA, Molenaar J, van Rappard JHA: The modeling of skin expanders, *Plast Reconstr Surg* 83:362, 1989.
4. Joss GS, Zoltie N, Chapman P: Tissue expansion technique and the transposition flap, *Br J Plast Surg* 43:328, 1990.
5. Mottaleb M, Wong RKM, Manders EK, Sasaki GH: Tissue expansion. In Riley WB, editor: *Instructional courses: Plastic Surgery Educational Foundation*, vol 1, St Louis, 1988, Mosby.
6. Radovan C: Tissue expansion in soft tissue reconstruction, *Plast Reconstr Surg* 74:482, 1984.
7. Sasaki GH: Tissue expansion. In Jurkiewicz MJ, Krizek TJ, Mathes SJ, Ariyan S, editors: *Plastic surgery: principles and practice*, St Louis, 1990, Mosby.
8. Shively RE: Skin expander volume estimator, *Plast Reconstr Surg* 77:482, 1986.
9. van Rappard JHH, Molenaar J, van Doorn K, et al: Surface-area increase in tissue expansion, *Plast Reconstr Surg* 82:833, 1988.
10. Morgan RF, Edgerton MT: Tissue expansion in reconstructive hand surgery, *J Hand Surg* 10A:754, 1985.
11. Gibney J: Tissue expansion in reconstructive surgery. Paper presented at annual meeting of the American Society of Plastic and Reconstructive Surgeons, Las Vegas, October 1984.
12. Manders EK, Schenden MJ, Furrey JA, Hetzler PT: Soft tissue expansion: concept and complications, *Plast Reconstr Surg* 74:493, 1984.
13. Nordstrom REA: "Stretch-back" in scalp reductions for male pattern baldness, *Plast Reconstr Surg* 73:422, 1984.
14. Sugihara T, Ohura T, Kim C, et al: The extensibility in human skin. Paper presented at PSEF International Tissue Expansion Symposium, San Francisco, October 1987.
15. Stark HL: Directional variations in the extensibility of human skin, *Br J Plast Surg* 30:105, 1977.
16. Ohura T, Sugihara T, Honda K: Post-operative evaluation in plastic surgery using the Bio-skin Tensiometer, *Ann Plast Surg* 5:74, 1980.
17. van Rappard JHA, Bauer FW, Grubben MJAL, et al.: Epidermopoiesis in controlled tissue expansion. In van Rappard JHA, editor: *Controlled tissue expansion in reconstructive surgery*, Nijmegen, Netherlands, 1988, SSN.
18. van Rappard JHA, Sonneveld GJ, Boughouts JMHM: Geometric planning and the shape of the expander. In van Rappard JHA, editor: *Tissue expansion in facial plastic surgery*, vol 5, New York, 1988, Thieme.
19. Zide BM, Karp NS: Maximizing gain from rectangular tissue expanders, *Plast Reconstr Surg* 90:500, 1992.

3 Reaction Patterns and Dysfunctional Changes in Expanded Tissue

Although tissue expansion has been applied clinically for more than 35 years, only a few articles have addressed the histomorphology of expanded skin in humans[1-5] and experimental animals.[6-13] No attempt has been made to correlate these consistent histomorphologic alterations in response to expansion with specific early or delayed functional changes`or to suggest a therapeutic management plan to address these concerns. Some of these changes may be either temporary or insignificant to the patient and therefore may not warrant medical or surgical intervention.

PATIENTS AND METHODS IN FOLLOW-UP

From 1979 to 1995 the author inserted 1026 expanders in 986 patients (57% females, 43% males; mean age, 27.5 years). A questionnaire was sent to 500 patients requesting a follow-up visit for an appraisal of their expanded tissue and their experience with this technique (Table 3-1). Only 176 (35%) of the queried patients responded, and 112 came for a follow-up visit. Fifty-eight patients agreed to a biopsy before expander insertion and immediately after completion of their procedures at 6 to 12 weeks (mean, 11.2 weeks), as shown in Table 3-2. Only 11 patients could have a biopsy 6 to 12 weeks after their reconstruction, and 21 were available for long-term follow-up biopsies at 1 to 4 years postoperatively. The age range of these 58 patients was 3 to 60 years (mean, 21.9 years). Standard commercial expanders were used, and their volume after expansion ranged from 375 to 850 cc (ml) (mean, 597.8 cc). The biopsy specimen from each patient was fixed in formalin, embedded in paraffin, cut at a thickness of 5 μm, and examined with various stains, including hematoxylin-eosin and azan-Mallory preparations. In 10 patients a control biopsy specimen was taken from normal tissue adjacent to the expanded area or from a body area opposite the expanded site. Seven expanders were inserted in the scalp region, 15 in the head and neck area, 13 in the breast, 8 in the trunk, and 15 in the extremities.

RESULTS OF FOLLOW-UP

Epidermis (Figure 3-1 and Table 3-3)

The epidermis is the thinnest, outermost portion of the skin, varying in thickness from 40 μm on the eyelids to 1600 μm on the palms. The average thickness for most of the epidermis is 100 μm, compared with 1500 to 4000 μm for full-thickness skin. The epidermis rests on and attaches to the basal lamina, which serves as a structural support and an imperfect barrier.

The major cells in the epidermis are the ectodermally derived *keratinocytes.* Keratinocyte differentiation occurs in 28 to 45 days, progressing from the basal proliferative germinal layer to the spinous layer, granular layer, and dead cornified layer. Under normal circumstances the epidermis is a renewing cell population in which cell production equals constant cell loss, thus preventing any change in overall tissue size. The tough cornified layer forms a barrier to water loss and penetration by external physical, chemical, and biologic insults.

Interspersed among the keratinocytes are three immigrant cells that enter the epidermis during embryonic development or continuously repopulate it during postnatal life. *Melanocytes,* derived from the neural crest, retain their ability to divide within the basal cell layers. Melanocytes produce melanosome pigments that protect the skin from harmful ultraviolet radiation. *Merkel cells,* derived neural crest cells, also reside among the basal keratinocytes and are

■ **Table 3-1**   Tissue Expansion Questionnaire

Name _____   Age _____   Date _____

Reason for Surgery   Date(s) of Surgery

_____   _____
_____   _____
_____   _____
_____   _____
_____   _____

Number   Location   Duration of Expansion

_____   _____   _____
_____   _____   _____
_____   _____   _____
_____   _____   _____
_____   _____   _____

Please comment on any side effects or complications during expansion:

_____
_____
_____
_____
_____
_____
_____
_____

Please comment on any side effects or complications after completion of expansion:

_____
_____
_____
_____
_____
_____
_____
_____
_____
_____

found in glabrous areas of the body (e.g., digits, lips, oral cavity). Merkel cells function as slow-adapting type I touch mechanoreceptors. Skin expansion rarely involves skin from glabrous areas. In contrast, changes in touch receptors after expansion of nonglabrous skin may be caused by alterations of free nerve endings and specialized corpuscular receptors in the dermis. *Langerhans cells* are located in the spinous layer and may constitute 4% of the total epidermal cell population. Langerhans cells are mesenchymal in origin, derived from precursor cells in the bone marrow. As with cells of the monocyte-macrophage lineage, Langerhans cells probably play a role in various immune processes, including allergic contact dermatitis and immune tolerance and surveillance against neoplasia.

Histomorphologic Epidermal Changes

In the patient population previously identified, epidermal reaction to long-term tissue expansion resulted in a quantitative increase in skin thickness at completion of expansion (6 to 12 weeks), with maximal thickness achieved 6 to 12 weeks later (Table 3-4 and Figure 3-2). The epidermal thickness returned to preexpansion levels in 1 to 4 years. In all specimens the stratum spinosum thickened slightly, but no significant differences were seen in the distinguishable layers (Figure 3-3). The rete peg ridges flattened throughout expansion but slowly recovered within 2 years. Microscopic evaluations did not reveal an increase in epidermal mitotic activity or any significant changes in the specialized melanocyte, Langerhans, and Merkel cells. Table 3-5 summarizes these responses.

■ **Table 3-1** Tissue Expansion Questionnaire—*Continued*

Please compare your expanded skin to adjacent or nonexpanded skin:

_____

Please evaluate your experience with tissue expansion technique (inconveniences, office and hospital visits, pain or discomfort during and after expansion, personnel, expectations, and final results):

_____

Please describe the quality of your expanded tissue 1-4 years after your reconstruction was completed:

1. Texture: _____
2. Color: _____
3. Dryness: _____
4. Scaliness: _____
5. Suntan/burn: _____
6. Swelling: _____
7. Numbness/itching: _____
8. Pain: _____
9. Malignancy: _____
10. Benign growths: _____
11. Stiffness: _____
12. Stretch marks: _____
13. Thinning hair: _____
14. Perspiration: _____
15. Skin allergies: _____
16. Skin infections: _____
17. Skin elasticity: _____
18. Depression at reconstructed site(s): _____
19. Changes in blood flow at reconstructed site(s): _____
20. Muscle weakness or tightness at reconstructed site(s): _____

Clinical Response to Epidermal Changes

Patients' responses to the questionnaire regarding epidermal changes indicated minimal long-term detrimental effects from the expansion process (Table 3-6). Except for dryness and hyperpigmentation, none of the responses indicated changes in epidermal instability, barrier integrity, melanocytic protection, or tumor formation.

Three (African American, Asian, and Hispanic) of the 176 patients (1.7%) indicated that their expanded skin remained darker than adjacent nonexpanded skin up to 4 years after surgery (Figure 3-4). No patient complained of hypopigmentation of their expanded skin. Clinical skin lightening or darkening may also result from vascular changes or dermal scarring.

Ten of the 176 patients (5.7%) complained of skin dryness after surgery that required daily application of skin lotions. The etiology of dry skin after expansion is unclear but may be related to postsurgical reduction of ground substance or decreased functional lubrication of skin from the remaining sweat and sebaceous glands. Skin dryness is most often related to excessive loss of moisture from the horny keratin layer of the stratum corneum.

■ **Table 3-2** Summary of Tissue Expansion and Biopsies in 58 Patients

Patient number	Gender	Age (yr)	Location of tissue expansion	Duration of procedures (wk)	Volume of expander (cc)
1	F	5	Scalp[†‡]	10	800
2	F	46	Breast	12	690
3	M	7	Head[*†‡]	9	650
4	F	32	Extremity	6	525
5	F	51	Breast[*†]	12	780
6	M	8	Head	10	500
7	F	11	Back[†‡]	12	550
8	F	33	Neck	10	450
9	M	9	Extremity[†‡]	8	390
10	F	34	Breast[†‡]	12	750
11	F	41	Scalp[*]	11	850
12	M	15	Extremity	10	650
13	F	36	Neck[†]	12	630
14	M	5	Back[*‡]	11	750
15	F	19	Head[†‡]	12	635
16	M	7	Extremity	12	450
17	F	36	Breast	11	750
18	F	5	Head[*]	11	435
19	M	7	Extremity	10	375
20	M	39	Scalp[†]	11	660
21	F	12	Extremity	10	445
22	M	15	Extremity	9	525
23	F	56	Breast	11	650
24	F	58	Breast	12	660
25	M	11	Back[†]	11	575
26	M	10	Scalp	12	600
27	M	24	Neck	9	450
28	M	21	Extremity[*†]	10	475
29	F	8	Head	12	435
30	F	12	Extremity	9	380
31	M	6	Head	12	575
32	F	38	Breast	12	700
33	M	11	Head	11	750
34	F	12	Back[*]	11	650
35	F	39	Breast	12	650
36	M	10	Extremity[†]	10	550
37	F	46	Breast[†‡]	12	675
38	F	41	Scalp	10	700
39	M	9	Head	10	575
40	M	7	Back	10	600
41	M	8	Scalp[*†]	12	770
42	F	42	Breast[†]	11	850
43	F	11	Extremity	10	390
44	M	7	Head	12	475
45	F	43	Breast[†]	11	750
46	M	9	Head[*†‡]	12	525
47	F	3	Back	10	600
48	M	21	Neck	10	450
49	M	8	Back	11	600
50	M	21	Scalp	12	700
51	F	39	Breast	12	725
52	M	11	Extremity[†]	9	515
53	F	7	Head[†‡]	10	535
54	M	25	Extremity	11	575
55	F	60	Breast[*†]	12	690
56	F	13	Back	12	600
57	F	41	Extremity[*†]	12	550
58	F	10	Extremity	10	475

*Patient biopsied 6 to 12 weeks after procedures completed.
†Patient biopsied 1 to 4 years after reconstruction completed.
‡Patient had control biopsy sample taken from tissue adjacent or opposite to expanded site.

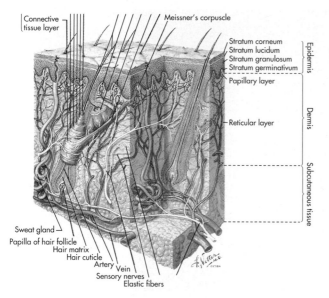

Connective tissue layer
Meissner's corpuscle
Stratum corneum
Stratum lucidum
Stratum granulosum
Stratum germinativum
Epidermis
Papillary layer
Dermis
Reticular layer
Subcutaneous tissue
Sweat gland
Papilla of hair follicle
Hair matrix
Hair cuticle
Artery Vein
Sensory nerves
Elastic fibers

Figure 3-1 The skin and its contents consist of layers that contain a network of vessels and nerves and specialized cells and appendages. The outer epidermal layer varies in thickness depending on its functional needs, from 40 μm (eyelid) to 1600 μm (palm), and consists of keratinocytes and three immigrant cells (melanocytes, Merkel cells, Langerhans cells). The deeper dermal layer is a complex amalgam of cells, filamentous and amorphous tissues, neurovascular networks, and epidermal appendages. Collagen and elastic fibers are the principal fibrous tissue within the dermis, and the glycosaminoglycans and glycoproteins form its ground substance. The upper papillary dermis below the epidermis averages 100 μm in thickness. The deeper reticular dermis represents the bulk of the dermis and extends 2000 to 2500 μm in depth. The amount and distribution of dermal appendages within the dermis differ according to the skin site. Scarpa's fascia divides the hypodermis into a superficial layer and a deep fat layer. The muscles under the adipose tissue are not shown.

Dermis (see Table 3-3 and Figure 3-1)

The dermis is an integrated system of cells; fibrous, filamentous, and amorphous connective tissues; neurovascular networks; and dermal appendages. Fibroblasts, macrophages, and mast cells are indigenous to the dermis, while other cells, such as lymphocytes and plasma cells, may enter the dermis in response to various stimuli. In contrast to the epidermis, no clear sequence of dermal cell differentiation parallels keratinocyte maturation.

Collagen and *elastic fibers* are the principal types of fibrous connective tissue of the dermis. About 80% to 85% of adult collagen is type I, and 15% to 20% is type III. Type IV collagen is confined to structures surrounded by basal lamina, such as in the basement membrane zone between the epidermis and dermis. Elastic fibers return the skin to its normal configuration when it is stretched or deformed. These fibers, when undisturbed, are in a contracted form but are capable of reversible extension to about twice their resting length. Elastic fibers account for about 4% of the dermal protein by weight. The collagen and elastic fibers are synthesized by fibroblasts and organize themselves according to a structural hierarchy from molecules to fibrils, fibers, and bundles. The bundles of collagen are the dominant structural pattern in the skin, with the elastic bundles bordering this main network.

The nonfibrous, connective tissue in the dermis includes the *glycosaminoglycans* (GAGs) and the finely filamentous *glycoproteins* (GPs) of the ground substance. In adult dermis the major GAGs are hyaluronic acid and dermatan sulfate, with chondroitin 4-sulfate and chondroitin 6-sulfate present in smaller amounts. Although the ground substance constitutes only 0.2%

■ **Table 3-3** Functional Units of Skin and Subjacent Tissue

	Cells	Appendages	Functions/responses
Epidermis	Keratinocyte		Protective barrier
	Melanocyte		Pigmentation
	Langerhans cell		Immunity
	Merkel cell		Touch reception
Dermis	Fibroblast		Collagen/elastic fiber, ground substance
	Macrophage		Scavenger
	Mast cell		Allergic response
		Hair follicle	
		Sebaceous gland	Sebum
		Eccrine sweat gland	Thermoregulation
		Apocrine sweat gland	Sweat
		Naked nerve fiber	Pain
		Meissner's, Pacini's and Krause's corpuscles	Pressure, temperature
		Blood vessel	
		Lymph vessel	
Hypodermis	Adipocyte		Insulation, energy
Muscle	Striated muscle cell		Movement

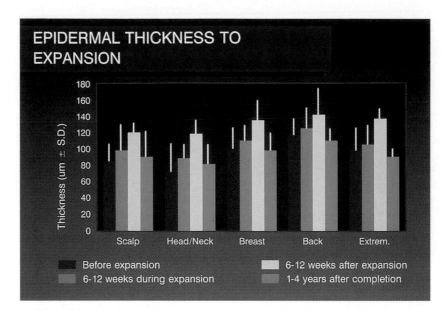

Figure 3-2 Histomorphologic changes in the epidermis to long-term expansion are predictable and result in a quantitative increase in thickness during expansion. Skin attains maximal thickness 6 to 12 weeks after expansion is completed. Within 4 years the epidermal reaction returns thickness to preexpansion levels. This response occurs in skin from all examined regions of the scalp, head and neck, breast, trunk, and extremities.

■ **Table 3-4** Histomorphologic Epidermal Thickness (μm±SE) Response Patterns to Long-term Skin Expansion*

	Before expansion	End of expansion (6-12 wk)	After expansion	
			(6-12 wk)	(1-4 yr)
Scalp	85 ± 30 (7)	97 ± 31 (7)	121 ± 15 (2)	92 ± 28 (3)
Head/neck	75 ± 31 (15)	89 ± 16 (15)	117 ± 18 (3)	84 ± 21 (5)
Breast	101 ± 27 (13)	111 ± 19 (13)	133 ± 24 (2)	98 ± 19 (6)
Back	115 ± 23 (8)	125 ± 24 (8)	142 ± 31 (2)	110 ± 15 (2)
Extremities	97 ± 25 (15)	105 ± 23 (15)	135 ± 13 (2)	88 ± 10 (5)

*Numbers in parentheses indicate number of patients. *SE,* Standard error.

■ **Table 3-5** Histomorphologic Epidermal Response Patterns to Long-term Skin Expansion*

Epidermal factor	Response
Thickness (acanthosis)	Increase
Rete ridges	Decrease
Keratinocytic maturation/mitotic index	No change
Hyperkeratosis (rare)	
Parakeratosis (rare)	
Spongiosis (rare)	
Atrophy (rare)	
Number and distribution of melanocytes/ Langerhans cells/Merkel cells	No change

*Epidermal results from 58 biopsied specimens.

■ **Table 3-6** Clinical Epidermal Response Patterns to Long-term Skin Expansion in 176 Queried Patients

Epidermal changes	Patients affected
Epidermal instability	
Scalding	0
Blistering	0
Dermatitis	0
Swelling	0
Dryness	10 (5.7%)
Barrier integrity	
Water loss	0
Entry of noxious material	0
Melanocytic changes	
Sunburn increase	0
Hyperpigmentation (freckles, suntan)	3 (1.7%)
Hypopigmentation	0
Oncologic resistance	
Benign lesions	0
Malignant lesions	0

of the skin's dry weight, it accounts for most of the volume of the dermis because it holds water in volumes up to 1000 times its own volume. On routine histologic stains, ground substances appear microscopically as empty spaces between collagen bundles.

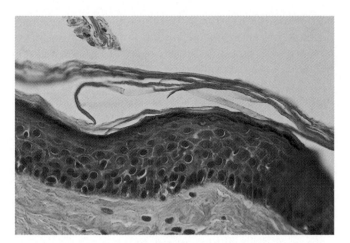

Figure 3-3 In a small number of biopsied specimens from the patients studied, reactive layering of the stratum corneum occurred during the expansion process. The stratum spinosum became thicker than the other epidermal layers. Flattening of the rete peg ridges was observed throughout expansion, with the ridges slowly returning within 2 years after expansion. No distinguishable changes in the immigrant cells (melanocytes, Langerhans cells, Merkel cells) and no increase in the keratinocytes' mitotic index were observed in the specimens.

Dermal Organization

The *papillary dermis* begins at the basement membrane zone below the epidermis and is about the same thickness as the epidermis (average, 100 μm). It contains a high content of type III collagen and a lesser amount of type I collagen. Collagenase activity is almost exclusively confined to the papillary dermis. Fibroblasts, macrophages, and mast cells are greater in number and have a higher proliferation and synthetic capability than cells in the reticular layer. Mature elastic fibers are usually absent in the normal papillary dermis. Overall the papillary dermis reflects few changes in structure even with significant structural changes in the reticular dermis. This phenomenon suggests that factors other than the connective tissue itself (e.g., the epidermis) may have a more prominent role in modulating the structure and function of the papillary dermis.

The *reticular dermis* represents the bulk of the dermis (average thickness, 2000 to 2500 μm) and extends from the papillary dermis deep to the hypodermis. The reticular dermis is composed primarily of type I collagen organized in large fibers and interwoven bundles. Large, mature, bandlike elastic fibers extend between the collagen bundles. In normal dermis, the elastic and collagen bundles of the reticular dermis increase in size progressively toward the hypodermis.

Dermal Appendages

Hair follicles. Hair performs no vital physiologic function in humans, whose bodies could be depilated

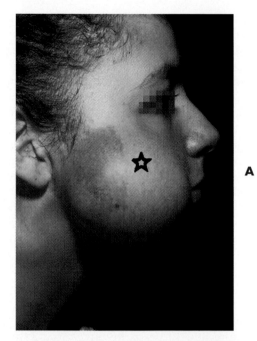

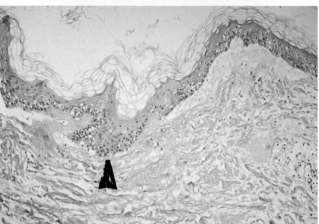

Figure 3-4 **A,** This 16-year-old Hispanic female observed a darkening of her expanded skin late in the 8-week expansion period. This slight degree of hyperpigmentation persisted for about 1 year postoperatively. The expansion experience revealed no complication that would stimulate the skin to darken. The patient was advised against significant sun exposure and used a 30 SPF (sun protection factor) sunscreen. Star indicates biopsy site on the patient's midface away from the nevus. **B,** Skin biopsy of the hyperpigmented "normal" skin was obtained at the end of the 8-week expansion period. Melanosome deposition *(arrow)* is increased in the lower epidermal layers after expansion compared with the melanosome pigment concentration in a preexpansion biopsy of "normal" skin. (magnification $\times$40.)

without any disadvantage. On the other hand, its psychologic function as a major social and sexual feature of the human body is apparent.

Each hair follicle begins by a crowding of nuclei in the germinal layer of the epidermis. This epidermal structure then penetrates downward as a solid column into the dermis. Finally, its base envelops a papilla of dermis and becomes a matrix from which the hair and its inner root sheath grow.

Postnatal hair can be divided into *vellus hair*, which is soft, unmyelinated (unmedullated), unpigmented, and seldom more than 2 cm (⅘ inch) long, and *terminal hair*, which is longer, coarser, myelinated, and pigmented. At puberty, vellus hair is replaced by terminal hair in the pubic, axillary, and facial areas and in the remainder of the body. Pubertal hair growth is androgen dependent. Later androgen stimulation may produce male-pattern baldness, in which terminal hair is replaced by fine, short hair resembling vellus.

The growth of hair is cyclic, consisting of the growing phase *(anagen)*, involuting phase *(catagen)*, and resting phase *(telogen)*. Hair follicles in humans are normally lost randomly and inconspicuously because adjacent follicles are in different phases of the hair cycle. Hairs in different regions of the body spend different amounts of cycle time in anagen, resulting in the characteristic variations in hair length. Scalp hair grows from 3 to 10 years, involutes in a 2- to 3-week period, and rests for 3 to 4 months. In adults at least 85% of all scalp hair follicles are in the anagen phase at any moment. Of the approximate 100,000 follicles in the average scalp, about 70 to 100 telogen hairs are shed daily.

Sebaceous Glands. The sebaceous gland is a lipid-producing structure that develops embryologically from the epithelial bud arising from the hair follicle. Sebaceous glands are found in all areas of the skin with the exception of the palms, soles, and dorsa of the feet. They are most numerous and productive in the scalp and face and largest in the forehead, nose, and back. The vast majority of the sebaceous glands are connected to a hair follicle. The ducts of the large glands join the hair canal about 500 μm below the skin surface. The body of the gland extends to twice this depth.

The sebaceous gland is a holocrine gland because of the sebum-secreting process. The entire sebaceous cell and its contents are cast off into the sebaceous duct. Sebum contains a mixture of lipids whose major components include triglycerides, wax, esters, squalene, and cholesterol. Maturation of sebaceous glands occurs predominantly within the reticular dermis. Sebaceous secretion is continuous rather than intermittent, with the amount and rate of sebum excretion onto the skin surface regulated by androgens.

Eccrine Glands. The true sweat glands in humans are the eccrine glands, which secrete a hypotonic solution that flows to the skin surface and cools the body by evaporation. They are most highly concentrated on the palms, soles, axillae, and forehead. Embryologically, eccrine sweat glands are derived from the surface epidermis, arising independently from the pilosebaceous units and descending to about the junction between the reticular dermis and subcutaneous fat. About 3 million eccrine glands are present at birth, with no additional formation later.

Histomorphologic Dermal Changes

Histomorphologic changes appear more frequently and more permanently in the reticular dermis than in the papillary dermis. After expansion surgery, quantitative analysis demonstrated that the reticular dermis was thinner at the end of expansion (6 to 12 weeks), but was significantly diminished 6 to 12 weeks after the procedure, and partially recovered 1 to 4 years later (Table 3-7 and Figure 3-5). In contrast, the papillary dermis did not change in compactness during expansion or postoperative recovery (Table 3-8 and Figure 3-6).

During and after expansion the collagen bundles within the reticular and papillary dermis were thickened, compacted, and oriented almost parallel to the skin surface (Figure 3-7). Elastic bundles and fibers within the dermis appeared thicker and longer. Occasionally, elastic fibers had a disrupted and fragmented appearance (Figure 3-8). Distribution and orientation of the collagen and elastic bundles of the expanded skin approached that of the normal dermis after 1 to 4 years but still retained a degree of compact thickness. Number and distribution of fibroblasts, mast cells, and macrophages did not change significantly. Melanin-filled macrophages in the papillary dermis did not increase in most patients. In patients with hyperpigmentation after expansion, however, melanosomes were increased.

■ **Table 3-7** Histomorphologic Reticular Dermal Thickness (μm±SE) Response Patterns to Long-term Skin Expansion*

	Before expansion	End of expansion (6-12 wk)	After expansion	
			(6-12 wk)	(1-4 yr)
Scalp	1753 ± 53 (7)	1360 ± 82 (7)	1244 ± 57 (2)	1543 ± 71 (3)
Head/neck	2004 ± 89 (15)	1484 ± 111 (15)	1385 ± 63 (3)	1740 ± 81 (5)
Breast	2187 ± 115 (13)	1644 ± 115 (13)	1588 ± 44 (2)	1874 ± 56 (6)
Back	2543 ± 285 (8)	1909 ± 125 (8)	1894 ± 37 (2)	2215 ± 34 (2)
Extremities	2355 ± 189 (15)	1649 ± 225 (15)	1687 ± 75 (2)	1963 ± 47 (5)

*Numbers in parentheses indicate number of patients. *SE*, Standard error.

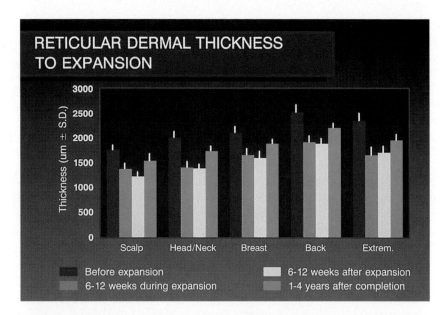

Figure 3-5 Changes in the thicker reticular dermis from expansion are depicted in biopsied expanded skin from the scalp, head and neck, breast, trunk, and extremities. The reticular layer became thinner at the end of expansion but was significantly diminished 6 to 12 weeks later.

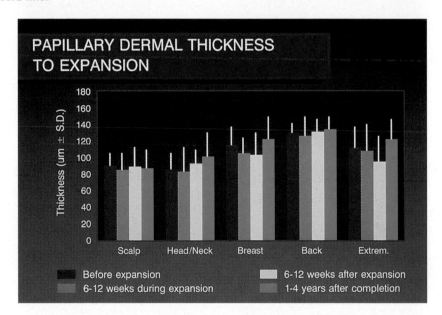

Figure 3-6 In contrast to the reticular dermis, the papillary dermis did not change in compactness during or after the expansion process. Although the papillary dermis in skin biopsied from the extremities was slightly reduced 6 to 12 weeks later, this response was not statistically significant.

■ **Table 3-8** Histomorphologic Papillary Dermal Thickness (μm±SE) Response Patterns to Long-term Skin Expansion*

	Before expansion	End of expansion (6-12 wk)	After expansion	
			(6-12 wk)	(1-4 yr)
Scalp	91 ± 15 (7)	85 ± 21 (7)	95 ± 24 (2)	87 ± 28 (3)
Head/neck	85 ± 18 (15)	84 ± 28 (15)	94 ± 17 (3)	181 ± 38 (5)
Breast	116 ± 23 (13)	185 ± 17 (13)	183 ± 23 (2)	124 ± 27 (6)
Back	127 ± 11 (8)	126 ± 24 (8)	134 ± 15 (2)	134 ± 17 (2)
Extremities	118 ± 26 (15)	188 ± 33 (15)	95 ± 31 (2)	121 ± 24 (5)

*Numbers in parentheses indicate number of patients. *SE,* Standard error.

Dermal appendages such as hair follicles, sebaceous glands, and sweat glands within the reticular dermis occasionally demonstrated compression, blockage, or atrophy (Figures 3-9 to 3-11). These degenerative changes were usually observed in the tissues subjected to greater expansion volumes. Seven patients with scalp reconstructions noted a decrease in their hair density after expansion (Table 3-9); their ages ranged from 5 to 56 years. Scalp expansion was useful for problems of burn alopecia, congenital giant hairy nevi, and male-pattern baldness (Figure 3-12). Interfollicular distances spread from 0.3 to 0.5 mm before surgery up to 1 to 2 mm after expansion and final flap advancement. New hair formation was not observed, but hair color occasionally changed, returning to normal within a year. A few

■ **Table 3-9** Hair Density Changes with 7 Scalp Expansions

	Before expansion	End of expansion (8-12 wk)	After expansion (6 mo)
Hair density (follicles/cm^2)	80-100	50-60	40-50

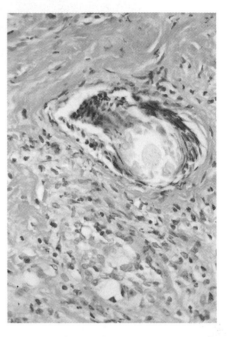

Figure 3-9 Hair follicle has undergone replacement fibrosis in facial skin that was expanded over 10 weeks to replace a burn scar contracture. Hair follicles are sensitive to pressure ischemia, which causes changes in their maturation phases or hair loss. (magnification ×40.)

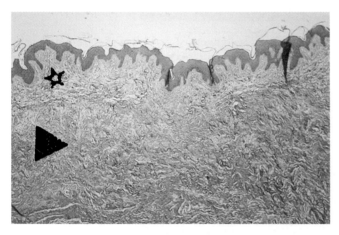

Figure 3-7 Collagen bundles within the papillary (star) and reticular dermis (arrow) appeared to become thicker, more compacted, and oriented parallel to the skin surface (25× magnification). The higher-powered view (40×) of the collagen bundles confirms these observations.

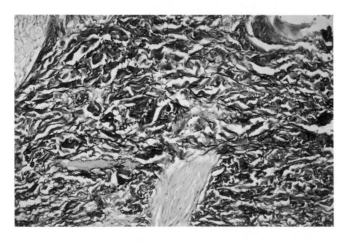

Figure 3-8 Elastic fibers appear to be thicker and occasionally disrupted in "normal" thigh skin that has been expanded for 12 weeks in a 26-year-old with an adjacent burn scar. The fragmented elastic fibers did not result in the clinical findings of striae. (40× magnification.)

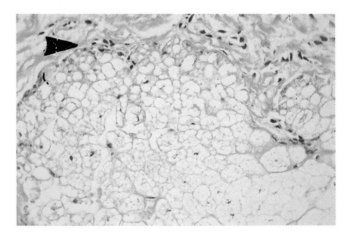

Figure 3-10 Sebaceous gland demonstrates infiltration of inflammatory cells (arrow) and early fibrous replacement in forehead skin that has been expanded for 8 weeks to resurface an adjacent nevus. A significant loss of sebaceous gland function can result in lack of sebum coverage to the overlying skin.

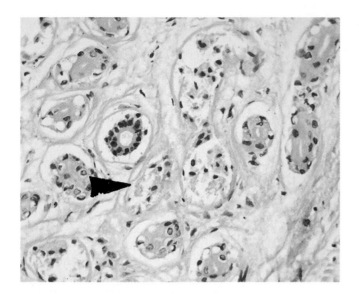

Figure 3-11 Sweat gland shows interseptal fibrosis *(arrow)* and loss of acinar cells in facial skin that has been expanded for 11 weeks to resurface a burn scar contracture. Clinical evidence is insufficient to show that a partial loss of sweat gland function in expanded skin is detrimental to the gland's integrity. (40× magnification.)

patients noticed an increased rate of hair growth. Rarely, the arrectores pilorum muscles adjacent to the hair follicles underwent replacement fibrosis.

Capillary loops from subpapillary plexuses and deeper reticular dermis were dilated, ectatic, and slightly increased in number during expansion but returned to a more normal architecture after expansion.

The exposed nerve network rarely underwent histologic changes during and after expansion (Figure 3-13). In addition, the number and distribution of Meissner's and pacinian corpuscles within the reticular dermis did not decrease after expansion and did not show signs of degeneration.

Clinical Response to Dermal Changes

Patients recorded additional long-term observations possibly related to dermal changes with expansion surgery. Fourteen percent (25 of 176) of the patients said their skin felt stiff and firm for more than 1 year after surgery. This subjective finding may partly result from the compactness of collagen and elastic bundles within the dermis. Almost 6% (10 of 176)

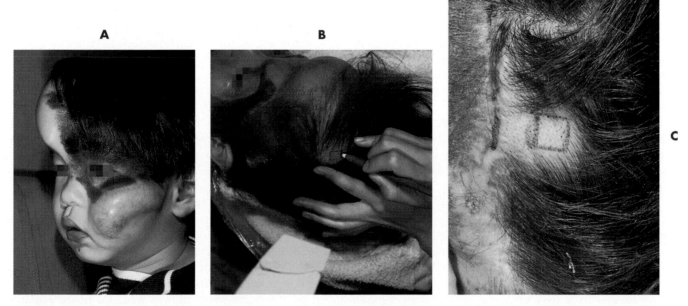

Figure 3-12 A, This 4-year-old Asian male had a giant, pigmented congenital nevus on the left periorbita, hemiforehead, and frontoparietal scalp. The number of hair follicles within a square centimeter of normal scalp destined for expansion was counted and an average of interfollicular distances recorded. The forehead, cheek, and scalp expansion was a two-stage procedure to remove this premalignant, distractive lesion. A 100 cc rectangular expander was inserted under the subcutaneous fat of the left midface. A 500 cc rectangular expander was positioned under the periosteum of the right forehead and extended caudally under the midline of the scalp to its vertex. A third 250 cc rectangular expander was positioned around the lesion's posterior limits and in the scalp's occipital area. The expanders were serially inflated over 3 months to provide sufficient tissue to resurface the scalp, forehead, and cheek. **B** and **C,** At completion of the 3-month expansion the hair follicles within a square centimeter of the expanded normal scalp were recounted and the interfollicular distances again recorded. Similar measurements were repeated 3 months after excision of the nevus and insertion of the expanded flaps. In general, interfollicular distance increased from 0.3 to 0.5 mm before surgery up to 1 to 2 mm, and hair density decreased from 80 to 100 follicles/cm² before surgery to 40 to 50 follicles/cm² after 6 months.

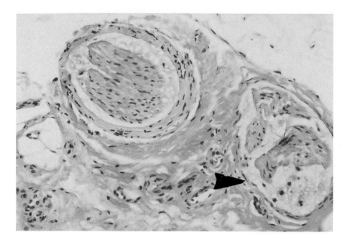

Figure 3-13 Round 400 cc expander was slowly inflated over 3 months under normal skin adjacent to a burn scar contracture on the thigh. Perineural fibrosis *(arrow)* was observed around a sensory nerve fiber in the subcutaneous fat layer of the expanded flap. In contrast, no histologic changes were observed within sensory organelles (Meissner's and pacinian corpuscles) during the expansion process. After 3 years the expanded skin still contained areas of numbness and slight paresthesias, which were of minimal concern to the patient. (magnification ×40.)

of patients developed striae after expansion, usually in skin of the buttocks (3), extremities (4), breast (2), and back (2). Most striae occurred in skin expanded more than once and with higher volumes of saline. No striae were observed in facial skin that underwent multiple expansions. Striae formation is believed to occur after ruptured elastic fibers undergo fibrous replacement.

Nine percent (16 of 176) of patients observed erythroderma on their expanded skin because of increased vascularity. Capillary spiders were most frequently noted in thin, expanded facial skin in children and older patients.

Seventy-seven percent (7 of 9) of patients who had scalp expansion noted thinning of their hair at least 1 year after surgery. Thinning hair may be caused by increased follicular atrophy. Such factors, acting simultaneously on many follicles, have the effect of synchronizing follicular growth cycles. This results in a loss of large numbers of telogen hairs when the synchronized hair follicles enter their anagen phase.

Forty-eight percent (84 of 176) of patients said their expanded skin had less sensation than adjacent normal skin 1 year after surgery. After 2 to 4 years, patients with abnormal sensations of pain, pressure, touch, and temperature decreased to 15% (26 of 176). These findings could not be related to the normal number and distribution of sensory corpuscles observed in expanded skin.

Most patients could not distinguish significant changes in perspiration from the expanded skin after physical or emotional activities. Hypofunction of sebaceous glands is not associated with any recognized pathologic state; specifically, it is not an important factor in skin dryness. No patients observed hyperfunction or greasiness of their expanded skin.

Hypodermis
(see Table 3-3 and Figure 3-1)

The hypodermis lies beneath the reticular dermis and is predominantly composed of *adipocytes,* which are organized into lobules defined by septae of fibrous connective tissue. Nerves, vessels, and lymphatics are located within the septa. Hair follicles and eccrine sweat glands extend into the subcutaneous fat.

The hypodermis insulates the body, serves as an energy reservoir, and cushions and protects the skin. The mean thickness of the hypodermis varies from patient to patient and in different regions of the body.

Histomorphologic Hypodermal Changes

The fatty layer is very intolerant to standard expansion regardless of the body site (Table 3-10). Histologic examination showed that subcutaneous fat responded by undergoing compression atrophy and fibrosis during expansion, 6 to 12 weeks later, and up to 1 to 4 years after reconstruction. The adipocytes initially become flattened and smaller and then lose their fat content, leaving empty shells of cells. Later, replacement fibrosis occurs, diminishing the thickness of the hypodermis by up to 30% to 50% (Figure 3-14).

Clinical Response to Hypodermal Changes

A consistent group of patients observed a significant loss of bulk under their expanded flaps 1 to 4 years after reconstruction, with concave depressions noted in midfaces (25%), breasts (25%), backs (20%) and extremities (64%) (Table 3-11). In some patients, bony prominences became more apparent under the expanded flaps because of loss of the fatty cushion.

Ten of 16 patients (62%) requested secondary procedures (e.g., liposuction of adjacent normal tissue, lipoinjection of depressed expanded tissue) to provide improved symmetry to the reconstructive sites (Figure 3-15). The technique for liposuction to harvest fat cells for lipoinjection employs the syringe technique or a suction pump at reduced negative atmospheric pressure (15 inches/mm Hg). A large-bore cannula is

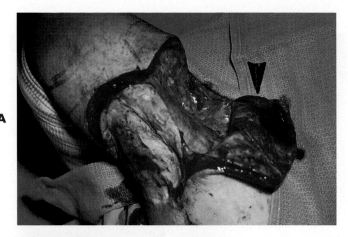

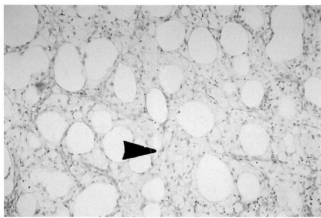

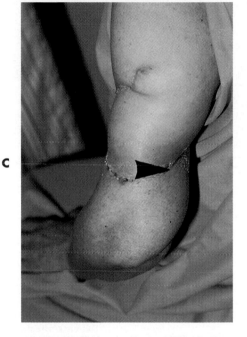

Figure 3-14 **A,** Round 500 cc expander was inserted under the deep subcutaneous fat layer of normal skin on lateral aspect of the left upper extremity. Conventional slow expansion was performed every week to tissue and patient tolerance. At the end of 12 weeks the depressed skin graft (10 × 12 cm) was excised, but its dermal scar bed was retained for autogenous fill. The undersurface of the expanded flap contained a large area of central fat necrosis that probably resulted from expander pressure. **B,** Histologic findings from the area of fatty necrosis *(arrow)* demonstrated replacement fibrosis of adipose cells and interseptal migration of inflammatory cells. The remaining adipocytes appeared to be normal. **C,** Patient's extremity is shown 6 weeks after the expanded flap was transposed and inserted over the dermal scar bed of the skin graft. The degree of depression *(arrow)* was expected to become more evident as healing progressed because of further injury to adipocytes under the expanded flap.

■ **Table 3-10** Histomorphologic Hypodermal Thickness (μm±SE) Response Patterns to Long-term Skin Expansion*

	Before expansion	End of expansion (6-12 wk)	After expansion	
			(6-12 wk)	(1-4 yr)
Scalp	453 ± 27 (7)	249 ± 50 (7)	233 ± 75 (2)	252 ± 93 (3)
Head/neck	1549 ± 300 (15)	929 ± 77 (15)	876 ± 113 (3)	928 ± 281 (5)
Breast	3775 ± 1508 (13)	1084 ± 253 (13)	1004 ± 219 (2)	1114 ± 471 (6)
Back	2884 ± 563 (8)	1306 ± 158 (8)	1117 ± 291 (2)	1225 ± 547 (2)
Extremities	3595 ± 1743 (15)	2035 ± 315 (15)	1832 ± 447 (2)	1978 ± 572 (5)

*Numbers in parentheses indicate number of patients. *SE,* Standard error.

recommended to reduce injury to the delicate adipocytes. The aspirate is strained by gravity through a gauze dressing. The retrieved fat is immediately injected into separate tunnels within the depressed area (Figure 3-16).

Muscle Layer

Histomorphologic Muscle Changes
Skeletal muscles were subjected to stretch or compression during the expansion process. Tissue expanders were inserted under the frontalis muscles in the

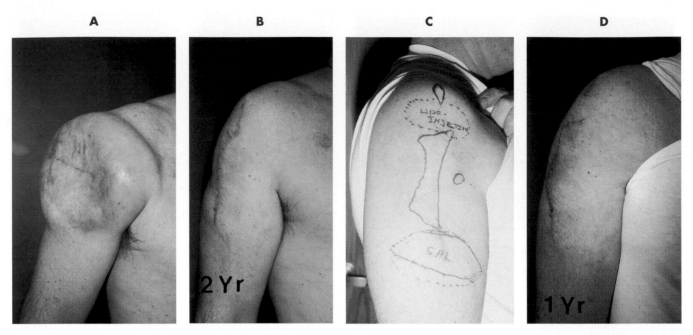

Figure 3-15 A, This 56-year-old patient requested removal of a scarred site over his right upper extremity; salubrasion had been attempted to soften the pigmentation of a large tattoo over the deltoid area. The abrasion scarred the skin, which still contained the pigmentation. Two crescent expanders (300 cc) were inserted around the square-shaped scar bed (10 × 10 cm) and slowly expanded over 3 months. The entire pigmented area was able to be removed, leaving a vertical scar. **B,** After 2 years, the new scar matured, with less pigmentation and thickening. The patient's concern related to the areas of depression in the upper and lower portions of the upper extremity. Touch sensation to the overlying skin was near normal. **C,** Patient was scheduled for lipoinjection of autologous fat into the upper depression, suction-assisted lipectomy from the areas of prominence around the lower depression, and a revision of the central widened scar. **D,** Patient's reconstructed site 1 year after the revision surgery. Areas of depression are less clinically apparent, and the widened central scar improved to a thinner line.

■ **Table 3-11**   Clinical Hypodermal Response Patterns to Long-term Skin Expansion in Queried Patients

Area of concavity/depression	Patients affected
Midface	3 of 12 (25%)
Breast	5 of 25 (20%)
Back	1 of 5 (20%)
Extremities	7 of 11 (64%)

■ **Table 3-12**   Clinical Muscle Response Patterns to Long-term Skin Expansion in Queried Patients

Response	Patients affected
Brow ptosis on donor side	2 of 5 (40%)
Facial muscle paresis	2 of 12 (16%)
Back/extremity/chest wall complications	None

forehead or the pectoralis major muscle during breast reconstruction (Figure 3-17). These muscles were examined during and after expansion. Smaller muscles in the head and neck (facial muscles, platysma muscles) and larger muscles in the back and extremities were compressed during expansion. A few of these muscles were examined histologically for microscopic changes during and after expansion. Similar to fat, these muscles are intolerant to compression injury and undergo atrophy.

In general, significant histologic findings of fibrous scar replacement occurred more frequently in smaller muscles (facial) than in larger muscles (trunk, extremity). Muscle size was a more important factor than the expander location or the rate or duration of expansion in predicting the degree of muscle cell injury. The stri-

ated pattern was lost, leading to hyalinization and subsequent necrosis (Figure 3-18).

Clinical Response to Muscle Changes

Forty percent of patients who underwent skin expansion involving the subgaleal frontalis muscle had reduced eyebrow elevation 1 to 4 years after surgery (Table 3-12). It was unclear whether primary muscle injury or frontalis nerve injury resulted in brow ptosis. One patient required a secondary procedure (static fascia lata suspension, or "brow lift") to correct the ptosis.

Compression of facial muscles by expansion of midface or neck skin resulted in muscle weakness and facial asymmetry during movement in 16% of patients with midface reconstructions. None of these patients,

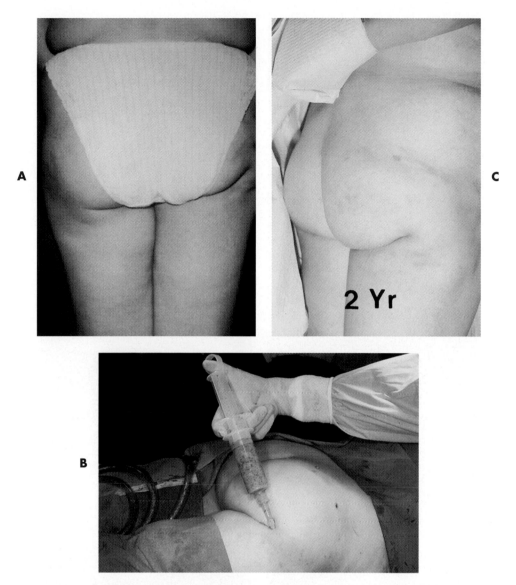

Figure 3-16 A, This 35-year-old patient underwent tissue expansion to her left lateral thigh for removal of a traumatic scar. After 8 weeks of serial expansion the scar was removed and the expanded tissue advanced to cover the defect. This resulted in an area of depression lateral and inferior to the gluteal scar line. **B,** Liposuction of fat from the abdomen by syringe technique (2.4 mm cannula) resulted in about 100 cc of fat aspirate. This was immediately strained through gauze and the fat emptied into a 30 cc syringe. The fat was gently injected into separate tunnels within the depressed site. **C,** Lipoinjection has corrected the depressed area and improved the contour. The reconstruction continued more than 2 years from the initial fill.

however, required secondary procedures to correct this problem. Expansion of the pectoralis major muscle or compression of the larger muscles of the trunk and extremity did not produce clinical complaints of muscle weakness or tendon adhesions.

Capsule

A reactive capsule was present around every tissue expander. Although no statistical correlation was found between the histomorphology of the capsule (Figure 3-19) and the rate or duration of expansion, capsules surrounding textured expanders were thinner than those formed against smooth-surfaced im-

plants. Thickness of capsules ranged from 300 to 1500 μm in 58 patients.

At surgery the rim of thick reactive capsules accentuates the postoperative depression produced by the force of the expander on bone or soft tissue. This contour defect has been referred to as a "dishlike well" deformity. Although resorption of the capsule's remaining rim and floor may eventually occur, surgical removal of the elevated rim around the expander base can significantly "improve" the contour of the reconstructed site and lessen a temporary depression of the calvaria (Figure 3-20).

Thicker capsules were found whenever a significant hematoma or seroma persisted postoperatively.

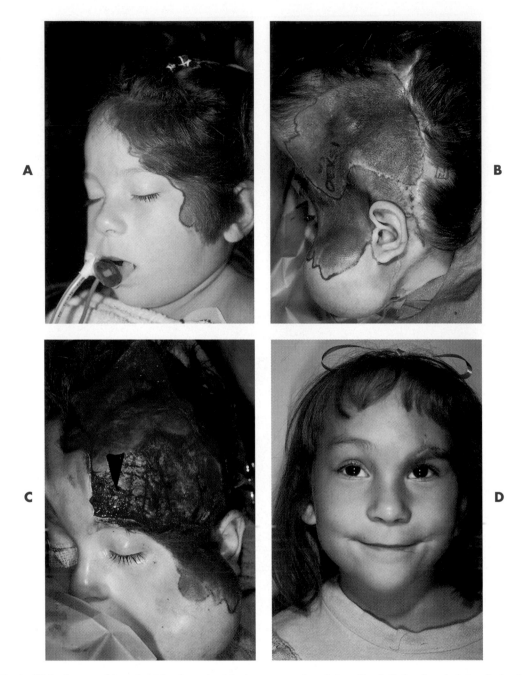

Figure 3-17 **A,** This 5-year-old patient had a giant hairy nevus involving the left forehead, lateral cheek, and frontal-temporal-occipital areas of the scalp. A round 200 cc tissue expander was inserted under the cheek's subcutaneous fat. Two 600 cc rectangular expanders were positioned end-to-end under the galea aponeurotica of the normal forehead and scalp tissue. **B,** The expanders were inflated slowly for 3 months to tissue and patient tolerance. No hair loss was observed during stretching, but the normal excursion of the left frontalis muscle became less apparent as the expander progressively compressed both the frontal branch and the frontalis muscle above it. At the end of expansion the cheek expander contained 180 cc (ml) of saline, and each of the rectangular expanders was filled more than 500 cc. **C,** The nevus was removed at the level of the frontalis muscle fascia in the forehead and to the galea aponeurotica in the scalp. Preservation of the frontalis muscle and its nerve *(arrow)* was possible because the nevoid cells rarely penetrate to the muscle's fascial level. **D,** The expanded forehead skin was advanced over the frontalis muscle. The remainder of the expanded scalp skin resurfaced the left-side scalp that was excised. One year after reconstruction the frontal muscle recovered only partial function, which contributed to brow ptosis.

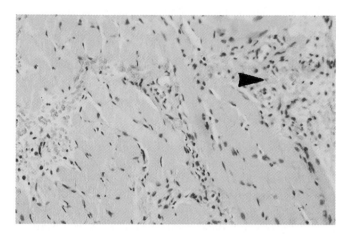

Figure 3-18 At surgery a biopsy of the expanded frontalis muscle from the patient in Figure 3-17 demonstrated hyalinization of the striated muscle fibers with replacement fibrosis *(arrow)*. Direct observation or biopsy of the frontal branch of the facial nerve was not possible at surgery to determine the extent of neuropraxia from balloon compression. (40× magnification.)

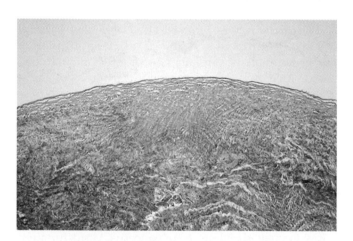

Figure 3-19 Reactive capsule around a smooth-surfaced tissue expander was removed to unfurl the expanded tissue. The expander was filled slowly over 3 months to produce extra tissue to resurface a skin graft site. The capsule consisted of a glistening inner fibrous layer with thick bundles of collagen in parallel alignment. The outer layer contained more loosely aligned collagen fibers within a vascular matrix. Macrophages, fibroblasts, and foreign-body giant cells were interspersed throughout this outer amorphous layer.

Capsules examined at the end of expansion (6 to 12 weeks) had progressed to an inner fibrous layer with thick bundles of collagen and an outer layer containing loosely dispersed collagen and an established vascular network (see Figure 3-19, *B*). Macrophages, fibroblasts, and foreign-body giant cells were present throughout the capsules. Remnants of capsule were still identifiable 1 year after the procedure.

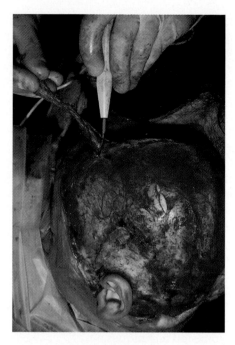

Figure 3-20 Patient in Figure 3-17 during surgery. Pressure on the calvaria by the scalp expanders produced a "welling" effect that was accentuated by the buildup of thickened capsule at the expander base and the depression of the bony floor. If this elevated rim of scar tissue and capsule is left in place, a visible outline may persist for more than a year. This thickened reactive tissue should be removed to lessen the depression before skin closure.

MANAGEMENT PLAN

Although the skin excretes wastes, receives sensory stimuli, and helps regulate body temperatures, its principal function is to be a protective barrier against external intrusions of microbes, chemicals, and various forms of radiation and to be a containment barrier for blood, fluids, and tissue.

The principal resistance to permeation of most noxious substances resides in the thin outer *stratum corneum*, or horny layer. This compact layer consists of dried, dead, elongated cells that contain keratin, which provides strength and chemical resistance. Most of the lipoidal deposits are found between the compressed cells in the form of neutral lipids. Transport through the horny layer depends on the properties and arrangement of its hydrophilic and hydrophobic membranes and their thickness. Alternate pathways for diffusion are located in the shunts provided by the hair follicles, sweat and sebaceous glands, and their intercellular matrices.

Expanded soft tissue appears clinically unchanged after expansion, except for occasional dry skin, hyperpigmentation, erythroderma, decreased hair density, paresthesia or numbness, striae formation, subcutaneous depression, or muscle weakness. However, microscopic changes are observed up to 4 years after completion of the procedure. All layers, with the exception of the epidermis, seem to be transiently or permanently altered during and after the expansion process. It is difficult to distinguish, however, between the direct influences of stretch or compression forces of expansion and indirect influences such as reactive scarring or postsurgical maneuvers.

Most of the 176 patients who responded to the questionnaire were satisfied with the overall results of their expanded-tissue reconstruction. However, the questionnaire did reveal certain transient or permanent changes that could be related to histomorphic alterations with the expanded tissue. Some could be improved with medical and surgical treatments. Other problems have no known satisfactory therapeutic means to correct them. Optimal treatment for these complications remains prevention through improved selection of patients and judicious and effective surgical and expansion techniques.

Epidermal Changes

The initial epidermal reaction to expansion was temporary, with thickening (possibly hyperplasia and hyperactivity of proliferation) and crowding of the cells at the basal layer. Light microscopy showed no increase in the mitotic index of the keratinocytes and no differences in the melanocyte, Merkel cell, or Langerhans cell systems within the epidermal layer. Microscopically the epidermis appeared to return to its normal state within 1 to 4 years after surgery. Despite the temporary changes, the principal functions of the epidermis (excretion, temperature regulation, protective barrier, containment) were not compromised. In addition, no increase occurred in the development of benign or malignant lesions within the expanded skin.

On the basis of this brief clinical experience, the author recommends that a skin moisturizer and general deep skin conditioner be applied to the expanded skin site. Replenishment of hydration to the traumatized expanded skin may reduce the annoyances of dry scaly skin during and after the procedure. Hydration of the stratum corneum may enable skin expansion to proceed more rapidly because of changes in skin resistance.

The importance of controlled-release drugs (loaded liposomes) or tretinoin (Retin-A) to the epidermis during the expansion process has yet to be investigated. The author recommends that a broad-spectrum sunscreen lotion or cream be applied to the expanded tissue for at least 3 months to protect against photosensitivity and photoaging. A sun protection factor (SPF 15+) appears to be adequate and should absorb both UVB (290 to 320 nm) and UVA (320 to 400 nm) ultraviolet light. This protection should reduce the incidence of deepening color in the skin of pigmented patients, retard degeneration of connective tissue in the dermis, and prevent the depletion of Langerhans cells, which influence the immune system.

Dermal Changes

In contrast to the epidermis, the dermis continued to demonstrate microscopic and clinical traces of the expansion process years later. Histologic examination of expanded dermis demonstrated thickened and compacted collagen bundles and elastic fibers that often had focal areas of fragmentation and elastosis. The initial thinness of the stretched reticular dermis partially recovered to its original dimensions 1 to 4 years later. A favorable finding was the global recovery or tolerance to expansion forces shown by the numerous dermal appendages and adnexal structures. Thus the occasional findings of atrophy to hair follicles, sebaceous glands, and sweat glands had no significant clinical repercussions for patients.

Hair density was reduced after stretching because of follicular dropout and fibrosis, asynchronization of the growth phase, and increased interfollicular distance. Increased vascularization during mechanical stretching of tissue usually disappeared after the stress stimulus was removed. Nerve tissue and corpuscular organelles appeared to withstand the expansion process. Occasionally, fibrosis and inflammatory cell infiltrates involved exposed nerve endings.

These microscopic dermal findings may account for the clinical side effects of skin stiffness (14%), striae formation (5%), erythroderma (9%), hair thinning (77%), and decreased sensation (15% to 48%), which patients viewed as long-term concerns. Unfortunately, no effective means exist to prevent or correct these problems, even with judicious slow expansion and meticulous surgical skill.

Hypodermal Changes

A primary patient concern relates to the permanent loss of fat in the subcutaneous layer from the pressure and compression of the expander units. This concave depression can mar an otherwise excellent reconstructive result. Unfortunately, slow and low-volume expansions still produce a significant loss of this intolerant tissue. Surgical attempts to fill the deficient area by the preservation of fatty layers under the reconstructive site inadequately address this problem. Because of the high incidence of postoperative depressions, especially in areas of high fat content, one in two patients may request surgical correction. Liposuction of adjacent normal areas can improve the overall contour to some extent. Repeated lipoinjection of fat offers an alternative means to fill the depressed area, but long-term results vary.

Muscle Changes

Expansion injury to striated muscles can occur with the expander either above or below the muscle units. Direct-pressure necrosis with subsequent fibrosis occurs more frequently with muscles of smaller bulk, such as those in the facial area. The frontalis muscle is especially prone to paresis resulting in brow ptosis. Surgical suspension of the brow may be necessary to improve the aesthetic functional results.

SUMMARY

Tissue expansion remains an established method of reconstruction providing ideal tissue replacement with minimal scarring. Long-term changes in the expanded tissue, however, need to be emphasized to patients. An attempt to correlate histomorphologic changes to clinical changes in expanded tissue represents a simplistic approach to emphasize a causal relationship. Some of these deleterious patient concerns can be prevented or reduced by careful preoperative selection, pretreatment plans, judicious expansion, and skilled surgical techniques. Other problems are inherent to the expansion process; some may be improved through remedial procedures, but for the remainder, no effective means of improvement may be available.

REFERENCES

1. Argenta LC, Marks MW, Pasyk KA: Advances in tissue expansion, *Clin Plast Surg* 12:159, 1985.
2. Grossman JAI, McGraw JB, McDougal HD, et al: Histopathology of human skin expansion, *Plast Surg Forum* 7:85, 1985.
3. Rees RS, Nanney LB, Fleming P, et al: Tissue expansion: its role in traumatic below-knee amputations, *Plast Reconstr Surg* 77:133, 1986.
4. Pasyk KA, Argenta LC, Hassett C: Quantitative analysis of the thickness of human skin and subcutaneous tissue following controlled expansion with silicone implant, *Plast Reconstr Surg* 81:516, 1988.
5. Sasaki GH: Refinements in tissue expansion. In Jurkiewicz MJ, Krizek TJ, Mathes SJ, Ariyan S, editors: *Plastic surgery: principles and practice*, St Louis, 1990, Mosby.
6. Austad ED, Rose GL: A self-inflating tissue expander, *Plast Reconstr Surg* 70:588, 1982.
7. Brobmann GF, Huber H: Effects of different-shaped tissue expanders on transluminal pressure, oxygen tension, histopathologic changes, and skin expansion in pigs, *Plast Reconstr Surg* 76:731, 1985.
8. Diaz P: Nerve elongation. Paper presented at the Tissue Expansion Today symposium, Hershey, Penn, September 1986.
9. Francis AJ, Marks R: Skin stretching and epidermopoiesis, *Br J Exp Pathol* 58:35, 1977.
10. Leighton WD, Russel RC, Marcus DE, et al: Experimental expansion of cutaneous and myocutaneous free flap donor sites: anatomical, physiological and histological changes, *Plast Surg Forum* 9:262, 1986.
11. Pasyk KA, Austad ED, McClatchey KD, et al: Electron microscopic evaluation of guinea pig skin and soft tissues "expanded" with a self-inflating silicone implant, *Plast Reconstr Surg* 70:37, 1982.
12. Pasyk KS, Austad ED, Cherry GW: Intracellular collagen fibers in the capsule around self-inflating silicone expanders in guinea pigs, *J Surg Res* 36:125, 1984.
13. Stark GB, Hong C, Narayanan K, et al: The use of a tissue expander to elongate axial blood vessels, *Plast Surg Forum* 9:151, 1986.

4 Complications in Soft Tissue Expansion

Complications in soft tissue expansion range from minor side effects to life-threatening problems.[1-2] The author estimates that more than 125,000 tissue expansion surgeries were performed from 1956 to 1995 without any expansion-related deaths. In the late 1970s and early 1980s, surgeons reported complication rates as high as 40% to 50% because of improper patient selection, limited experience, evolving techniques, and the use of first-generation expander units and valve systems.[3-7] As surgeons became more sophisticated about tissue expansion techniques in the late 1980s and into the 1990s, the rates and types of complications have decreased to 3% to 5%.[8,9]

Major complications are defined as those that alter the original surgical plan and include closed infections, exposure and extrusion of the expander system, implant failure with deflation, and induced flap ischemia that may lead to skin necrosis. The more frequent *minor complications* include valve turnover, improper valve location or placement, inadequate tissue expansion, and valve and tubing exposure, and usually reflect inexperience with the technique.

This chapter discusses the frequencies and types of major and minor complications in relation to the expansion site and its influence on the desired outcome. Some of these complications can be prevented, whereas others appear to be inherent to the procedure.

PATIENT AND EXPANDER CONSIDERATIONS

This discussion is based on 1505 tissue expansions the author performed in 1086 patients between 1979 and 1995. Follow-up studies ranged from 1 to 12 years and patients' ages from 1 to 76 years.

Tissue expansion was indicated when adjacent skin was insufficient to provide a primary closure for an optimal functional and aesthetic result. Noncandidates included those who (1) could not comply with the protracted course and psychologic embarrassment of expansion, (2) lacked enough available donor skin, or (3) exhibited unstable or infected donor tissue.

The patient's psychologic stability should be evaluated because of the progressive changes in body image that expansion induces during later phases. Goin[10] conducted a limited psychologic study on patients undergoing tissue expansion and concluded that most patients adapted to and tolerated the inconveniences of this procedure. Although a psychologic disturbance is not an absolute contraindication to expansion surgery, the surgeon should consider other techniques that can equally satisfy the reconstructive needs and do not rely on patient acceptance.

Higher complication rates in expansion surgery result from many factors. One of the most important factors involves expansion in unstable or infected tissues. Radovan's early experience was expanding a cross-leg flap for coverage of an exposed tibial fracture.[11] To gain experience with this new technique, Radovan and other surgeons performed these initial cases in clinical situations of infection, exposed tendons and bones, and poor circulation from diabetes mellitus.

All expanders used in the author's experience were conventional products designed with remote injection port systems or incorporated valves within the expander units. Custom-designed units were used in several cases because of unusual anatomic considerations. No attempt was made to exteriorize a reservoir valve away from the expander balloon unless infection occurred around a prosthetic valve. If this minor complication was discovered, partial unroofing of the valve above the skin was done to permit drainage but maintain the valve within its pocket. This simple surgical maneuver, however, does not prevent progressive bacterial invasion around the balloon.

Periprosthetic infections tend to occur when the exposed valve is located above the balloon. In these cases, effective drainage around the balloon cannot occur, creating a pooled fluid medium for bacterial growth. The problem is further complicated when an autogenous graft or silicone prosthesis is to be inserted after expansion. In these situations the entire expander system should be removed when infection is present.

The skin flap is then advanced and allowed to heal for at least 4 months, with delayed insertion of the graft material under the expanded tissue.

Early aggressive surgical management of an impending valve exposure, rather than passive management of an exposed valve, is strongly recommended, including valve and balloon removal and replacement into another pocket. The author has inserted a few expanders with an externalized valve to avoid possible pain during percutaneous needle insertion into a buried valve. However, topical treatment of the skin over the valve port with anesthetic agents before needle insertion can minimize this painful aspect of the expansion experience.

The author prefers a completely buried system because of hygienic concerns of a draining port, contamination of the lining capsule around the tubing and balloon, problems with alloplastic or autogenous graft exchanges, and inflammatory fibrosis of the residual capsule surrounding the tubing and balloon. Salvage of an exposed balloon through thinning of the overlying tissue becomes a more complicated management problem than valve exposure. Continued balloon expansion will increase the skin opening and lead to full exposure and possible bacterial invasion of the capsule.

TISSUE EXPANSION PROTOCOL

Perioperative assessment of expansion factors includes defect size; available donor tissue; number, size, shape, and placement of expander units; anticipated scar lines; estimated duration and frequency of expansion; and possible need for secondary expansions (see Chapter 2).

Surgical protocols include the following:

- Small incisions distant from flap borders to prevent wound dehiscence and implant exposure
- Creation of adequate subcutaneous or subgaleal pockets
- Intraoperative antibacterial coverage: parenteral cefazolin (Ancef), 1 g, and gentamicin (Garamycin), 1.0 to 1.5 mg/kg body weight; irrigation solution of bacitracin wash, 50,000 U/500 ml saline
- Intraoperative filling of expander unit with the bacitracin wash containing a small volume of methylene blue

The introduction of bacitracin solution within the expander unit is an attempt to prevent prosthetic contamination and infection. Antibacterial agents in saline are not used during filling procedures in the office. Methylene blue–stained solution can more easily detect leakage from the expander unit during insertion and helps target the proper valve chamber for injections. Expanders are filled intraoperatively to tissue tolerance to reduce the incidence of hematomas and seromas and to avoid the creation of stubborn implant folds that may later erode through the skin.

Postoperatively, initial expansion begins 1 week after insertion and continues each week or every 2 weeks. Strict aseptic technique is used when filling the expanders. The amount of filling is determined by the patient's comfort level, tissue blanching, and degree of the expander's palpable firmness. The end of expansion is determined when the final width of the domed flap reaches 2.5 to $3.0\times$ the defect's width (cm).

At surgery, expansion is performed for 3 to 5 minutes to gain additional tissue before expander removal. An anatomic elevation of the flap is done to preserve the integrity of significant functional structures (e.g., muscles, nerves) in the area. Forward advancement of the expanded flap is preferred to protect sensory nerves within the flap. Capsulotomy and capsulectomy are usually required to unfurl and maximally utilize the extra tissue. Surgical drains are inserted if significant wound fluid is present or anticipated.

COMPLICATIONS

The author inserted 1505 expanders in 1086 patients from 1979 to 1995. Twenty percent (217) of patients required insertion of two or more expanders at the first stage for either large or anatomically complicated defects. Fifteen percent (163) of patients required multiple expansion periods (two to four surgeries for insertion and subsequent tissue advancement) to convert partial reductions into a completed reconstruction. The outcome was evaluated as a success when sufficient tissue was made available to complete the preoperative reconstructive plan.

In the 1505 inserted expanders, 125 major complications (8.3%) occurred that required implant removal, altered surgical treatment, or additional reparative procedures. Major complications included closed infections or cellulitis, balloon and valve exposures, implant failure, and induced flap ischemia or necrosis. The rate of complications progressively decreased from 1979, which illustrates that a learning curve occurs in this seemingly simple but technically demanding procedure. From 1979 to 1985, 87 major complications (13.5%) occurred in 645 inserted expanders. The number of major complications in the 10 years from 1986 to 1995 decreased to 33 in 860 cases (3.8%). These major complications occurred in all areas of the body, where surgery either produced compromised blood flow

to the tissues or created thin and unstable flaps (Table 4-1).

The site of expansion adversely affected the expansion process. Major complications less frequently involved the forehead and nose; more frequently the scalp, breast, and upper extremity; and most often the ear, midface and neck, and lower extremity (Figure 4-1).

Closed Infections and Cellulitis

Thirty (2%) closed infections or cellulitis occurred in 1505 prosthetic insertions. This complication was most frequently observed in the scalp (4.9%), trunk (5%), and ear (8.3%) (Table 4-2). The incidence was lower in the midface and neck (0.4%), upper extremity (0.8%), breast (1.5%), and lower extremity (2.3%). No closed infections occurred in the lateral forehead or in the midforehead with a glabellar flap for nasal reconstruction.

The causes of closed infections were identified in three main areas: (1) perioperative contamination, (2) cellulitis from folliculitis or abscesses, and (3) port (valve) infections (Table 4-3). The one perioperative infection probably occurred from a break in sterile technique at surgery. Parenteral, local, and intraprosthetic antibiotics have helped minimize bacterial growth after inadvertent contamination. Cellulitis played a role in one third of closed infections, possibly because of contamination from infected hair follicles (midface, neck, scalp), abscesses around sutures and under scabs, or

■ **Table 4-1** Major Complications in 1505 Tissue Expanders

Complication	Number of cases	Incidence rate (%)
Closed infections/cellulitis	30	2.0
Balloon/valve exposure	42	2.8
Implant failure	15	1.0
Induced ischemia/necrosis	38	2.5
TOTAL	125	8.3%

■ **Table 4-2** Site and Incidence of 30 Closed Infections or Cellulitis in 1505 Inserted Expanders

Site	Infections/ insertions	Incidence per site (%)
Lateral forehead	0/64	0
Midforehead*	0/30	0
Midface/neck	1/244	0.4
Upper extremity	2/250	0.8
Breast	7/461	1.5
Lower extremity	4/173	2.3
Scalp	7/144	4.9
Trunk	4/79	5.0
Ear	5/60	8.3

*Glabellar flap for nasal reconstruction.

■ **Table 4-3** Etiology of 30 Closed Infections

Cause	Cases (%)
Perioperative contamination	1 (3.3)
Cellulitis (folliculitis, scab/suture abscess)	10 (33.3)
Valve port contamination (delayed)	19 (63.3)

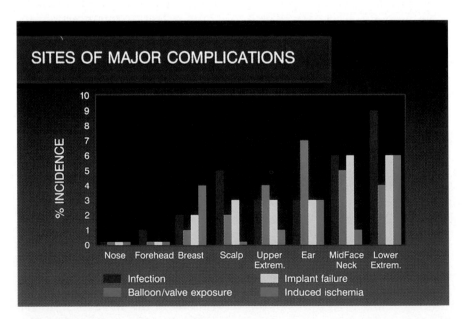

Figure 4-1 The four types of major complications occurred more frequently, in ascending order, in the breast, scalp, upper extremity, ear, midface and neck, and lower extremity. Whenever an implant system is positioned under intrinsically thin skin (ear, midface), hair-bearing tissue (scalp), surgically injured tissue, and tissues with reduced circulation (upper and lower extremities), major complications are more likely to occur.

poor blood supply (lower extremity). The primary cause of closed infections, however, was port (valve) contamination (63.3%) from a break in sterile technique during expansion. Cultures from infection sites most often revealed *Staphylococcus epidermidis* and *aureus*, *Streptococcus*, *Pseudomonas aerogenes*, and gram-negative bacilli.

Balloon and Valve Exposures

Forty-two balloon or valve exposures occurred in 1505 inserted expanders (2.8%). The highest rate of exposure occurred in reconstruction of the ear (6.7%), midface and neck (4.9%), and upper (4%) and lower (4%) extremities (Table 4-4).

Table 4-5 summarizes the most common etiologies for prosthetic exposures. One third of implants protruded through adjacent incision sites located within the lesions or at their borders. Most of these complications either occurred early in the series or when distant incision sites were not available. Implant folds or the firm backer under the expander produced resistant points leading to skin erosion despite maneuvers to remove or displace them (31%). This complication can be eliminated if the balloons are designed without backing and filled quickly to the fill volume. Insertion of balloons and valves under the unstable and thinner skin of scars (21.4%), skin grafts (9.5%), and radiated tissue (4.7%) continues to be a source for implant erosion.

■ Table 4-4 Incidence of 42 Balloon/Valve Exposures in 1505 Expanded Sites

Site	Exposures/insertions	Incidence per site (%)
Lateral forehead	0/64	0
Midforehead*	0/30	0
Breast	4/461	0.9
Scalp	3/144	2.1
Trunk	2/79	2.5
Upper extremity	10/250	4.0
Lower extremity	7/173	4.0
Midface/neck	12/244	4.9
Ear	4/60	6.7

*Glabellar flap for nasal reconstruction.

■ Table 4-5 Etiology of 42 Balloon/Valve Exposures

Cause	Cases (%)
Dehiscence of intra/paralesional incisions	14 (33.3)
Implant fold or backer	13 (31.0)
Unstable skin	
Scars and thin skin	9 (21.4)
Skin grafts	4 (9.5)
Radiated skin	2 (4.7)

Implant Failures (Deflation)

Implant failures, which resulted in an insignificant amount of retained fluid within the prosthesis, occurred in 15 of 1505 expanders (1.0%) (Table 4-6). Implant failures were most frequently recorded in the scalp (2%), midface and neck (2%), ear (1.7%), and lower extremity (1.7%).

The most common causes of deflations were iatrogenically induced, related to misdirected needle sticks into the valve, tubing, or balloon (60%) (Table 4-7). Other causes were disruption at implant joints and seals (26.7%) and slippage of the tubing off the in-line connector (13.3%).

The repeated entry of a large-bore needle (18 gauge or larger) into the port can produce significant back-pressure leakage as the implant volume rises. Nonperpendicular needle entry may not allow the gel sealant to occlude the exit site. An inadvertent puncture of the tubing or balloon will lead to continuous leakage and deflation. Iatrogenic accidents are avoidable with improved techniques. Most needle sticks, however, occurred in children, who tend to move more during needle insertion.

Disruption of the implant at its weak points around joints and seals results from an implant flaw that is accentuated with high volumes and pressures. Pretesting the implant with methylene blue–stained fluid at insertion may reduce this problem. Disruption of tubing at the in-line metal connector can occur when the tubing is not secured to the connector with a suture. On the other hand, a tightly secured knot may cut through the tubing and cause disconnection. Several cases of this

■ Table 4-6 Incidence of 15 Implant Failures in 1505 Expanded Sites

Site	Failures/insertions	Incidence per site (%)
Lateral forehead	0/64	0
Midforehead*	0/30	0
Breast	1/461	0.2
Upper extremity	1/250	0.4
Trunk	1/79	1.3
Ear	1/60	1.7
Lower extremity	3/173	1.7
Scalp	3/144	2.0
Midface/neck	5/244	2.0

*Glabellar flap for nasal reconstruction.

■ Table 4-7 Etiology of 15 Implant Failures

Cause	Cases (%)
Iatrogenic (needle stick)	9 (60)
Disruption at implant joints/seals	4 (26.7)
Disruption at in-line connector	2 (13.3)

■ **Table 4-8** Incidence of 38 Cases of Induced Ischemia in 1505 Expanded Sites

Site	Number/insertions	Incidence per site (%)
Lateral forehead	0/64	0
Midforehead*	0/30	0
Trunk	0/79	0
Scalp	0/144	0
Midface/neck	2/244	0.8
Upper extremity	3/250	1.2
Ear	2/60	3.3
Breast	21/461	4.6
Lower extremity	10/173	5.8

*Glabellar flap for nasal reconstruction.

■ **Table 4-9** Etiology of 38 Cases of Induced Ischemia

Cause	Cases (%)
High volume/high pressure	3 (7.9)
Thin skin (atrophic/infantile)	5 (13.1)
Compromised skin (diabetes mellitus, radiation, previous expansion)	6 (15.8)
Traumatic skin dissection	24 (63.2)

type of disruption occurred when the valve was placed across an active joint such as the knee or elbow.

Induced Flap Ischemia (Necrosis)

The expander produced flap ischemia in 38 of 1505 expansions (2.5%) (Table 4-8). Flap ischemia leading to necrosis occurred most often in the lower third of the lower extremity (5.8%) because of the paucity of blood supply to the skin in this area. Flap ischemia was next most common in primary or immediate breast reconstruction (4.6%). Perfusion of the thinly dissected flap after a mastectomy may be further compromised by the expander unit. The thin skin of the postauricular region also can undergo necrosis during ear reconstruction with the expander (3.3%).

The most common cause of induced ischemia was traumatic skin dissection (63.2%), followed by compromised skin resulting from radiation injury, diabetes mellitus, and previous expansions (15.8%); atrophic and infantile thin skin (13.1%); and excessive expansion (7.9%) (Table 4-9).

MANAGEMENT OF COMPLICATIONS

Closed Infections and Cellulitis

Closed infections of prostheses or cellulitis of the skin should be aggressively treated by early antibiotic and surgical intervention if systemic symptoms are present

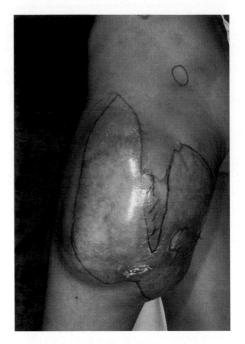

Figure 4-2 Perioperative implant infection occurred within 4 days of expander insertion. Two balloons were filled to tissue tolerance at surgery. Infection was documented by erythema, shiny appearance of edematous skin, blisters, tissue warmth, low-grade temperature (99° to 100° F [37.2° to 37.7° C]), anorexia, and localized pain. The expanders were removed on the fifth postoperative day and autoclaved before reinsertion after the pockets were irrigated with antibiotic solution. Perioperative parenteral antibiotics were given, and the expanders were refilled with bacitracin solution. Surgical drainage with an enclosed bulb system removed fluid for 5 days. Cultures showed *Staphylococcus epidermidis* and streptococci. The expansion process was successfully salvaged by early aggressive intervention.

and a permanent implant is anticipated on completion of expansion. Perioperative infections are usually caused by a break in sterility involving the surgeon, surgical field, and prosthesis (Figure 4-2). These infections become clinically evident within a week after surgery and are associated with flap erythema, blisters, and local tenderness. Cellulitis of the overlying skin and port infections occur much later during the expansion process and may result from suture line infections, folliculitis, and scabs (Figure 4-3) or a break in aseptic technique during filling of the expanders (Figure 4-4).

Because compromised aseptic technique represents 60% of closed infections, emphasis focused on reducing port infections by establishing a protocol (Table 4-10). From 1979 to 1985 in the author's series, a strict aseptic technique was followed for port injections. The skin was swabbed three times with alcohol, followed by three times with Betadine paint. Sterile gloves were used to withdraw sterile saline with a 30 cc syringe. A 23-gauge butterfly needle was inserted perpendicularly into the valve (Figure 4-5). After filling the butterfly needle was removed and the

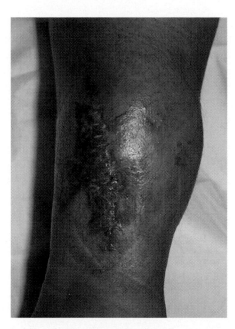

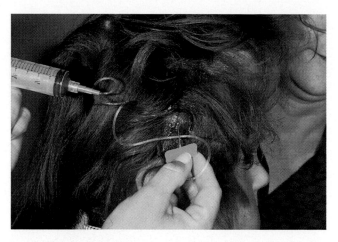

Figure 4-3 Suture line infection occurred 2 weeks after insertion of a 200 cc rectangular expander to the posterior calf for removal of a tattoo. Skin bacteria entered around the suture material, producing cellulitis in the lower extremity. Exploration demonstrated deep tissue bacterial invasion of the capsule by *Staphylococcus* and *Streptococcus*. The expander was removed with a partial excision of the tattoo.

Figure 4-5 A 23-gauge butterfly needle is inserted perpendicular to the plane of the valve after skin preparation with alcohol and Betadine paint. Sterile gloves are used to withdraw saline from a 30 cc (ml) vial in a 30 cc syringe and should be used throughout the filling procedure (photo does not show proper sterile technique with gloved hands, as observed in Figure 4-6).

■ **Table 4-10** Preparation of Port Site for Injection (Author's Series, 1979-1991)

Phase	Protocol
Preinjection	70% alcohol swabbing—3 times
	Betadine paint—3 times
	Garamycin cream 0.1%*
Injection	Sterile gloves
	23-gauge butterfly needle
	30 cc disposable syringe
	100 cc sterile normal-saline vial(s)
Postinjection	Garamycin cream 1%*
	Occlusive dressing technique (Band-Aid)

*Since 1986.

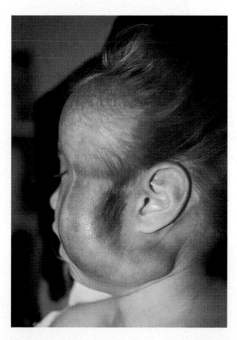

Figure 4-4 Port infection from a break in sterile technique during expander filling in the office (8 weeks) resulted in retrograde infection to the cheek and forehead expanders. A periprosthetic infection that begins at the valve rapidly progresses to the balloon. Once deep invasion of the capsule occurs within 3 to 4 days, the expansion procedure is usually terminated. In this case, expansion had provided sufficient tissue to resurface the forehead and preauricular defect despite the extent of the port infection. Culture of the deep capsule revealed *Pseudomonas aerogenes* and *Staphylococcus aureus*.

entry skin site covered with a Band-Aid. Eleven delayed port infections (2.0%) were observed in 615 expander cases (1979 to 1985) on this protocol, used from 1979 to 1985 (Table 4-11). From 1986 to 1995, Garamycin cream was applied over the skin site after needle withdrawal to prevent skin bacteria from entering through the needle tract and producing a periprosthetic infection (Figure 4-6). With the addition of an antibiotic cream to the standard protocol, the number of delayed valve infections was reduced to 8 documented closed infections in 890 expander cases (0.1%).

Occasionally, early detection of an infected port can be effectively managed by exteriorizing the valve. Periprosthetic infections usually result in removal of the implant system (Figure 4-7), because the established capsule camouflages physical changes to the overlying skin and prevents early detection of infection. Progressive infection develops until the patient complains of lethargy, loss of appetite, and pain with a low-grade fever.

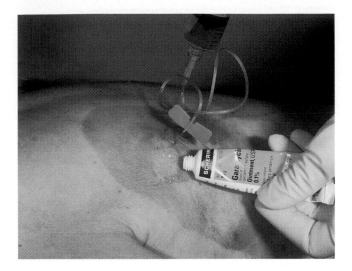

Figure 4-6 Application of 1% Garamycin ointment over the needle penetration site on the skin has significantly reduced port infections. Garamycin cream may be placed on the skin before and after needle penetration into the valve. The antibiotic cream may reduce bacterial contamination during both needle entry and backflow of saline from the valve.

The optimal management of infectious complications is to prevent them. Intraoperative parenteral antibiotics, antibacterial irrigations and expander filling solutions, strict aseptic surgical techniques, autoclaving of expander systems, control of hematoma collections, and early drain removal have reduced perioperative infections. During expansion, local wound infections (e.g., scabs, incisional crusting, suture abscess, folliculitis) should be constantly monitored and, if present, treated appropriately with local or systemic antibiotics, ointments, and débridement. Aspiration

■ **Table 4-11** Influence of Antibiotic Cream on Port Infections in 1505 Expander Cases

Treatment	Infections	Number of expanders	% of Cases
No antibiotic ointment (1979-1985)	11	615	2.0
Garamycin cream 0.1% (1986-1995)	8	890	0.1

Figure 4-7 **A,** Periprosthetic valve infection occurred about 10 weeks into the expansion process. Rapid retrograde infection involved its balloon and contaminated adjacent scalp expanders that were continuous with the forehead expander. **B,** At surgery, deep capsular bacterial invasion was noted around the valve, tubing, and balloon located in the forehead. **C,** Bacterial invasion of the other scalp pockets in continuity with the forehead expander was noted. Complete capsulectomy with flap advancement permitted resurfacing of the calvaria after excision of the giant nevus.

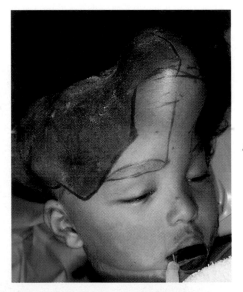

A

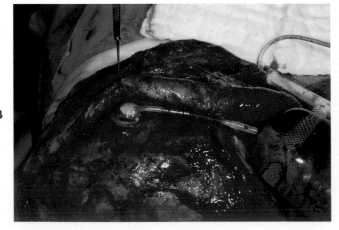

B

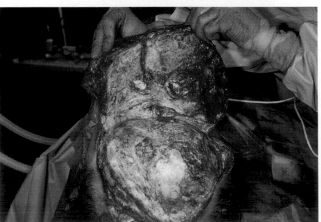

C

and culture of fluid immediately subjacent to the filling port can be useful to determine periprosthetic infection. No hematogenous spread of bacteria from a distant infected source to the prosthetic site has been recorded.

If an implant becomes infected shortly after insertion, an attempt should be made to salvage the prosthesis. This decision is based on whether the infection was detected early and the local tissue or capsule has not developed an established infection (deep invasion, granulating surface of the capsule). A *salvage management protocol* (SMP) for early, noninvasive infections includes the following:

- Systemic antibiotic coverage
- Removal of expander system implant(s)
- Culture and Gram stain of fluid and capsule
- Irrigation of pocket(s)
  2-3 L saline
  Betadine paint lavage
  Bacitracin solution
- Autoclaving or exchange of expander system
- Insertion of expander and valve
- Drainage

SMP was used for 28 expander systems exposed to early, noninvasive closed infections and salvaged 16 (57.1%) through early aggressive intervention.

If an infection occurs late in the course of expansion, the surgeon should proceed expeditiously to complete the procedure. In general, no attempt is made to retain the expander for additional expansions. A modified SMP is used, with the addition of a curettage and a capsulectomy as needed to complete the planned procedure, with excision and flap advancement when appropriate. A permanent implant should not be inserted when an established infection has occurred; insertion can be considered 6 to 12 months later. In all cases of established infections that occurred early or late in the expansion course, the expanders were removed to control the infection. Wound management was similar to that for late occurrence of noninvasive infections.

Balloon and Valve Exposures

Exposed balloons and valves are contaminated by definition. Contamination may develop into deep invasive infections. On the other hand, closed infections of the expander system may secondarily produce exposure from thinning of skin over the prosthesis. Prevention of implant exposure from an inappropriate incision site remains the best management to avoid this complication.

Incisions for implant insertion may be located intralesionally, paralesionally, or away from the pocket or defect in a cosmetically acceptable area. The direction of the incision should be radial or perpendicular to the expander pocket to decrease the risk of wound dehiscence (Figure 4-8). The decision to select an incision site distant from the location of implant or valve insertion significantly reduces the incidence of dehiscence (Figure 4-9). The selection of low-profile valves and balloons without backers minimizes thinning of the overlying skin (Figure 4-10).

Smoothing out the implant folds is achieved by filling the balloon to the specified volume. Full inflation of an implant often is not possible because of the pocket's confinement. Attempts to massage away the implant folds or to move the implant to another position usually are unsuccessful (Figure 4-11). These maneuvers become more difficult when textured implants are present because of the envelope's firmness and inflexibility. Balloon deflation will temporarily reduce implant pressure against the skin, but the implant fold will return when expansion is resumed. Capsular flaps may be created to reinforce weakened skin areas but usually do not form an effective barrier. A simple method that can provide some support to thinnedout skin is applying layers of steri-strips over imperiled sites.

At times the only solution in infection management is to remove the implant and permit the tissues to heal. Improved selection of donor sites remains an important preventive measure. Placement of implants and valves away from scars, skin grafts, and thin skin should reduce the incidence of impending and frank bacterial exposures (Figure 4-12).

Once balloon exposure occurs, the defective area becomes larger with further expansion. The implant must be removed because attempts to salvage the balloon are usually futile. When valve erosion and exposure occur, exteriorizing the valve may be an effective solution. However, retrograde periprosthetic infection may develop if drainage is not effective.

Implant Failures (Deflation)

Implant systems that deflate in the early phases of expansion require replacement of the defective part(s). Although implant integrity cannot be guaranteed once the system is inserted, the surgeon is responsible for inserting an intact expander system. Instillation of a small amount of methylene blue–stained saline solution into the expander unit can determine leakage during pretesting and after insertion.[12,13] The defective part of the system can be replaced or corrected before skin closure. If deflation occurs any time after skin closure, the site of failure can be determined either by removing the entire system or by inspecting and replacing the defective system with endoscopic assistance (see Chapter 17). The most common cause for deflation

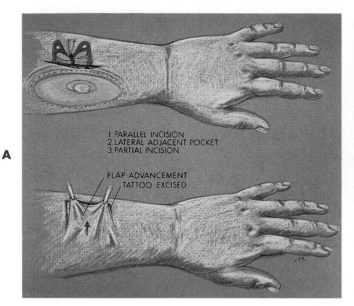

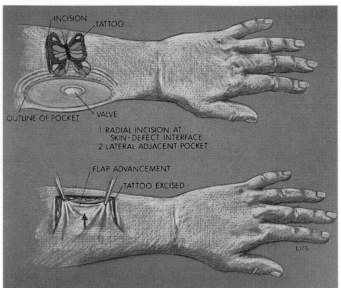

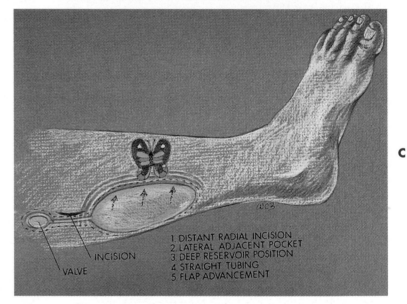

Figure 4-8   **A,** Incision parallel and adjacent to the balloon can result in early wound dehiscence. Partial excision of the defect during balloon insertion increases the likelihood of dehiscence because of tension across the line of closure. **B,** Incision radial and away from the balloon reduces the incidence of dehiscence during early expansion. **C,** Incision distant from the balloon and valve significantly decreases the chances for premature dehiscence of the incision with later implant contamination.

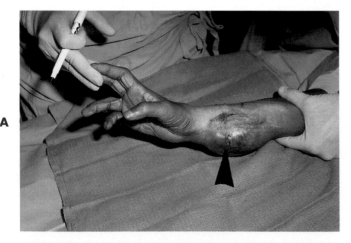

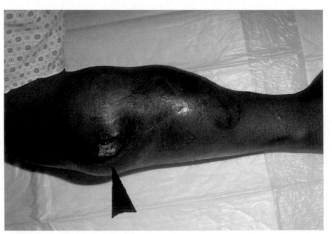

Figure 4-9   **A,** Balloon contamination occurred with dehiscence *(arrow)* of the incision over the expander unit. Expansion of normal skin of the forearm was planned to replace an adjacent skin graft. **B,** Implant exposure resulted from a dehiscence of the incision placed within the tattoo *(arrow),* which was inadvertently stretched during the eighth week of expansion.

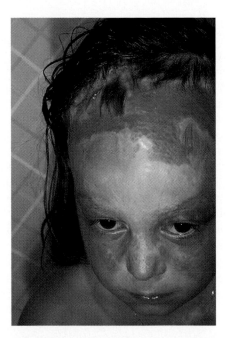

Figure 4-10 Implant exposure occurred along the border of the hairline (precapillary) incision during the fifth week of expansion. The hard backing of the expander eroded through the healing scar.

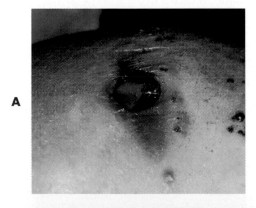

A

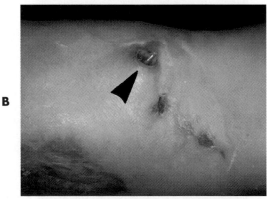

B

Figure 4-11 **A,** Implant fold or "knuckle" eroded through a previous scar during tissue expansion on the back. Contamination of the implant resulted in termination of the procedure. **B,** Implant fold *(arrow)* eroded through the expanded flap of the calf. This complication aborted the process because further expansion would increase the opening.

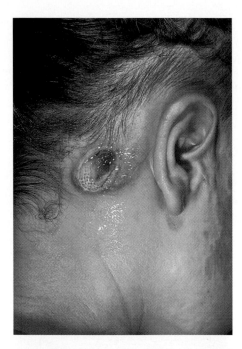

Figure 4-12 Firm valve eroded through the thin postauricular skin. Expansion of the adjacent scalp balloon continued without contamination of the main unit. The valve was exteriorized, permitting periprosthetic dependent drainage.

is inadvertent needle perforation of the balloon or tubing. Imperfect sealing of a needle perforation at the valve site can lead to slow leakage. Replacement of the system's defective portion will correct the problem.

Implant failure may also be caused by separation of tubing at the in-line metal connector or by an overturned valve. Clinical, radiographic or endoscopic examination can identify an overturned valve. Repositioning is easily accomplished by righting the upside-down valve. The disrupted tubing can be diagnosed by endoscopy or direct vision and reconnected.

Induced Flap Ischemia (Necrosis)

Flap ischemia should be aggressively managed because of the expected contamination and infection of the underlying expander unit. Although sudden reduction of perfusion pressure during expansion can lead to irreversible tissue death, this is a relatively infrequent cause of flap ischemia. Tissues undergoing expansion possess an increased blood supply induced by the expansion process.[14,15] Despite this advantage, the blood supply within expanded skin may be compromised during aggressive expansion and result in flap demise. Most surgeons do not exceed this limit during serial expansion. Clinically, the findings of local pain, skin blanching, and high tissue tension are obvious and avoided by the surgeon.

The thin skin from senile atrophy in elderly patients and the skin of infants are more likely to undergo further thinning during expansion. Judicious expansion must be done in these patients and in those whose skins are compromised by diabetes mellitus, radiation dermatitis, collagen disorders, and prior expansions (Figure 4-13).

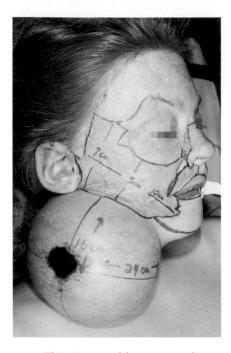

Figure 4-13 This 11-year-old patient underwent two expansions to the neck skin to resurface the skin graft covering his right midface. During the second expansion the expander eroded through the apex of the flap made thin from the previous expansion process. The expanded flap was advanced to the midface with a horizontal closure of the débrided area.

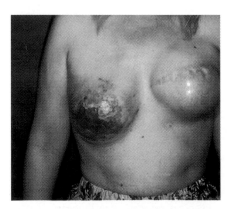

Figure 4-14 Skin loss to the right breast occurred after a prophylactic subcutaneous mastectomy and insertion of an adjustable permanent tissue expander. This patient had insulin-controlled diabetes mellitus. The left breast underwent a modified radical mastectomy with insertion of an anatomic expander. A split-thickness skin graft successfully covered the right breast. Later the left breast mound was lowered during implant exchange with a textured, adjustable saline-gel prosthesis.

A traumatic skin dissection remains the most common cause of skin loss. This complication can be observed after mastectomy because of the presence of thin flaps in addition to the tissue expander (Figure 4-14). Total muscle coverage of the expander unit in primary breast reconstruction is therefore desirable not only to prevent implant exposure, but also to control the lateral "gutter" and prevent implant migration into the axillary region.

The management of impending skin loss during the early perioperative period involves reducing the volume within the expander to allow maximum tissue perfusion. The clinical benefits of vasoactive drugs to reduce tissue injury and increase local blood flow are currently under investigation (Figure 4-15). If this is unsuccessful, early débridement of the necrotic skin is completed before infection occurs. The expander may be reinserted under the newly closed skin, or it may be removed and inserted later when the wounds have healed.

SUMMARY

Tissue expansion remains an exceptional reconstructive technique because of its ability to provide ideal tissue replacement. As expected, this technique has resulted in various complications during its development. The novice surgeon may experience complication rates as high as 40%, primarily because of improper patient selection, limited experience, and

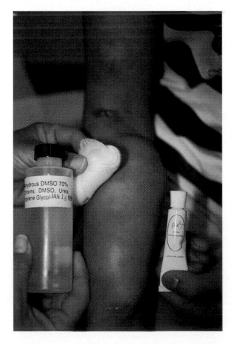

Figure 4-15 Use of 50-75% dimethyl sufoxide (DMSO) on compromised skin increases blood flow, possibly through the mechanism of histamine and prostaglandin release. DMSO solution also reduces edema and local pain.

rudimentary implant designs. As surgeons become more sophisticated with the technique, the rates of major complications should decrease to 3% to 5%.

An optimal approach to manage these major complications is prevention, using aseptic surgical techniques, attention to surgical details, and sterile port-filling procedures. A salvage management protocol (SMP) to overcome major complications of early, non-invasive wound infections and implant exposures can result in a high success rate. Early implant failures may be managed by replacing the defective portion of the expander unit. Late failures may require surgery, at which time intraoperative expansion is beneficial to gain additional tissue. Flap ischemia may be best managed by surgical débridement and flap closure before implant contamination.

REFERENCES

1. Austad ED: Contraindications and complications in tissue expansion, *Facial Plast Surg (Int Q Monogr)* 5:379, 1988.
2. Ashall G, Quaba A: A hemorrhagic hazard of tissue expansion, *Plast Reconstr Surg* 79:627, 1987.
3. Manders EK, Schenden MJ, Furrey JA, et al: Soft tissue expansion: concepts and complications, *Plast Reconstr Surg* 74:493, 1984.
4. Sasaki GH: Principles of expansion technique. Paper presented at First International Tissue Expansion Symposium sponsored by the Plastic Surgery Educational Foundation, San Francisco, October 1987.
5. Sasaki GH: Complications in soft tissue expansion. Paper presented at Third International Tissue Expansion Symposium sponsored by the Aesthetic Plastic Surgery Society of Japan, Sopporo, Japan, October 1991.
6. Austad ED: How I prevent complications. Paper presented at First International Tissue Expansion Symposium sponsored by the Plastic Surgery Educational Foundation, San Francisco, October 1987.
7. Argenta LC, Marks MW, Pasyk KA: Advances in tissue expansion, *Clin Plast Surg* 12:159, 1985.
8. Sasaki GH: Complications and management of soft tissue expansion. Paper presented at Fourth International Tissue Symposium sponsored by the Brazilian Society of Plastic Surgery, Sao Paulo, Brazil, October 1993.
9. Sasaki GH: Refinements in tissue expansion. In Jurkiewicz MJ, Krizek TJ, Mathes SJ, Ariyan S, editors: *Plastic surgery: principles and practice*, St Louis, 1990, Mosby.
10. Goin M: Psychological aspect of tissue expansion. Paper presented at Educational Foundation of the American Society of Plastic and Reconstructive Surgeons Symposium, Pasadena, Calif, November 1984.
11. Radovan C: Tissue expansion in soft-tissue reconstruction, *Plast Reconstr Surg* 74:482, 1984.
12. Goldstein RD, Schuster SH: Methylene blue: a simple adjunct to aid in soft tissue expansion, *Plast Reconstr Surg* 80:452, 1987.
13. Sasaki GH: Avoidance of complications in soft tissue expansion. Paper presented at Tissue Expansion Symposium sponsored by the American Society of Plastic and Reconstructive Surgeons, Pasadena, Calif, November 1985.
14. Sasaki GH, Pang CY: Pathophysiology of skin flaps raised on expanded pig skin, *Plast Reconstr Surg* 80:452, 1987.
15. Cherry GW, Austad E, Pasyk K, et al: Increased survival and vascularity of skin flaps elevated in controlled, expanded skin, *Plast Reconstr Surg* 72:680, 1983.

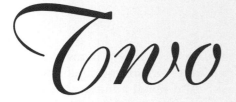

PART *Two*

CLINICAL EXPERIENCE

5 Scalp and Forehead Reconstruction

Diseases and defects of the hair-bearing scalp and contiguous forehead present some of the most complicated psychologic, pathologic, and wound-healing challenges to patients. The resulting disfigurements are not only difficult to hide because of their visibility and erratic patterns, but also possess a predilection either to degenerate into a malignancy (e.g., congenital giant nodular nevus) or to develop an infection (e.g., atrophic skin grafts). Since the forehead is the anterior extension of the scalp, acquired or congenital defects frequently involve both sites.

Various conventional methods exist to correct such problems as hereditary male-pattern baldness, acquired alopecia (e.g., from burn scar contractures, radiation dermatitis, skin graft coverage), and diseases of the scalp (e.g., congenital nevus, malignancies). These established procedures include hairpiece replacement, microplug transplantation, strip grafts, fractional excisions, local flaps, and free-flap transfers. In the last 20 years, tissue expansion has become recognized as a primary or adjuvant procedure for the correction of inherited alopecia and primary or secondary defects that result from scalp loss.

ANATOMIC CONSIDERATIONS

The scalp proper consists of the soft tissues above the bony calvarium (calvaria) from one temple to the other and from the eyebrows to the superior nuchal line behind. The scalp may be conveniently divided into five distinct layers to form the acronym SCALP (Figure 5-1), as follows:

Skin
Connective tissue (dense)
Aponeurosis
Loose connective tissue
Periosteum (pericranium)

Skin

The skin of the scalp is extremely thick, nonpliable, and firmly attached to the underlying dense connective tissue layer. The skin contains numerous hair follicles, which extend to significant depths within the dermal fat layer. Additional adnexal structures, such as sweat glands and sebaceous glands, contribute to the unyielding nature of scalp skin. The skin of the forehead, however, is thinner and more pliable but still abundantly supplied with sebaceous and sweat glands.

Connective Tissue

The dense connective tissue layer is the *superficial fascia*, through which course the smaller nerves, lymphatics, and major arteries and veins of the scalp. This layer holds the vessels firmly in place and acts as a union between the skin and aponeurosis below. The temporoparietalis fascia, containing the superficial temporal artery and vein, represents a portion of this layer.

Aponeurosis

The aponeurotic layer, frequently referred to as the *epicranial aponeurosis* (galea aponeurotica), contains both the two frontalis and two occipitalis muscles and the intervening aponeurosis. The occipitalis muscles originate from the outer half of the superior nuchal bones, surrounded by the anterior and posterior leaflets of the galea aponeurotica, and insert into this layer. The galea also extends itself between the origins of the occipitalis muscles as a tongue of tissue directly on the central nuchal prominence. The frontalis muscles, on the other hand, possess minimal bony origins and originate from the skin's undersurface at the level of the eyebrows. Stray fibers of the frontalis muscles advance downward and may insert into the frontal bones' periosteum at the level of the supraorbital rims. The frontalis muscles are similarly incorporated by the galea aponeurotica and insert into this broad fascial sheet. The galea proper is a dense, strong fibrous layer that is connected to the frontalis muscles anteriorly and occipitalis muscles posteriorly.

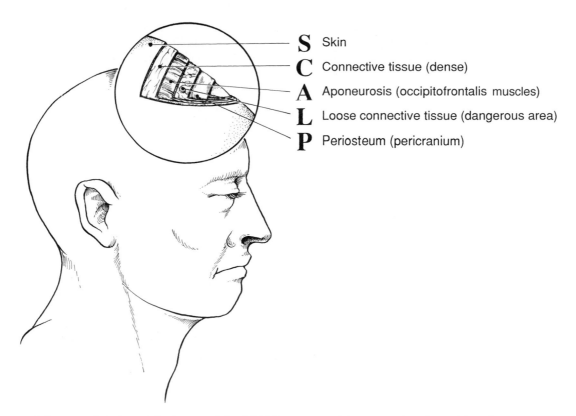

S Skin

C Connective tissue (dense)

A Aponeurosis (occipitofrontalis muscles)

L Loose connective tissue (dangerous area)

P Periosteum (pericranium)

Figure 5-1 Schematic drawing of the layers of the SCALP acronym: *s*kin, *c*onnective tissue (dense), *a*poneurosis, *l*oose connective tissue, and *p*eriosteum.

Loose Connective Tissue

The loose connective tissue permits free movements of the scalp and is frequently referred to as the *scalping plane.* This potential space allows large collections of blood to accumulate. This space is closed posteriorly by the superior nuchal line and laterally by the superior temporal crest line. Since no anterior attachments exist, bleeding in this space will appear in the tissue of the upper and lower lids. Because of this anatomic relationship, swelling and ecchymoses can be anticipated within the eyelids and at times in the infraorbital tissues after insertion of forehead and scalp expanders.

Tissue expanders are localized preferentially in this loose connective tissue space, which represents an accessible surgical plane in a nearly bloodless field. The rigid galea aponeurotica does not present a physical barrier against expansion and gradually succumbs to the force of expansion. In the forehead region, tissue expanders may be located either under the skin or beneath the frontalis muscle layer, depending on the requirements for tissue replacement.

Periosteum

The periosteum is loosely attached to the surface of the calvaria, except along coalescent sites at suture lines,

temporal crest lines, and orbital rims. The *arcus marginalis* represents the firm union of the frontal periosteum and the periorbita at the orbital rims. At suture lines the periosteum dips between the bones and blends with the periosteum of the inner skull, which is the outer layer of the dura. The periosteum on the frontal bones becomes especially adherent along the superior temporal crest lines. At this location the superficial temporoparietalis fascia and the deep temporal fascia (covering the temporalis muscle) coalesce with the periosteum of the frontal bones.

Vessel and Nerve Distributions

The numerous vessels of the scalp and forehead form an extensive anastomotic network (Figure 5-2, *A*). The five major vessels are derived from both the internal and the external carotid arterial systems. Anteriorly, the supraorbital and supratrochlear arteries, accompanied by their nerves, travel over the forehead and scalp as branches of the ophthalmic arteries from the internal carotid system. Their terminal branches anastomose with their twins from the opposite side and with the superficial temporal arteries (external carotids). Laterally, the superficial temporal artery ascends from under the zygomatic arch in front of the ear, traveling along with branches of the auriculotemporal nerve. The terminal anterior (frontal branch) and posterior (parietal ranch) vessels supply the largest area of the scalp and anastomose with the corresponding vessels of the opposite side. The posterior auricular artery (external carotid) arises from behind the ear and distributes itself to the adjacent scalp along with its sensory nerve. The occipital artery (external carotid) courses over the occipital area, and continues forward to the scalp vertex, accompanied by the greater occipital nerve.

All nerves of the scalp are sensory (Figure 5-2, *B*), except for the motor facial nerve branches (cranial nerve VII) to the frontalis, occipitalis, and auricularis muscles and the motor branches of the trigeminal nerve (cranial nerve V) to the temporalis muscles. The supratrochlear, supraorbital, and auriculotemporal sensory branches are derived from the sensory portion of the trigeminal nerve. The greater auricular and greater occipital nerves are sensory and of spinal ori-

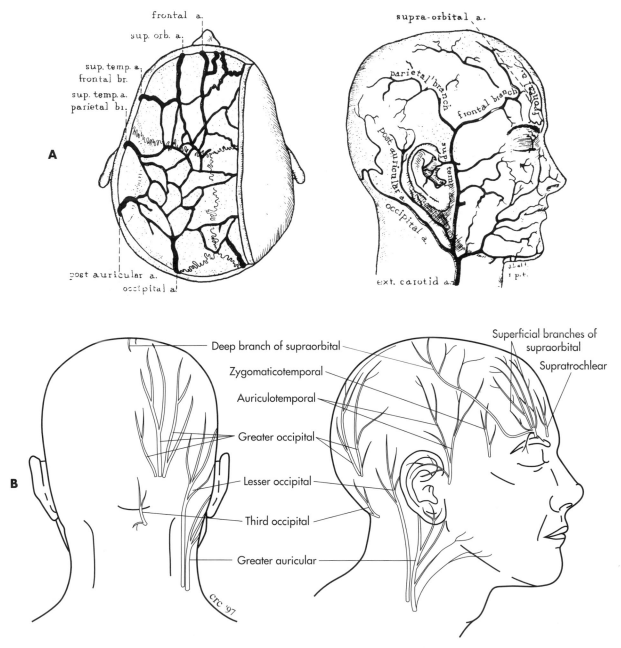

Figure 5-2   **A,** Schematic drawing of the vast anatomic network of terminal arterial vessels from the external and internal carotid arteries. These identified vessels have accompanying venous tributaries. The five major arteries are the (1) supratrochlear and supraorbital vessels (ophthalmic artery from internal carotid system), (2) frontal branch of superficial temporal artery (external carotid system), (3) parietal branch of superficial temporal artery (external carotid), (4) posterior auricular artery (external carotid), and (5) occipital artery (external carotid). **B,** Cutaneous nerves of the scalp.

gin. Any of these sensory nerves may be subject to neuralgic pain after expansion surgery, especially the occipital and supraorbital nerves.

CLASSIFICATION

Hair-bearing Scalp Defects

The hair-bearing scalp (excluding the forehead) may be artificially divided into separate zones to aid in locating lesions and in turn to determine the donor areas of expansion (Figure 5-3), as follows:

Zone I   Right temporal scalp is bounded anteriorly by the frontal hairline, posteriorly by a line drawn from the ear's posterior aspect upward for 7 cm, caudad by the upper portion of the helical rim, and cephalad by a horizontal line drawn 7 cm above the ear.

Zone II   Central scalp is bounded anteriorly by the frontal hairline, extends laterally on each side within the horizontal cephalic lines of zones I and III, and is bounded posteriorly by the anterior border of zone IV. Zone II is subdivided into II-A and II-B by a coronal line drawn from the midear to the opposite side.

Zone III   Left temporal scalp is bounded anteriorly by the frontal hairline, posteriorly by a line drawn from the ear's posterior aspect upward for 7 cm, caudad by the upper portion of the helical rim, and cephalad by a horizontal line drawn 7 cm above the ear.

Zone IV   Posterior occipital scalp is bounded cephalad by an extension of the horizontal anterior borders of zones I and III, anteriorly on each side by the posterior borders of zones I and III, and caudad by the inferior hairline.

The donor sites for expansion usually surround the involved zones to provide sufficient hair-bearing scalp to complete the coverage. Because defects rarely fit neatly into the previously described zones, the "best-fit" concept of expander placement into available donor sites takes precedent. If a congenital nodular nevus involves primarily zone I, for example, expanders would be inserted under the galea aponeurotica of zones II-A, II-B, and IV. If a burn scar contracture occupies primarily zone II, expansion would occur under zones I, III, and IV. In these cases the surgeon must consider the long-term consequences of including hair-bearing scalp that may eventually be part of the distribution of hereditary baldness.

Forehead Defects

The forehead may also be subdivided into three zones to facilitate planning the surgical approach for expansion surgery (Figure 5-3), as follows:

Zone F-I   Right forehead is bounded laterally by the frontotemporal hairline, superiorly by the hairline of zone II-A, inferiorly by the browline, and medially by a vertical line through the midpupil reference point.

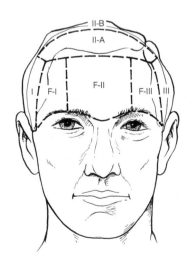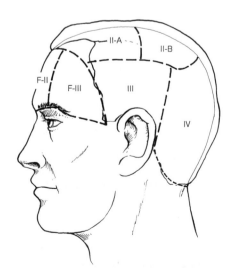

Figure 5-3   The hair-bearing scalp can be subdivided into five regions, each of which may represent a defective area and the adjacent donor sites. Similarly, the forehead may be divided into three subsections, which may represent either a defective area or a donor site.

Zone F-II   Midforehead is bordered laterally on each side by the medial boundaries of zones F-I and F-III, superiorly by the hairline of zone II-A, inferiorly by the browline, and medially by a vertical line through the midpupil point.

Zone F-III   Left forehead is bounded laterally by the frontotemporal hairline of zone II-A, inferiorly by the browline, and medially by a vertical line through the midpupil point.

Forehead expansion can be considered when the lesion involves an isolated part of the anatomic forehead or, more often, a combination of the hair-bearing scalp and forehead. Expanders may be inserted under normal areas adjacent to the defect. For example, if a scar is located in zone F-I, an expander may be located under zones F-II and F-III. The area of a skin graft in zone F-II may be resurfaced by expansion within zones F-I and F-II. If a lesion such as a giant hairy nevus occupies the hair-bearing scalp skin in zone III and extends onto the left forehead (zone F-III), a single expander is inserted under the galea of the forehead (zone F-II) and the adjacent unaffected scalp (zones II-A, II-B, and IV). If the entire forehead skin is involved, no useful donor tissue may be available for expansion.

One of the goals of forehead reconstruction is to locate the final scar along the frontal hairline, along the browline, or in the vertical midline of the forehead. In addition, the surgeon has the option of expanding only forehead skin or the skin–frontalis muscle complex, depending on the requirements for tissue replacement. Dissection in a plane above the frontalis muscle is often bloodier and risks skin ischemia from surgical trauma. Expansion of such compromised skin can result in eventual skin necrosis. Expansion of the frontalis muscle and stretching of the facial nerve's frontal branch may result in a poorly functioning frontalis muscle. Therefore, if one of the reconstructive goals is to provide frontalis muscle function, expansion of this muscle must be performed slowly to preserve as much activity as possible. Despite this precaution, brow elevation may be compromised, leading to a less than optimal result of brow ptosis.

STRATEGIC CONSIDERATIONS

After completion of the expansion process in the hair-bearing scalp, a more natural direction of flap advancement facilitates an easier and more effective reconstructive result. Straight advancement of temporally based flaps toward the scalp's sagittal line covers more of the scalp defect than flaps located in the frontal or occipital areas that are moved in a cephalad or caudad direction. Side-to-side advancement of flaps has a greater chance for providing sufficient coverage after a single expansion than back-to-front reconstructions, which may require more than one procedure. The implementation of rotation advancement or transposition flap designs can overcome the limitations of simple advancement at the expense of increased scar length and possible addition of skin grafts. The type of flap design may also determine optimal hair density and direction of hair growth of the expanded flap in its new location.

In the forehead, similar advantages exist in selecting the best direction of expanded flap advancements. After expansion is completed in the forehead, side-to-side advancement of tissue is more effective than a cephalad or caudad advancement to provide enough skin coverage to complete the reconstruction. Vertical movement of skin may result in either insufficient skin after expansion or malposition of the frontal hairline or browline. Reexpansion of forehead skin that was initially advanced vertically may be required to address the limitations of vertical flap advancements.

The surgeon should always recognize that intraoperative expansion may be useful for coverage of small defects or in patients who are unable to tolerate the demands of long-term expansion. Intraoperative expansion may be preferable for the removal of small scalp or forehead defects whose diameter measures less than 2.5 to 5.0 cm.

Preoperative counseling and surgical planning are essential to complete the reconstruction and meet patient expectations and needs. The surgeon should emphasize that the enlarging expander will produce a physical deformity that may lead to a functional impairment. The surgeon should explore the possibility of a limited expansion period for the patient who cannot accept a temporary deformity. This patient must be informed before surgery that a second expansion period may be required to complete the reconstruction goals. In general, women may be able to disguise the expanded mounds better because of hair-styling techniques.

Type and Number of Expanders

The number and shape of expanders are determined by the size, shape, and location of the defect and the donor tissue. In the scalp the entire length of the donor tissue adjacent to the defect should be utilized in the expansion process. In the forehead either a round or a rectangular expander may be inserted under the galea aponeurotica next to the defect. If the defect is centrally located, an expander of appropriate size and shape may be positioned on each side of the forehead.

The largest commercially available rectangular expanders are 15 to 19 cm in length and 8 to 10 cm in width. Anatomic dimensions for round and crescent expanders are also available to help in selection of the most appropriate implant for a given defect. Custom-made expanders may be designed to fit unusual defect sizes and configurations but are expensive and may delay the procedure because of manufacturing concerns. The advantages of a textured surface over a smooth-walled implant are not yet defined. The formation of a thinner reactive capsule surrounding a textured implant has not significantly benefited the expansion process.

The author strongly advises against the use of expanders that possess firm corners or edges that may weaken and thin out skin during the expansion process. The constant pressure of these silicone reinforcements, backings, and corners on adjacent tissue quickly erodes skin, resulting in implant exposure and infection. In the scalp an area of alopecia from implant ischemia will mar an otherwise excellent reconstructive effort.

SURGICAL TECHNIQUE

The forehead or scalp is first infiltrated with lidocaine (Xylocaine) containing epinephrine (1 : 400,000) to provide local anesthesia and to reduce bleeding. The expanders may be inserted under either the galea aponeurotica or the periosteum. Dissection can be facilitated by using the Helper* instrument, which has a spoonlike end on a malleable handle that bends around the curvature of the rigid calvaria. The dissected pockets should be large enough to permit the implants to lie comfortably in a flattened position to avoid buckling. If multiple expanders are required, creation of a single pocket contains the expanders to prevent septae formation between them. The septae anchor the pocket, forming a bridge of tissue that is not included in the expansion process.

Expanders should be positioned adjacent to and at times under the defect for 1 to 2 cm to compensate for possible implant migration away from the defect's leading edge during expansion. An implant can be safely inserted partially or entirely under the defect only when the skin defect is stable enough to withstand the rigors of expansion. Placement of an expander directly under a skin lesion may be advantageous in special circumstances, such as the lack of adequate donor tissue to accommodate the expander's dimensions.

Incisions may be made within, adjacent to, or away from the defect to create the subgaleal pocket. The closer the incision is to the expander's final location, the greater the chance for implant exposure and infection. To minimize the risk of incision dehiscence, the access site is placed away from implant. Favored distant incision sites for insertion of scalp expanders include those around the hairline of the ear. Distant incision sites for insertion of forehead expanders may be located at least 3 cm within the temporal hair or 3 cm behind the midsagittal forehead hairline. Incision length varies from 1.5 to 3.0 cm. If a remote valve system is selected, the injection port is usually tunnelled away from the incision site in the opposite direction from the expander so that the port is under stable thick skin to prevent valve erosion and subsequent exposure.

After the surgical pockets have been developed, the expander, tubing, and remote valve system are examined for implant imperfections. The expander is partially inflated with saline containing bacitracin (50,000 U/500 ml normal saline) to determine whether any break exists in the closed system. The addition of a small amount of methylene blue to the filling solution improves detection of any leaks from the expander system before and during insertion. The surgeon can select an expander with an incorporated valve, which obviates potential problems with placement and function of a remote valve. After the incision is approximated in a standard layered closure, the expander is filled to tissue tolerance to reduce bleeding (tamponade effect), maintain the pocket size, and smooth out the partially filled envelope.

Inflation Technique

Serial inflation begins usually 1 week after insertion of the expander, depending on integrity of the overlying tissue and healing of the incision site(s). The filling process is treated as a minor surgical sterile procedure. The skin overlying the valve first may be anesthetized with the application of EMLA Cream* (lidocaine 2.5%, prilocaine 2.5%) for at least an hour before needle insertion. The valve site is prepared with Betadine paint. Sterile gloves are worn to fill the 30 cc syringe, using an 18-gauge needle to withdraw sterile saline from 100 cc disposable vials. A 23-gauge butterfly needle is introduced through the skin and punctures the soft spot in the valve's center. Aspiration of methylene blue–stained fluid from the valve indicates that the needle is positioned correctly. The volume of saline injected at each session depends on the patient's response to pressure pain, firmness of the expanded mound, and skin perfusion color; the most significant is the degree of patient discomfort during the active filling phase. Patients should not leave the session in pain, although they may experience pressure discomfort up to 12 hours later.

Inflation proceeds weekly or every 2 weeks until adequate expansion is achieved to complete the reconstruction. To ensure that enough tissue has been created to cover a defect, the dome of the expanded tissue should be about 2.5 to 3.0 times the width of the lesion. This amount of expansion is required, especially when the expanded flap must traverse the normal curvature of the calvaria. In general, most cases require about 10 to 12 weeks of expansion.

---

*Wells Johnson Co., Tucson, Arizona.

*Astra Pharmaceutical Products, Inc., Westborough, Massachusetts.

When sufficient tissue has been generated, the patient is returned to surgery for the final reconstruction. Intraoperative expansion is performed for about 5 minutes to gain 1 to 2 cm of additional tissue before opening the pocket. An incision is made at the defect–expanded mound interface and the balloon(s) removed. A trial advancement of the expanded flap determines adequacy for closure. If additional release and advancement are necessary, a combination of capsulectomy and capsulotomy unfurls the expanded flap. Surgical drains may be necessary for a few days, especially when a capsulectomy is performed. Sutures are removed 2 to 3 weeks postoperatively.

CASE RESULTS: SCALP EXPANSION

Scalp expansions for reconstructive problems are performed primarily to reestablish hair-bearing scalp skin in diseased or traumatized areas. Trauma may result in multiple or large areas of scar alopecia and may produce unstable skin subject to bleeding and ulceration. The trauma may have caused significant loss of scalp skin that required skin grafting to resurface the exposed calvaria. Skin grafts are areas of alopecia that may serve as temporary or permanent replacement tissues to cover traumatic loss of hair-bearing scalp. Diseased scalp may involve malignant or premalignant tumors that require excision and coverage. Malignancies, such as melanomas, basal cell epitheliomas, squamous cell cancers, and adnexal cell tumors, should be managed first by excision and skin grafting.

Reconstruction of the alopecic grafted sites may be performed later by expansion of adjacent hair-bearing scalp. Tissue expansion, however, may be compromised when the surgical site has been exposed to radiation injury. On the other hand, expansion techniques can be used to obtain hair-bearing scalp skin before excision of premalignant lesions such as severe actinic keratoses and giant hairy nevi. No evidence indicates that expansion either stimulates existing malignancies to spread or converts premalignant lesions into cancers.

Traumatic and diseased scalp defects usually result in loss of almost all scalp layers, from the hair-bearing skin down to either periosteum or bone. Expansion of adjacent tissue in the subperiosteal or subtemporoparietal planes can replace all layers of tissue loss. Since any part or all of the frontalis-galea-occipitalis muscle unit may be interrupted by excisional treatment of the primary lesion, the brow complex may need to be elevated and fixed. A primary concern during expansion reconstruction is to recreate the anterior frontotemporal hairline configuration and the direction of hair growth in the reconstructed sites.

Since 1979 the author has reconstructed 127 scalp defects (Table 5-1) that involved only the scalp or extended to the forehead. All required full-thickness resurfacing with expanded scalp flaps. For larger lesions, expansion of donor tissue was repeated up to three times to obtain complete coverage. In 27 cases (21%) a single expander was able to create sufficient scalp coverage. In 47 cases (37%) two expanders were necessary to obtain tissue, and three expanders were required in 53 cases (42%). The duration of expansion for each phase varied from 6 to 14 weeks.

Thirty-five reconstructions involved zone I (right temporoparietal area) (Table 5-2). Expanders were inserted under the periosteum of tissue adjacent to the lateral defect. Thirty-one reconstructions were in zone III (left temporoparietal area), with expansion under donor tissue adjacent to the defect. Advancement of expanded scalp tissue in a lateral direction was easier to provide coverage of temporal defects than in a cephalad-to-caudad direction. Thirty-two reconstructions involved zone II-A (anterior midscalp) and required stretching tissue from the posterior midscalp. Eleven lesions were located primarily in zone II-B (posterior midscalp) and covered by expanded tissue from the anterior midscalp. Eighteen reconstructions

■ **Table 5-1**   Types of Scalp Lesions in 127 Scalp Reconstructions

Type	Number
Trauma	
Scar alopecia	7
Unstable scar	5
Radiation injury	5
Skin graft alopecia	31
Premalignancy	
Diffuse actinic changes	7
Sebaceous nevus (nevus sebaceus of Jadassohn)	11
Giant hairy nevi	54
Malignancy	
Skin graft after excision	6
Turban tumor (cylindromas)	1

■ **Table 5-2**   Sites of 127 Scalp Reconstructions

Zone	Site	Number
I	Right temporoparietal scalp	35
II-A	Anterior midscalp	32
II-B	Posterior midscalp	11
III	Left temporoparietal scalp	31
IV	Occipital scalp	18

were situated in zone IV (occipital scalp) and resurfaced by expansion of zone II tissue. Repeat stretching of expanded tissue usually involved lesions in zones II and IV that required major advancement of tissue in a forward-to-backward direction.

The 27 minor complications (21%) involved implant malposition, implant failure, exposure, and incision dehiscence (Table 5-3). These required a corrective procedure but did not result in ending the expansion process. Eight major complications (6%), however, terminated the procedure because of infection or flap necrosis. Complication rates increased in the pediatric population and in previously expanded tissue.

■ **Table 5-3** Complications in 127 Scalp Reconstructions

Type	Number
Minor (21%)	
Malposition	2
Implant failure	4
Exposure	
Balloon	6
Tubing	2
Valve	5
Incision dehiscence	8
Major (6%)	
Infection	7
Flap necrosis	1

CASE REPORTS AND ANALYSES: Scalp Reconstruction

CASE 1: Alopecia of Right Temporoparietal Scalp (Zone 1)

History (Figure 5-4, A)

This 45-year-old patient sustained a scalp avulsion injury from a motor vehicle accident. A split-thickness skin graft covered the 14 × 14 cm defect. The problems included (1) reconstructing the right anterior frontal and temporal hairline in symmetry with the opposite side, (2) providing hair-bearing scalp skin with similar hair density and direction, and (3) correcting ptotic right brow (1 cm lower than left brow).

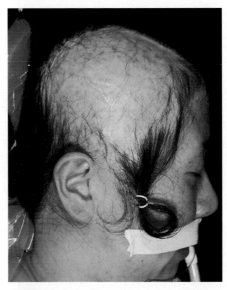

5-4A

Surgical Procedure (Figures 5-2, *B* and 5-4, *B, C*)
Two 800 cc rectangular expanders (8 × 20 cm) were inserted in the subperiosteal plane under normal hair-bearing scalp skin (zones II-A, II-B, and IV) adjacent to the defect. The expanders were positioned on-end to each other in a continuous single pocket. A single 2.5 cm incision along the postauricular hairy boundary of the left ear permitted dissection of the pocket with the Helper instrument. The two remote valves were located in their own pockets on the left parietal scalp area.

Serial expansion progressed weekly for 16 weeks until sufficient scalp tissue was produced. For a defect 14 cm wide, each hemispheric dome attained a final measurement of 28 to 35 cm wide (2.0 to 2.5 × 14 cm) to advance the flaps 14 to 17.5 cm.

After excision of the skin graft, a total capsulectomy was performed on the expanded flaps to unfurl their domed shape. Base capsulotomies released the flaps to permit further advancement. Meticulous flap approximation was performed in a layered closure of the galea aponeurotica (3-0 absorbable sutures), subdermis (4-0 absorbable sutures), and skin (6-0 nonabsorbable sutures).

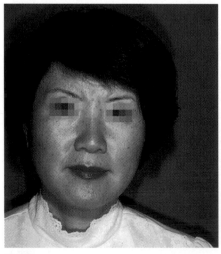

5-4B

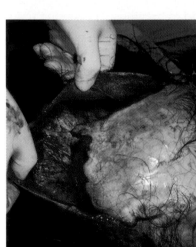

5-4C

Results (Figure 5-4, *D* and *E*)
A year after surgery the entire area of alopecia has been replaced with expanded scalp skin from donor zones II-A, II-B, and IV. The anterotemporal hairline has been reestablished in symmetry with the opposite side. Brow ptosis was partially corrected by elevation of the right forehead with a series of permanent sutures from the caudal edge of the galea aponeurotica, enveloping the frontalis muscle, to the proximal border of the inserted expanded flap. The right forehead was elevated in the subperiosteal plane down to the orbital rim with a horizontal release of the arcus marginalis. Hair density and direction are identical to the opposite side. Sensation returned to near-normal levels within 1 year after surgery. Minimal scar alopecia developed along the seam lines.

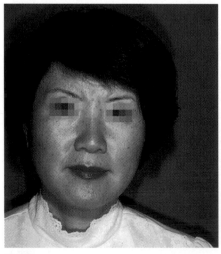

5-4D

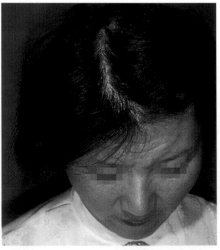

5-4E

CASE 2:   Alopecia of Central Scalp (Zones II-A and II-B)

History (Figure 5-5, *A*)

This 4-year-old patient sustained a full-thickness burn to the central scalp that required an 11 × 11 cm split-thickness skin graft coverage. The large defect, involving zones II-A and II-B, produced significant psychologic impairment for the patient in his preschool environment. The goals of reconstruction were to (1) recreate an anterior frontal hairline and (2) provide stable sensory hair coverage that was dense and growing in an appropriate direction.

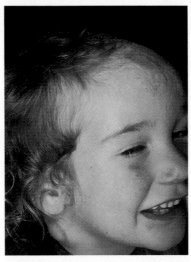

5-5A

Surgical Procedure (Figure 5-5, *B* to *E*)

Two 1000 cc rectangular expanders were inserted in the subperiosteal planes in zones I and II. The ends of each expander entered zone IV to wrap around the caudal edge of scalp alopecia in a single continuous pocket. A 2.5 cm incision along the posterior hair interface of each ear permitted dissection of this large subperiosteal pocket with the Helper instrument.

Serial expansion began 2 weeks after insertion and continued weekly for 4 months. Since each flap was responsible for half the measured 11 cm–wide defect, each flap was stretched until its dome attained a diameter of 11 to 13.75 cm (2.0 to 2.5 × 5.5 cm defect width = 11.0 to 13.75 cm dome diameter).

At surgery a complete capsulectomy unfurled each dome-shaped flap. A capsulotomy along the base of each flap enhanced further tissue advancement. Any thickened capsular buildup on the calvarial surface was removed with a cutting cautery to create a smooth surface for the expanded tissue. Minimal depression of the skull beneath the expanders was observed. The flaps were advanced toward the sagittal midline and in a cephalad direction to create the new anterior frontal hairline. Small "dog-ear" deformities in the occipital scalp were ignored and allowed to flatten out over time. Large dog-ear defects were occasionally excised in other cases but created larger areas of scar alopecia.

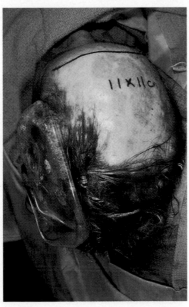

5-5B

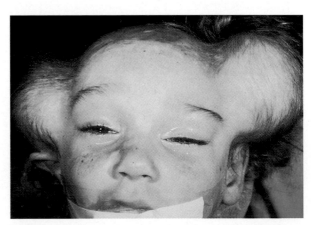

5-5C

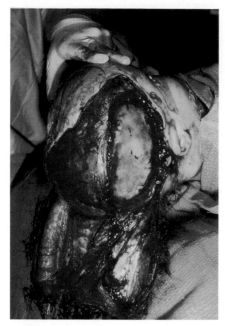

5-5D

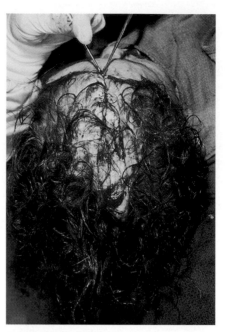

5-5E

Results (Figure 5-5, *F* to *I*)

Six years after surgery the patient has a stable, sensory hair coverage of the scalp. The anterior frontal hairline measures 5.5 cm from the brow and is in symmetry with the lower two thirds of the face. Frontalis muscle function remains intact without brow ptosis or asymmetry. The development of central male-pattern baldness at a later age is not anticipated because the reconstructed tissue was derived from the temporal areas.

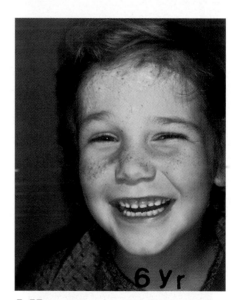

5-5F

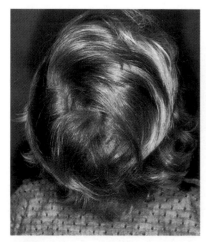

5-5G

5-5H

5-5I

CASE 3: Congenital Giant Hairy Nevus of Left Temporoparietal Scalp (Zone III)

History (Figure 5-6, *A*)

This 7-year-old patient had a 7 × 15 cm giant hairy nevus on the left temporoparietal area of his scalp. Because of the small incidence of malignant degeneration, total excision was planned. The goals of surgery included (1) complete removal of the congenital benign tumor and (2) coverage with stable scalp tissue.

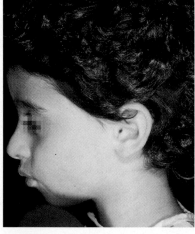

5-6A

Surgical Procedure (Figures 5-2, *B* and 5-6, *B, C*)

A 640 cc crescent-shaped expander was inserted in the subperiosteal plane under normal scalp tissue located in zones II-A, II-B, and IV. The pocket for the single expander was developed from a 2.5 cm incision behind the left ear. The remote valve was positioned in the occipital scalp area.

After weekly serial expansions for 4 months, sufficient tissue was generated to complete the reconstruction. The diameter of the expanded domed flap was 14 to 17.5 cm to permit at least a 7 cm forward advancement to cover the defect (2.0 to 2.5 × 7 cm defect width = 14.0 to 17.5 cm dome diameter).

At surgery a complete capsulectomy opened the flap for effective coverage. A capsulotomy at the base of the flap allowed further forward movement. Any capsular deformation on the calvarial surface was smoothed down to reduce irregularities.

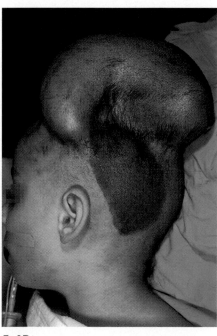

5-6B

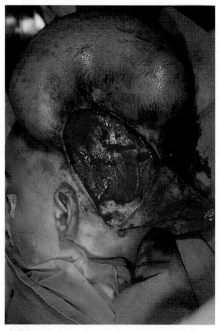

5-6C

Results (Figure 5-6, *D* and *E*)

One year after surgery the patient demonstrates complete coverage of the defect. Sensation has slowly returned, and the seam scar is acceptable. The final pathology report showed no evidence of malignant degeneration, with all borders free of nevoid cells. It is not known whether a male-pattern site of alopecia may form in the temporoparietal area from this expanded tissue, with development of central baldness.

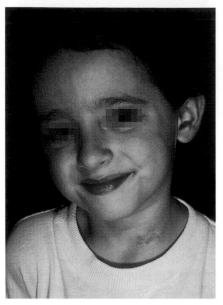

5-6D

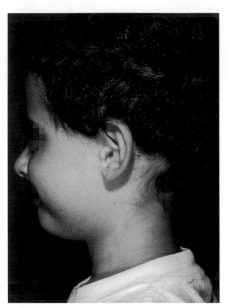

5-6E

CASE 4: Congenital Giant Hairy Nevus of Left Parieto-Occipital Scalp (Zones III and IV)

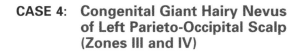

History (Figure 5-7, *A*)

This 5-year-old patient had a 10 × 17 cm congenital giant hairy nevus of the left parieto-occipital area of her scalp (zones III and IV). The goals of surgery were (1) to excise completely this area of benign tumor and (2) to resurface the defect with normal expanded scalp from adjacent sites (zones III, II-A, II-B, and IV). The final tissue advancement is mainly in a cephalad-to-caudad direction.

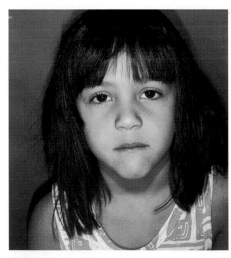

5-7A

Surgical Procedure (Figure 5-7, *B*)

Two 800 cc rectangular expanders were positioned in the subperiosteal plane under noninvolved scalp skin in zones III, II-A, II-B, and IV. The single pocket was developed from a 3.0 cm incision along the hair interface of the superoposterior border of the right ear. The dissection was facilitated by the flexible Helper instrument. The expanders were positioned front-to-back to each other around the lesion's circumference. The remote valve systems were located under the right temporal scalp.

Serial expansion was begun 3 weeks after insertion. Expansion was performed weekly over 12 weeks, generating domed flaps with a diameter of 12 to 15 cm. This amount of expansion permitted only 6 to 7.5 cm of forward advancement of tissue after capsulectomies and capsulotomies, leaving residual nevus behind.

Three months after the first expansion-advancement procedure, a second expansion by the same two implants was performed for 10 weeks, creating dome diameters of 10 to 12 cm on the reexpanded flaps. This expansion period permitted 5 to 6 cm of advancement in a cephalad-to-caudad direction to complete the reconstruction. Scalp advancement in either a cephalad or a caudad direction is more limited than in a side-to-side direction.

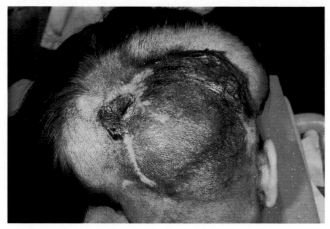

5-7B

Results (Figure 5-7, *C* and *D*)

Two years after reconstruction the patient demonstrates elimination of the benign nevus and preservation of her aesthetic hair units. Sensation returned after a year to near-normal levels. Hair density was acceptible to the patient despite two expansions (leapfrog technique).

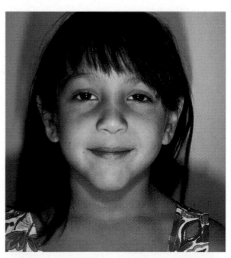

5-7C

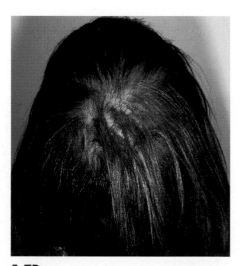

5-7D

CASE 5: Syringoma of Middle Scalp and Forehead

History (Figure 5-8, *A*)

This 56-year-old patient had a syringoma resected from his midscalp and upper half of the forehead and resurfaced with a split-thickness skin graft. Within a year of surgery the tumors recurred in zones II-A and II-B. The reconstructive goals were to (1) excise residual tumor, (2) resurface with hair-bearing scalp skin localized in the bitemporal and occipital areas, and (3) reestablish a functioning forehead unit.

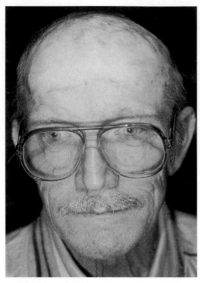

5-8A

Surgical Procedure (Figure 5-8, *B* to *G*)

Two 800 cc rectangular expanders were inserted under hair-bearing skin located in zones I, III, and IV (Figure 5-8, *A* and *B*). The single subperiosteal pocket for the expanders was elevated from a 2.5 cm postauricular incision behind each ear. After serial expansions over 10 weeks, the stretched flaps were advanced as far cephalad as possible. The remaining scalp defect measured about 7 × 20 cm, while the top half of the forehead consisted of a 3 × 20 cm strip of skin graft (Figure 5-8, *C*).

Six months later a single 800 cc rectangular expander was reinserted under the previously expanded scalp flap, along with two 3 × 10 cm rectangular expanders in the suprabrow position under functioning frontalis muscles (Figure 5-8, *D*).

After 8 weeks of scalp and forehead expansion, the expanded flaps were able to cover most of the remaining right side of the scalp defect. The lower half of the expanded forehead was elevated to reconstruct a 6 cm forehead with functioning frontalis muscles (Figure 5-8, *E* and *F*).

A third expansion to the hair-bearing area of the left scalp was performed 6 months later. Forward advancement of this tissue completed the scalp reconstruction (Figure 5-8, *G*).

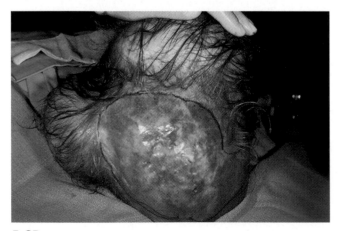

5-8B

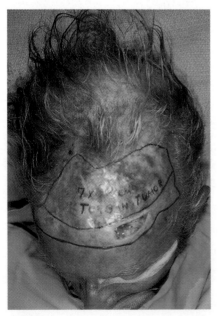

5-8C

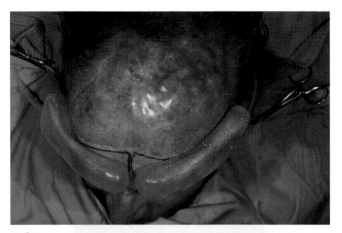

5-8D

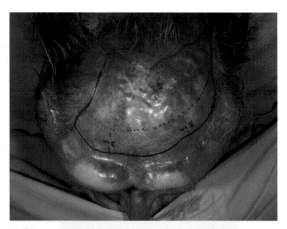

5-8E

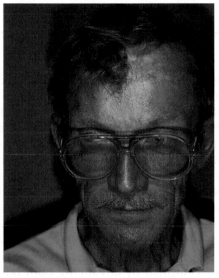

5-8F

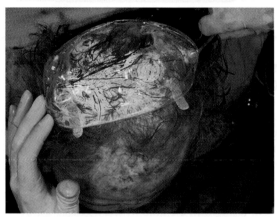

5-8G

Results (Figure 5-8, *H* to *K*)

Four years after his surgeries, the patient's hair density is acceptable but sparser than his original cover (Figure 5-8, *H* and *I*). Sensation had not re-

turned to a normal level. At 10 years (Figure 5-8, *J* and *K*), hair density is less but sufficient to provide satisfactory coverage. There has been no tumor recurrence.

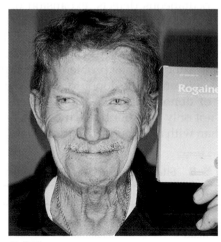

5-8H

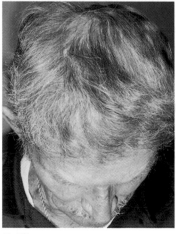

5-8I

Continued

Surgical Procedure (Figure 5-9, *B* and *C*)

Two 100 cc round expanders were inserted under the periosteum of the forehead through a single 2.5 cm vertical incision 5 cm behind the frontal hairline in the midsagittal line. Each remote valve system was positioned in the parietal scalp area. Each expander was filled intraoperatively with 25 ml of saline. After 10 weeks of slow expansion (10 to 15 ml saline/week),

each balloon was intraoperatively expanded with about 50 ml of saline to stretch the tissue further to gain 1 to 2 cm of "extra" tissue. The irregular 5 × 8 cm skin graft and midline scar were removed with preservation of the frontalis muscles. The central procerus muscle and origins of the corrugator muscles were destroyed from the accident. The expanded flaps were advanced toward the forehead midline in a zigzag closure.

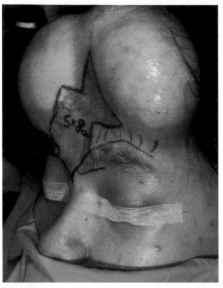

5-9B

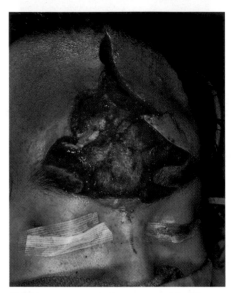

5-9C

Results (Figure 5-9, *D*)

Five years after his reconstruction the patient has functioning frontalis muscle units, an acceptable scar, and an aesthetic frontal forehead hairline. The medial heads of the eyebrows have drifted symmetrically apart because of the absence of the corrugator muscle attachments on the medial aspect of each superciliary arch.

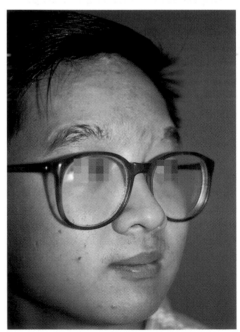

5-9D

CASE 2: Right Paramedian Forehead Scarring (Zones F-I and F-II)

History (Figure 5-10, *A*)

This 12-year-old patient had macerations to her right paramedian and midline forehead skin in a motor vehicle accident. The goals of surgery were to (1) resurface the damaged scarred skin with adjacent skin, (2) maintain the interbrow distance and relationship to the frontal hairline, and (3) preserve the muscle functions of the frontalis, procerus, and corrugator muscles.

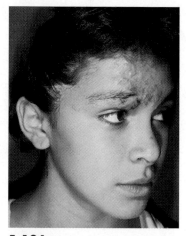

5-10A

Surgical Procedure (Figure 5-10, *B*)

A 100 cc round expander was inserted under the adjacent forehead skin through a 2.5 cm incision 5 cm behind the midsagittal forehead hairline. The pocket was dissected under the subcutaneous fat rather than under the subperiosteal or subgaleal plane because damage was confined to the skin and did not involve the functions or anatomic relationships of the deeper muscles. After 8 weeks of serial expansions (15 to 20 ml saline/week) the scarred tissue was removed. The defect was resurfaced with the expanded forehead skin, which was advanced toward the right with releasing incisions along the suprabrow and frontal hairlines.

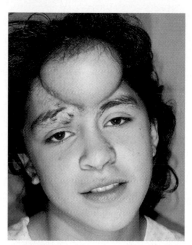

5-10B

Results (Figure 5-10, *C* and *D*)

Two years after her reconstruction the patient has normal frontalis, depressor corrugator, and procerus muscle function. The medial head of the brow did not retract toward the right, and the height of the right brow remained in symmetry with the opposite side. The irregular outline of the surgical scar has blended into the surrounding skin.

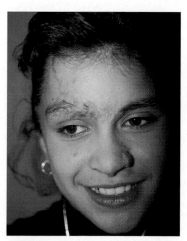

5-10C

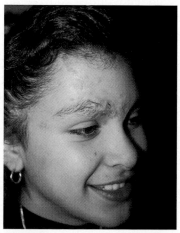

5-10D

6 Facial and Neck Reconstruction and Combined Procedures

Reconstruction of facial and neck disfigurements challenges the plastic surgeon's ingenuity and skill. The goals involve preservation of existing structures, correction of aesthetic or functional distortions, and provision of ideal tissue coverage with minimal and hidden incisional scars.

Reconstruction of facial features requires a dimensional approach to provide malar and chin prominences, aesthetic nasolabial folds and lower lip–to–chin sulcus, and symmetrically positioned lateral canthi, alar folds, and oral commissures. Facial and neck skin drapes over these natural or created topographic structures because of its mobility, thinness, and vascularity. Occasionally, however, expanded skin may not be ideal because of external (e.g., partial-thickness burn) or internal (e.g., fibrous tissue, restrictive capsule) scarring. In these patients the outcome may be compromised but can still be salvaged by overemphasizing the prominences and hollows with the use of autogenous tissue or alloplastic materials. Preservation of normal mimetic muscle activity produces symmetric facial expressions. Static suspension of mobile structures, such as the lower lid and oral commissure, may be required to overcome the gravitational effects of the replacement tissue, especially when normal muscle tension or action is absent.

Chronic tissue expansion of facial and neck skin provides the optimal tissue replacement for large disfigurements. Detailed attention in planning and implementing the expansion process will produce an improved result. For smaller defects less than 2.5 cm across, the technique of intraoperative expansion may provide additional tissue for skin replacement. Other conventional methods of reconstruction, such as skin grafts and local flaps, should always be considered during preoperative patient assessment. These methods may be more appropriate for a patient who may not accept the use of expanders, which may produce visible physical or functional deformities.

ANATOMIC CONSIDERATIONS

Midface

Skin

The skin of the midface is thin, vascular, mobile, and abundantly supplied with hair follicles and sebaceous and sweat glands. The inner half of midfacial skin is inherently mobile because of the absence of the deep fascia, permitting muscles to insert directly into the reticular dermis. The lateral aspect of the midfacial skin from the cheek to ear is more adherent to the underlying fascia and thus less able to be stretched or moved. The skin of the upper lip, lower lip, and chin has thickness similar to that of the scalp and is strongly affixed to the structures beneath. In the prepubertal male, advancement of anterolateral facial skin to a medial and cephalic position may later result in an abnormal beard pattern.

Tissue expansion of the entire midface skin is not significantly influenced by the anatomic differences between the inner and outer halves of facial skin. The skin over the malar eminence to the ear may initially demonstrate a greater resistance to expansion but soon yields to gradual progressive stretching. The mobile skin from the malar eminence to the nose expands in the same manner as the more adherent skin of the midface's outer half. The similar responses to expansion may be related to the surgical release of lateral skin from its adherent fascia during expander insertion.

Blood Supply

The vessels in the midface are an interconnecting system of free-flowing vascular anastomoses. The sympathetic vasomotor nerves from the superior cervical ganglia richly innervate the arterioles, accounting for blushing and blanching during emotional states. The facial artery is the midface's principal vessel and is derived from the external maxillary branch of the external carotid artery. The facial artery emerges in front of the masseter muscle at the base of the mandible and passes upward toward the angle of the mouth, along the side of the nose, and adjacent to the inner canthus of the eye. At that level the terminal branch of the facial artery anastomoses with the nasal branch of the ophthalmic artery. Communication exists between the vessels of each side of the face, including additional connections between the facial artery and the internal maxillary artery.

Branches from each of the facial arteries form an arterial ring, consisting of the superior labial artery around the upper lip and the inferior labial artery around the lower lip. The anterior facial vein is the companion vein of the facial artery. It originates near the inner angle of the eye by the union of the supraorbital and supratrochlear veins, takes a more superficial and less tortuous course than the artery, and terminates in the internal jugular vein. In contrast, tributaries from the superficial temporal vein, posterior facial vein, and posterior auricular vein empty into the external jugular vein, which communicates in a plexiform pattern with the internal jugular vein.

Tissue expansion has not been observed to compromise arterial perfusion within tissues. In fact, expansion represents a form of the *delay phenomenon,* which increases the number and size of perfusing vessels within the dome flap. Venous hypertension also has not been observed during expansion, which may collapse the thin-walled veins. Any partially obstructed vein during expansion probably decompresses its flow into an adjacent communicating vessel.

Nerves (Figure 6-1, *A*)

The two major nerves to the face are the *facial nerve* (cranial nerve VII) and *trigeminal nerve* (cranial nerve V). The facial nerve innervates all the muscles of expression, and the trigeminal nerve supplies the muscles of mastication (temporalis and masseter muscles). The entire sensation to facial skin is supplied by the three divisions of the trigeminal nerve, except for the area over the lower half of the mandibular ramus. The sensation to this isolated area is derived from the great auricular nerve (second and third cervical branches).

Cutaneous Sensation of Trigeminal Nerve.   The *ophthalmic,* or first, *division* of the trigeminal nerve divides into the following five cutaneous branches:

1. The *supraorbital nerve* exits the orbit through the supraorbital notch or foramen about two fingerbreadths from the median line. It supplies the central portion of the upper eyelid and then ascends to innervate the skin of the forehead and scalp as far back as the vertex.
2. The *supratrochlear nerve* emerges about one fingerbreadth from the median line and supplies the medial part of the upper eyelid and a small area of the forehead above the nasal root.

3. The *infratrochlear nerve* emerges from the orbit above the medial palpebral ligament and supplies a small area of skin between the upper eyelid and nose.
4. The *external nasal nerve* emerges on the face at the lower border of the nasal bone and supplies the skin of the nose as far down as the nasal tip.
5. The *lacrimal nerve* supplies the lateral part of the upper eyelid and the corresponding part of the conjunctiva.

The *maxillary,* or second, *division* of the trigeminal nerve divides into the following three branches:

1. The *infraorbital nerve* exits from the infraorbital foramen, passes under the levator labii superioris, and divides into the following terminal branches: palpebral branch for the posterior part of the nose, labial branch for the upper lip, and buccal branch for the cheek.
2. The *zygomaticofacial nerve* appears through a foramen as a twig and gives sensation to the skin over the malar eminence.
3. The *zygomaticotemporal nerve* supplies the skin of the anterior part of the temple.

The *mandibular,* or third, *division* of the trigeminal nerve innervates the muscles of mastication and also provides the following two branches to the skin:

1. The *mentalis nerve* exits through the mentale foramen and is deep to the depressor anguli oris muscle. Fibers distribute to the skin of the lower lip, chin, and mandibular body.
2. The *buccal nerve* appears at the anterior border of the mandible and provides sensation to the ear, temporal region, external auditory meatus, and scalp as high as the vertex.
3. The auriculotemporal nerve emerges from the upper border of the parotid gland and crosses the zygoma between the external ear and the condylar process of the mandible. Secretory fibers supply the parotid gland by way of communication from the otic ganglion. Auricular branches provide sensation to the skin on the anterior surface of the upper two thirds of the ear. Injury to this nerve can result in neuralgia and referred pain.

Sensation to facial skin is a complicated and intricate intermingling of various branches of the trigeminal and second and third cervical nerves. Since tissue expansion involves the insertion and inflation of balloons within the fatty areolar plane, sensory branches may be inadvertently injured by transection or stretching. After the expanded skin is advanced to cover a defect, the return of sensation varies depending on the degree of nerve loss or injury. In most patients, protective sensation returns within a year after surgery. Less frequently,

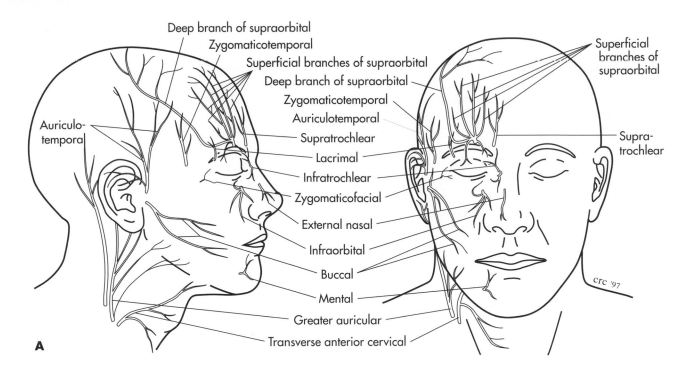

A

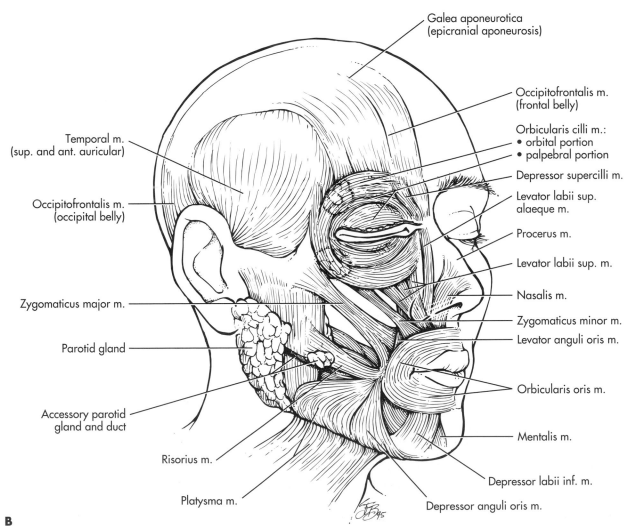

B

Figure 6-1 **A,** Cutaneous nerves of the face. **B,** Forehead, midface, and neck muscles of expression. Facial muscles originate from the facial bones but insert to the skin's undersurface. The development of a subcutaneous pocket to contain the expander unit therefore may temporarily disrupt the muscular insertions.

sensation within the expanded flap returns to presurgical levels. Although branches of the trigeminal nerve communicate with branches of the facial nerve in the face, reflex spasm involving the facial muscles (facial tic) has not been observed with injury to branches of the trigeminal nerve after expansion surgery.

Motor Functions of Facial Nerve (Figure 6-1, *B*). The facial nerve exits from the stylomastoid foramen and enters the parotid isthmus between the gland's superficial and deep lobes. The five terminal branches are as follows:

1. The *temporal branch* appears at the upper border of the parotid gland and supplies the frontalis and corrugator muscles.
2. The *zygomatic branch* emerges from the anterior border of the parotid above the parotid duct and supplies the orbicularis oculi, zygomaticus major and minor muscles, and the lip and nasal elevators.
3. The *buccal branch* passes below the parotid duct and supplies the buccinator and orbicularis oris muscles. It communicates with the buccal branches from the mandibular division of the trigeminal nerve.
4. The *mandibular branch* supplies the muscles of the chin and lower lip.
5. The *cervical branch* appears at the lower bottom of the parotid gland, passes within a fingerbreadth of the angle of the jaw between the platysma muscle and the deep fascia, and supplies the platysma and lower lip muscles.

Expansion surgery may occasionally alter the functions of muscles of facial expression in several ways. The author has observed paresis or paralysis in only a few patients who underwent expansion of a functioning frontalis muscle and skin unit for coverage of a contralateral forehead defect. In the forehead the level of dissection is usually in the subperiosteal or subgaleal plane. Thus no disruption of the galeal origin or dermal insertion of this brow elevator should occur. The mechanisms of injury therefore must include fibrous replacement of muscle fibers, axonotmesis or neurotmesis of the frontal nerve branches, or alteration of the muscle's direction of movement.

Since a subcutaneous pocket is developed always in the midface or neck during expander insertion, disruption of the insertions of the muscles (orbicularis oculi, orbicularis oris, upper and lower lip depressors) may result in an attenuation of facial expression postoperatively (see next section). If a significant injury occurs to a branch of a facial nerve (that enters on the undersurface of a facial muscle) during insertion, gradual expansion, or removal of the expander, muscle paralysis or paresis is anticipated.

Muscles

The facial muscles of expression lie anterior to the parotid gland; are located around the orifices of the eye, nose, and mouth; and act as sphincters or dilators. All mimetic muscles are innervated by the facial nerve.

The two dominant muscles are the orbicularis oculi and orbicularis oris sphincters. The *orbicularis oculi muscle* is composed of three parts: the orbital, palpebral, and lacrimal portions. The *orbital portion* passes in a circle from the medial palpebral ligament, above the brow, across the temple and cheek, and then back to the medial palpebral ligament. These fibers have no lateral attachments and are responsible for the "crow's feet" wrinkles at the eyes' lateral angles. The *palpebral portion* arises from the medial palpebral ligament and is contained within the lid proper, inserting into the lateral palpebral raphe. This muscle section usually acts involuntarily and closes the lids during sleep and in blinking. The *lacrimal portion* consists of fibers that pass medially behind the lacrimal tear sac and is attached to the posterior lacrimal crest. This part can also contract independently of the other two portions, wrinkling the skin around the eye and giving partial protection from wind or light.

The *orbicularis oris muscle* is the predominant sphincter of the mouth and forms the greater part of the lip substance. Its fibers encircle the mouth and extend upward to the nose and downward to the groove between the lower lip and chin. A complex arrangement of contributing suspensory fibers from the buccinator muscle, depressors, and elevators permits varied lip movements, such as closing, pursing, protruding, inverting, and twisting.

The two lip elevators are located lateral to the nose. The *levator labii superioris alaeque nasi* is a small muscle lying alongside the nose. It divides and inserts into the lateral ala and upper lip. This muscle dilates the nostril and elevates the upper lip. The *levator labii superioris muscle* lies lateral to the levator labii superioris alaeque nasi muscle and elevates the upper lip. Superiorly the muscle is overlapped by the orbicularis oculi muscle.

The *buccinator muscle* is located lateral and under the zygomaticus major and minor muscles. This wide muscle and its overlying buccal fat pad thicken the cheek. The buccinator muscle arises from the alveolar margins of the upper and lower jaws, external to the molars and posterior to the pterygomandibular raphe. Its uppermost and lowest fibers pass directly into the upper and lower lips, respectively, but the middle segment decussates, with the upper half entering the lower lip and the lower half the upper lip. The buccinator retracts the mouth angle and is therefore an antagonist of the orbicularis oris muscle. Other functions include pressing the cheek against the teeth during mastication, blowing, and sucking.

The *risorius muscle* lies above the buccinator and is opposite the corner of the mouth. Its fibers arise from the fascia covering the masseter muscle and converge at the angle of the mouth, where they insert into the skin. Its primary function is to draw the mouth in a lateral direction, producing a grin and smile.

The *depressor anguli oris (triangularis) muscle* is superficial and triangular in shape and lies below and medial to the risorius muscle. It contributes to depression of the angle of the mouth.

The *depressor labii inferioris muscle* is short and wide, lying below and medial to the depressor anguli oris muscle. Its medial border decussates with its opposite side, leaving a triangular space that is filled by the mentalis muscle.

The *mentalis muscle* passes from the lower incisor downward to the skin over the chin. It raises the skin over the area, accentuating the transverse groove or sulcus between the lip and chin.

Expander Insertion

In the lateral midface, expanders are inserted within the subcutaneous fat over the preparotid fascia, parotid gland, and subjacent masseter muscle. Injury to the intraparotid branches of the facial nerve and parotid (Stensen's) duct is unlikely to occur as long as the dissection is kept above the parotid's superficial fibrous capsule. The superficial layer is derived from the investing layer of the deep cervical fascia, which splits at the parotid's lower pole to ensheath it. The superficial parotid sheath passes from the gland's anterior border and continues over the masseter muscle to attach to the lower border of the zygomatic arch. Stensen's duct passes under the extension of the superficial parotid fascia directly on the masseter muscle one fingerbreadth below the zygoma. It is accompanied by the transverse facial artery above and the buccal branch of the facial nerve below. The duct bends abruptly around the anterior border of the masseter, pierces the buccinator muscle, and opens on a papilla opposite the upper second molar tooth.

The expander pocket in the medial midface region is in the subcutaneous fatty tissue. Since the plane of dissection is between the skin and the mimetic facial muscles, disruption of the insertions of the muscle elevators of the nasal ala, lip, and nasolabial fold may result in attenuation of facial expressions postoperatively, as noted earlier.

Facial muscle dysfunction may also occur because of nerve injury. Since branches of the facial nerve generally insert under the facial muscles of expression, the facial nerves are usually protected from injury in the dissection phase. Therefore tissue expansion of the face is not performed intentionally under mimetic facial muscles; irreversible damage to the delicate myoneural junctions, leading to muscle paralysis or paresis, is likely.

Fortunately, appropriate facial movement returns in almost every patient after separation of the insertions of facial muscles from the dermis. It is speculated that facial muscles reattach themselves into the dermis

or adjacent scar tissue (capsule) to permit effective movement after reconstruction.

The negative effects of expander pressure and weight on limitation of muscle action are unknown.

Neck

Skin

The skin of the neck extends from the anterior edge of the trapezius muscle across to the opposite side, bordered above by the mandible and a line drawn backward from its angle to the posterior boundary and below by the clavicles and sternal notch. The skin of the anterior neck is loosely attached, thin, and highly vascular. The skin of the posterior upper neck is thicker and more adherent than that over the posterior lower and anterior parts. The posterior neck skin contains numerous sebaceous glands and more hair follicles.

Blood Supply

The blood supply to the skin of the neck is abundant with numerous anastomoses, primarily from the external carotid artery and its major branches. The external jugular vein and its many tributaries have extensive collateral communications with the internal jugular vein. These major vessels lie deep to the superficial fascia and platysma muscle complex of the neck.

Superficial Fascia

The superficial fascia consists of a poorly defined thin layer of fat and connective tissue under the skin. The rhomboid-shaped *platysma muscle* lies in the superficial fascia of the neck and arises from the deep fascia covering the pectoralis major and deltoid muscles as low as the second rib. Platysma fibers pass upward and medially and insert into the lower border of the mandible. Some of its upper fibers reach the face and mingle with the risorius and other depressor muscles of the lower lip. The anterior border of the platysma decussates behind the chin, leaving the middle section of the neck and its lower part uncovered. Since it is a muscle of facial expression, the platysma is supplied by the cervical branch of the facial nerve, which extends into its deep surface. Between the muscle and the underlying superficial layer of the deep cervical fascia lies a clearly defined cleavage plane filled by loose areolar tissue, in which the external jugular vein is found.

Deep Cervical Fascia.   The superficial fascia of the deep cervical fascia lies under its thin subcutaneous fat layer. This investing layer splits to envelop two muscles (trapezius and sternocleidomastoid) and two salivary glands (submaxillary and parotid). It extends from the ligamentum nuchae posteriorly to the anterior midline of the neck, where it continues with its split half on the opposite side. This layer is attached above to the external occipital protuberance, the superior nuchal line, the mastoid process, the zygomatic arch, and lower border of the mandible. In the shoulder and neck the superficial fascia of the deep cervical fascia is attached to the acromion process and scapular spine, the clavicle, and manubrium sterni. As this fascia exits the ligamentum nuchae, it splits to invest the trapezius muscle, reuniting at the muscle's edge to form the roof of the posterior triangle.

The *posterior triangle* of the neck is demarcated by the posterior border of the sternocleidomastoid muscle, below by the middle third of the clavicle, and behind by the anterior border of the trapezius. The investing fascia divides again at the posterior border of the sternocleidomastoid muscle, and the two layers join at its anterior border to form the roof of the anterior triangle. The *anterior triangle* of the neck is described by the midline of the neck, which extends from the symphysis of the mandible above to the sternal notch below, and behind by the anterior border of the mandible and a line drawn backward from its angle to the posterior boundary.

The enveloping cover of the submaxillary gland is accomplished by a splitting of the fascia at the gland's lower border. The superficial layer attaches to the lower border of the mandible, and the deep layer adheres to the mylohyoid line of the mandible. Similarly, the parotid investment is created by a splitting of the fascia at the lower border of the parotid gland. The deeper layer passes below the gland and attaches to the base of the skull, and the superficial layer passes above the parotid and attaches to the zygomatic arch.

Nerves (Figure 6-2)

Four superficial nerves are associated with the posterior border of the mid–sternocleidomastoid muscle and supply the skin of this region. They are derived from the anterior primary rami of the second, third, and fourth cervical nerves through the branches of the cervical plexus, which lies under the muscle. The lesser occipital, greater auricular, anterior cutaneous, and supraclavicular nerves pierce the superficial investing layer of the deep cervical fascia.

The *lesser occipital nerve* (second cervical nerve) appears at the junction of the middle and upper thirds of the posterior border of the sternocleidomastoid muscle, where it hooks around the spinal accessory nerve. It passes upward and backward along the posterior border of the muscle to supply the skin over the lateral part of the occipital region. The spinal accessory nerve (cranial nerve XI) supplies the sternocleidomastoid and trapezius muscles. The spinal portion arises from the fifth or sixth segments of the spinal cord, and the cranial contribution is accessory through the vagus nerve. The spinal accessory nerve is located very superficially, lying beneath the investing layer of fascia.

The *greater auricular nerve* (second and third cervical nerves) appears at a slightly lower level than the lesser occipital nerve, runs parallel with the external jugular vein, and enters the nuchal region posterior to

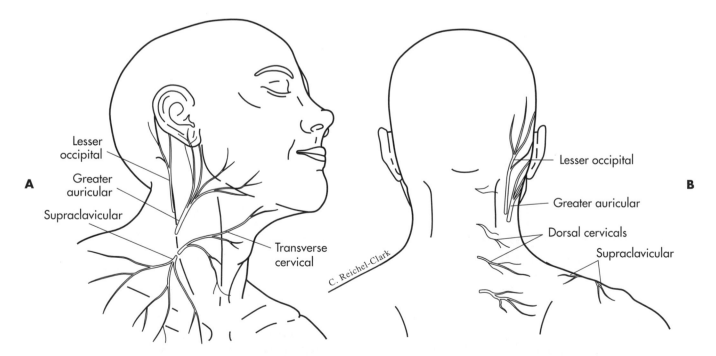

Figure 6-2 Cutaneous nerves of the neck.

the ear. It supplies the skin over the angle of the jaw, parotid gland, posteroinferior half of the lateral and medial aspects of the auricle, and skin of the mastoid region.

The *anterior cutaneous nerve* of the neck appears close to the greater auricular nerve and runs transversely forward across the sternocleidomastoid muscle. It divides into ascending and descending branches and supplies most of the skin of the side and front of the neck. In its course across the sternocleidomastoid muscle, it lies either superficially or deep to the external jugular vein.

The *supraclavicular nerve* (third and fourth cervical nerves) arises just below the anterior cutaneous nerve as a single trunk that divides into three branches. The medial (anterior) branch descends over the medial third of the clavicle and supplies the skin of the front of the chest down to the level of the sternal angle. The intermediate branch crosses the clavicle and descends on the thoracic wall as far as the second rib. The external (posterior) branch passes over the trapezius muscle and the acromion and innervates the skin on the upper and back parts of the shoulder region.

Expander Insertion

The skin of the anterolateral neck may be effectively expanded because of its thinness and excellent blood supply. The skin of the posterior neck region is more difficult to stretch because of its thickness and adherence to the underlying structures. Expanders are inserted under the skin within the thin subcutaneous fat layer of the superficial fascia. Although expanders may be inserted under the platysma muscle, it is safer to create a pocket over it. Injury to the motor branch of the platysma muscle, larger vessels, and the spinal accessory nerve is less likely to occur with a dissection above the superficial investing layer of the deep cervical fascia. It is unnecessary to identify the cutaneous branches of the superficial sensory nerves at the midposterior border of the sternocleidomastoid muscle during pocket dissection. In most patients, variable sensation returns to the expanded skin after flap advancement. Neither venous hypertension nor arterial ischemia has been observed during compression of the major vessels of the carotid and jugular vascular network.

CLASSIFICATION OF FACE AND NECK DEFECTS

The face and neck may be subdivided into zones to aid in highlighting the deformities and in turn selecting the donor sites for expansion (Figure 6-3, *A*), as follows:

Zone I   The lateral midface is bordered posteriorly by the anterior border of the auricle, inferiorly by a line drawn from the angle of the mouth to the ear lobe, and superiorly by a line extending from the lateral canthus of the eye to the helical root attachment to the face. Its medial border is determined by a vertical plumb line that drops at a point that bisects the distance from the lateral canthus to the helical root of the ear and ends at the inferior borderline.

Zone II   The medial border of the midface is determined by a vertical line dropped from the midpupil to the inferior end of the nasolabial line at the level of the angle of the mouth. The superior border is the subciliary border of the lower lid. The inferior boundary extends from the angle of the mouth to the ear lobe. The lateral border of zone II is coincident with the medial border of zone I.

Zone III   The inner third of the midface is bounded medially by the nasomaxillary and nasolabial fold, superiorly by the subciliary border of the lower lid, laterally by the coincident lateral border of zone II, and inferiorly by a line extending from the angle of the mouth to the ear lobe.

Zone IV   The lower third of the midface is triangular shaped. The base of the triangle follows the marionette fold, and the sides converge at the ear lobe. The upper border extends from the angle of the mouth to the ear lobe, and the lower border follows the mandibular edge.

Zone V   The upper half of the neck is bounded by the median neck line, mandibular edge, and a horizontal line from the superior border of the thyroid gland to the posterior hairline.

Zone VI   The upper lip segment is bounded by the nasal sills, vermilion borders of the lips, and nasolabial lines.

Zone VII   This area is delineated by the vermilion borders of the lips, marionette folds, and chin line.

The donor site for expansion is usually adjacent to the defect in order to replace skin with similar characteristics. In the midface and neck areas the available site is evident because of limited donor tissue. The direction of expanded-flap advancement, however, is determined by the aesthetics of the final scar. The optimal scar should be camouflaged in one or more of the aesthetic lines of the face (Figure 6-3, *B*). For example, if a burn scar contracture involves zone I, skin expansion of zones II and III will advance the flap, with closure along the preauricular aesthetic crease line. If a

ZONAL LESIONS OF MID-FACE AND NECK

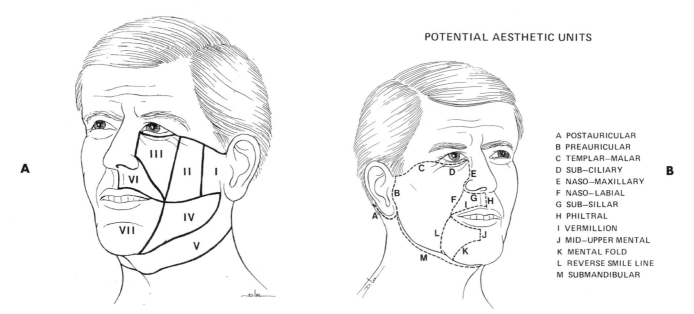

Figure 6-3 **A,** The face and neck may be subdivided into seven zones to aid in isolating location of the lesion and adjacent donor sites. The donor sites are selected on the basis of anatomic and aesthetic units. **B,** Skin closures are located along anatomic and aesthetic lines. Seam lines are camouflaged by hiding them within these anatomic borders.

congenital nevus is in zone II, it is preferable to expand both zone I and zone III and advance each flap toward the midline of the face, with an oblique vertical scar. If a skin graft scar is in zone III, the expanded skin of zones I and II is advanced and closed along the naso-maxillary and subciliary lines.

When a defect involves zone IV, the surgeon may expand above the mandibular margin (zones I, II, and III) or below it (zone V). An improved reconstructive result is achieved by advancing the expanded tissue in zones I, II, and III downward, with the final scar hidden at or slightly below the mandibular margin. When expanded neck tissue in zone V is advanced in a cephalad direction over the cervicomandibular angle onto zone IV, the surgeon can anticipate an un-natural tenting of tissue across this natural crevice. Lesions in zones VI and VII are optimally reconstructed by expanding lateral cheek flaps, which are advanced toward the midline of the lips or chin.

PRACTICAL CONSIDERATIONS

Although the surgeon approaches expansion reconstruction of the midface and neck primarily by evaluating the site and configuration of the defect and the available areas for donor tissue, other practical factors influence the outcome.

Expanded skin is always more efficiently used when tissue advancements are performed in a transverse direction. Thus the surgeon can anticipate that

a single expansion procedure may satisfy coverage when zones I, II, and III are involved either as the defect or the donor sites. Less tissue is available when expanded flaps are advanced in a cephalad or caudad direction. This tissue deficiency is especially apparent when vertical advancements traverse the sub-mandibular sulcus from the midface down or the neck up. The extra tissue obtained from expansion appears to be "swallowed up" in creating the sulcus. Thus the surgeon can anticipate perhaps two expansion periods to reconstruct defects in zones IV and V that require upward or downward movement of expanded flaps.

The same principles of efficient expansion and coverage apply to the neck. Transverse advancements can often resurface large midline defects after a single expansion either by stretching both lateral neck skins, with a midline closure, or by expanding skin from only one side of the neck, with a vertical midneck or lateral neck closure. Moving expanded flaps from the base of the neck up to the cervicomandibular angle, or vice versa, frequently requires two expansion periods, depending on the defect's size and location.

Small defects less than 2.5 cm in width may be reconstructed by an intraoperative expansion technique, especially when flaps are advanced in a transverse direction. Such a vertical closure takes advantage of the greatest amount of skin laxity. In contrast, intraoperative expansion may fail to provide enough tissue when flaps are advanced in a vertical direction with a horizontal scar.

SURGICAL TECHNIQUE

In the face and neck area, preoperative assessment and planning are critical because of the need to maintain aesthetic and functional units. The goals of reconstruction are not only to resurface the face and neck with stable and pliable skin, but also to (1) provide optimal sensation and color match, (2) maintain facial movement, (3) create natural facial prominences, hollows, and depressions, and (4) preserve eyelid and lip competence and appearance.

Sufficient and normal donor skin must be available for expansion to achieve these goals. Patient counseling must emphasize the physical deformities that will be produced during expansion. Occasionally these aesthetic deformities lead to transient functional deformities during the expansion process, such as eyelid ectropion or depressed angulation to the oral commissure. The patient must understand that these inconveniences may occur, but restoration of functional anatomy of these structures to their original status is anticipated once the second stage is completed. At times, however, secondary corrective procedures may be required because of continued deformity despite provision of sufficient skin during flap advancement.

The surgeon must visualize the anticipated scar configuration so that it follows as close as possible to the lines of facial and neck aesthetic units. Selection of the donor site for expansion is based on in which zone the defect is located and in which direction the expanded skin will be advanced to approach the aesthetic lines of closure. If the entire midface (zones I, II, and III) is deformed, for example, the only available donor skin is the neck (zone V), and the surgeon may anticipate two expansion surgeries. The first expansion period involves stretching the neck skin and advancing it upward conservatively to the lower half of the midface. At this first expansion the submandibular sulcus must be established rather than aggressively moving the flap upward to its farthest extent, thereby risking a tenting effect at this significant anatomic site. After the tissues have settled, the previously expanded midface skin is reexpanded and moved farther upward toward the subciliary, nasomaxillary, and nasolabial lines.

The surgeon also must carefully select the incision site for dissection of the surgical pocket. Improper location of the access site may produce a weakened area that delays expansion because of suture line dehiscence and implant exposure. An infected implant often requires removal, thus terminating the procedure (see Chapter 4).

A remote incision away from the expander reduces the chances for exposure and infection. In the facial and neck area the author favors a small incision (2.5 to 3.0 cm) at the posterior auricular sulcus or retrolobular site. This approach hides the scar and permits safe, efficient dissection above the preparotid fascia and platysma muscle. When a remote valve is used, the valve pocket can be rapidly developed under the scalp from the same incision site. The disadvantages of a distant incision include (1) creation of a new but hidden scar and (2) more difficult and extensive dissection to the site of the expander pocket. Special instruments, such as the Helper and Spreader,* facilitate the creation of precise but distant pockets for the balloon and its valve. An intralesional or paralesional incision is not recommended in facial and neck expansion because of possible implant exposure from fresh scars in thin skin.

An appropriate expander in size and shape is outlined on the donor skin adjacent to the defect. Pocket dissection is usually 1 cm larger than the expander's base dimensions to prevent implant buckling. If the defect is stable enough to be elevated and expanded, the expander pocket may intrude partially under this tissue to compensate for gravity-induced implant descent away from the defect's leading edge.

This implies that the lower margin of any created pocket must not be too large, relative to implant size, to reduce downward slippage. An expander that falls significantly away from the defect's border will not efficiently expand tissue. The surgeon may need to revise the pocket early in the expansion process by repositioning the expander closer to or under the defect's leading edge.

A sufficient amount of 0.25% lidocaine (Xylocaine) with epinephrine (1:400,000) is injected by insufflation technique, which balloons the donor tissue in a patient under general anesthesia. If the patient is awake, a buffered solution (9 ml 0.5% Xylocaine plus 1 ml sodium bicarbonate) is substituted to minimize the burning sensation of an acidic solution of Xylocaine. On completion of the procedure, the operative site is reinforced with 0.5% bupivacaine (Marcaine) with epinephrine for prolonged anesthesia and subsequent patient comfort. Subcutaneous insufflation of the anesthetic agents facilitates scissors dissection and reduces bleeding. Blood loss or hematoma development can be further reduced by a tamponading effect after filling the expander to tissue tolerance.

Dissection is begun in the subcutaneous fatty plane with a medium-length scissors, using a spreading action to minimize trauma. Longer scissors are useful to complete the most distant portion of the dissection. The Helper and Spreader instruments aid in eliminating resistant strands of tissue and defining the pocket's limits.

Before implant insertion, the expander, tubing, inline connector (if used), and valve are checked for

---

*Laroe Undermining Forceps, Robbins Instruments, Chatham, N.J.

imperfections. The addition of 0.5 ml of methylene blue into the expander with bacitracin solution (50,000 U/500 ml normal saline) helps detect fluid leaks before and during expander insertion.

The pocket for the remote valve should be developed in an opposite direction from the expander through the same incision. The partially filled balloon is inserted into its pocket and filled with saline through the noninserted valve to the pocket's capacity. The valve is then guided into its pocket in an upright position. The tubing should be taut so as to prevent curling, which can lead to partial or complete obstruction and pressure necrosis to the overlying skin. Displacement of the tubing away from the incision site by suture fixation reduces the risk of exposure. The valve itself should be placed under stable tissue to reduce the chances of skin necrosis from its prominent dome. It is strongly recommended that valves *not* be positioned under the thin postauricular skin. Selection of low-profile valves also reduces the opportunity for tissue erosion and exposure.

Expansion is begun about 1 to 2 weeks after insertion, when the overlying tissue and incision site have healed. Expansion is treated as a minor surgical procedure using sterile technique. After alcohol povidone-iodine (Betadine) solution, and gentamicin (Garamycin) ointment are applied to the valve site, sterile gloves are worn to fill the individual syringes (20 cc) from 50 cc (ml) vials of sterile saline. Small-volume disposable containers of saline should be used to minimize multiple needle entries into a large-volume container, which increases the chance for contamination. The author uses a 23-gauge butterfly needle to reduce the risk of tearing the valve, which can lead to saline leakage from back pressure.

Serial inflation continues weekly or every 2 weeks until sufficient tissue is obtained, when the expanded dome is two and one-half to three times the defect's width, usually within 10 to 12 weeks.

The patient then returns to surgery for completion of the reconstruction. Intraoperative expansion is performed to gain 1 to 2 cm of additional tissue. After removal of the expander system, trial advancement of the flap determines whether base or dome capsulotomies and capsulectomies are needed to open the expanded flap for maximum unfurling of the tissue.

Internal Sculpturing
(Figures 6-4 and 6-5)

The concept of internal sculpturing reinforces the need to create (1) midface and chin definition to match the contralateral side or (2) near-normal topography on the affected side. In reconstructive surgery, vascularized dermal fat mounds provide stable structures to accentuate the malar eminence and mental (chin) protuberance. This is accomplished by

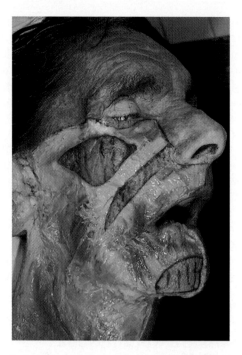

Figure 6-4 The concept of defining midface reconstruction involves augmenting prominences and creating natural furrows. This may be accomplished at the second stage of reconstruction by retaining vascular dermal mounds that accentuate the malar, mental, and nasolabial eminences, as shown in this cadaver. The tissue may be deepithelialized to create prominences. Deepening crevices adjacent to the mounds can reproduce normal sulci such as the nasolabial line.

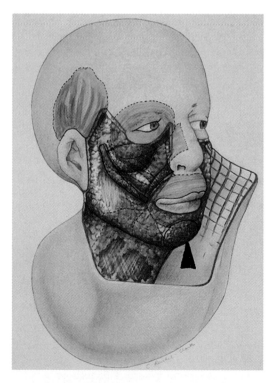

Figure 6-5 Dimensional reconstruction of the midface. Retained tissue mounds simulate the malar eminence, nasolabial fold, and mentum *(arrow)*.

removing the epithelium from a nonmalignant defect or scar over a normal prominence and shaping it to resemble a structure that will become visible under the expanded flap. Autogenous fat grafts, capsular scar tissue, and cartilage provide at best a temporary mound and cannot be relied on for a permanent dimensional reconstruction. Insertion of alloplastic implants to the cheek or mental prominence may substitute for autogenous tissue when minimal or no tissue remains after excision of the defect. Insertion of these implants can be accomplished in a subperiosteal position.

The surgeon may need to create appropriate depressions adjacent to these prominences to emphasize the nasolabial line, inframalar hollow, and chin-lip sulcus. This can be accomplished by resection of fat or scar tissue within these areas. Liposuction may not be successful in producing hollows and furrows because of an abundance of fibrosis.

Suspension Techniques
(Figure 6-6)

Suspension techniques may be considered during the reconstructive phase to support the lower lip and oral commissure. Flap ptosis is reduced by securing the flap's undersurface to floor structures with strategically placed sutures. Sutures are placed in a triangulated pattern to distribute the fixation and to

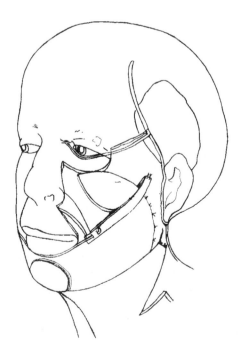

Figure 6-6 Passive suspensions using synthetic materials or autogenous tissue can stabilize and position the lower lid and oral commissure. This technique is beneficial to counter the downward forces present after reconstructive procedures.

maximize blood flow into and out of the flap. Absorbable 3-0 sutures should produce temporary fixation that will adhere the flap at a higher level to prevent skin ptosis.

Dermal grafts, fascia lata strip grafts, and alloplastic slings may provide internal scaffolding to reduce the incidence of lower lid bowing or ectropion as well as incompetency or deformation of the lips and oral commissure. In the lower lid the strips are wrapped around the medial canthal ligament, threaded along the subciliary margin, and interwoven laterally to the deep temporal fascia. This dissection is facilitated by threading a small, curved tendon retriever under the lower lid skin from a medial or lateral incision, grasping the strip, and pulling the graft through the tissues to the opposite side.

In the mouth the strip graft is partially divided in a longitudinal direction. A chevron-shaped incision at the commissure and two vertical incisions slightly beyond the lips' midline at the vermilion borders permit passage and dermal fixation of the strip graft. Again, a small, curved tendon retriever is threaded from the upper midlip incision to the commissure, with one end of the divided strip grasped and pulled out from the midlip incision. The other end of the split graft is then passed the same distance across the lower lip and retrieved beyond its midportion. The strands of the strip graft are fixed to the dermis of the middle upper and lower lip. The bifurcated portion of the graft is fixed to the dermis at the commissure. The single portion of the strip graft is interwoven around the zygomatic arch to provide a stabilized oral unit that resists downward distortion.

CASE RESULTS: MIDFACIAL EXPANSION

In clinical situations, discussion of tissue expansion often cannot be limited to the midface. Since many clinical problems (e.g., burns, trauma, benign and malignant tumors, birthmarks) involve the entire face, discussion of midface reconstruction usually includes the forehead, brows, eyelids, nose, ears, and neck. To aid the surgeon in planning midfacial procedures, the midface is conveniently divided into seven anatomic zones (see Figure 6-3, *A*). As in the forehead area, expanded skin is most easily advanced when moved in a side-to-side (nose to ear) rather than in a cephalad-to-caudad direction (lower eyelid to mandible).

The author has completed 109 midfacial reconstructions (Table 6-1). These involved the sequelae of trauma, port-wine stain hemangiomas, and premalignant lesions. Advancement of expanded flaps was more difficult to accomplish in the cephalad or caudad direction because of the gravitational restrictions of movement and the consequences of such mobilization of tissue (e.g., distortions to lower lids, nose, and lips). These situations may require two or more expansion phases to stabilize the gains of advancement without producing significant tissue distortions to facial structures. In general, the duration of expansion ranged from 6 to 14 weeks, depending on the defect's location and size.

Table 6-2 lists location of the defects in the author's series and the zones of expanded donor tissue in the midface.

The lateral or preauricular area (zone I) is most easily reconstructed by expansion of donor skin from the central (zone II) and paranasal (zone III) areas. Lesions located near the nose (zone III) are resurfaced by expansion of donor sites in zones I and II. The final incision closure lines should ideally follow the aesthetic lines along the subciliary groove, nasomaxillary junction, nasolabial fold, marionette fold, and mandibular border. Zone II defects are effectively removed by expansion of donor tissues in zones I and III, but the resultant midcheek scar will be more visible.

■ **Table 6-1** Types of Facial Defects in 109 Reconstructions

Type	Number
Trauma	
Scar	12
Burn contracture	21
Skin graft	37
Benign lesions	
Port-wine stain	5
Premalignancy	
Giant hairy nevus	32
Malignancy	
Skin graft	2

Expansion of donor tissue from the lower cheek and neck for replacement of large skin defects in the upper lip, lower lip, and chin is not recommended. Often the skin characteristics of the donor tissue do not match the recipient skin. Expanded reconstructive efforts may significantly distort these mobile structures.

Complications of midfacial expansion are more common than those in the forehead region (Table 6-3). Minor complications resulted in additional procedures to correct the problems but did not terminate the expansion process. The most common minor complications, such as implant exposure and incision dehiscence, were likely to occur in difficult wound environments, such as burn scar contractures and thin skin from more than one expansion process. Major complications terminated the procedures and usually required 6 months to a year before insertion of another expander unit.

■ **Table 6-2** Sites of 119 Midfacial Reconstructions

Zone	Site	Number
I	Preauricular	33
II	Midcheek	28
III	Paranasal	58

■ **Table 6-3** Complications in 109 Midfacial Reconstructions

Type	Number
Minor (12%)	
Malposition	2
Implant failure	1
Exposure	5
Incision dehiscence	4
Flap ischemia	1
Major (4%)	
Infection	4

CASE REPORTS AND ANALYSES: Midfacial Reconstruction

CASE 1: Large Preauricular Nevus (Zone 1)

History (Figure 6-7, *A*)
This 15-year-old patient had a large, 5 × 7 cm congenital nevus to the right preauricular region of her face (*Z-1*, zone I). Because of cosmetic disfigurement and the possibility of malignant change, the patient requested its removal. The goals of surgery were to (1) remove the entire nevus, (2) preserve the normal anatomic relationships and functions of the midfacial structures, (3) resurface the defect with normal skin, and (4) produce a cosmetically acceptable scar.

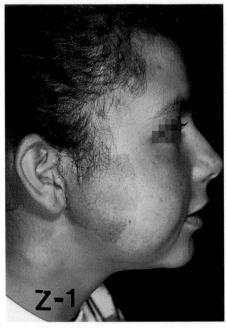

6-7A

Surgical Procedure (Figure 6-7, *B* and *C*)
A 200 cc rectangular expander was inserted under the subcutaneous tissue of the midface from a preauricular incision. The expander was located between the edge of the nevus to the paranasal region. After 10 weeks of expansion, 90% of the nevus was removed. The expanded midfacial skin was advanced laterally with releasing incisions along the lateral canthus.

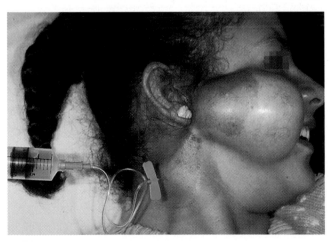

6-7B

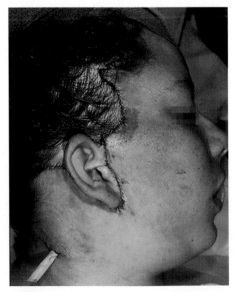

6-7C

Results (Figure 6-7, *D*)
Three years after completion of surgery the patient has preservation of the normal anatomic relationships and functions of the lateral canthus of the eyelid, nose, and right commissure of the lips. The final scar is placed in an aesthetic location acceptable to the patient. The scar extends from the temporal hairline, along the anterior edge of the nevus remnant, around the ear lobe, and behind the ear. The patient has declined secondary procedures to remove the remaining portion of the nevus.

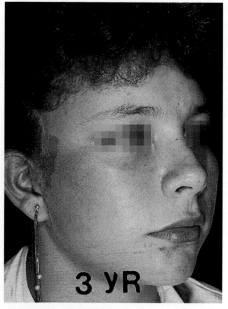

6-7D

CASE 2: Congenital Nevus on Left Midface (Zone II)

History (Figure 6-8, *A*)
This 3-year-old patient had a 3 × 4.5 cm nevus on her left midcheek (*Z-II,* zone II). The parents requested removal of the nevus because of the cosmetic deformity and the possibility of malignant degeneration. The goals of reconstruction were (1) excision of the entire nevus, (2) a cosmetically acceptable midface scar, and (3) preservation of midfacial structures and function.

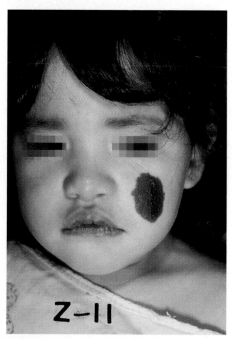

6-8A

Surgical Procedure (Figure 6-8, *B* and *C*)

A 100 cc round expander was positioned under the nevus in the subcutaneous plane through a 2.0 cm incision behind the left ear lobe. The valve system was located in the thicker postauricular scalp skin rather than under the thin retroauricular skin. The expander was filled with 50 ml of saline at surgery to reduce hematoma formation and to shorten the duration of expansion in this young patient. Expansion continued weekly for 8 weeks, creating a 10 cm dome (3 × 3 cm lesion width = 9 cm). This amount of expansion provided sufficient tissue to replace the defect.

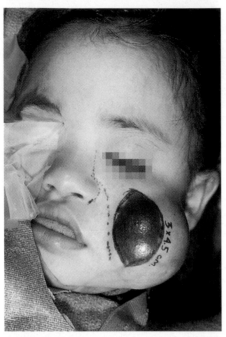

6-8B

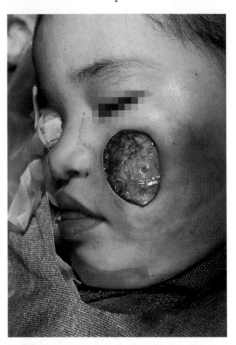

6-8C

Results (Figure 6-8, *D*)

Two years after her reconstruction the patient shows no recurrence of the nevus. In addition, the zigzag scar is barely noticeable, with preservation of midfacial structures and functions. The lower lid support has been maintained without malposition of the oral commissure. However, a slight depression exists in the area of expansion.

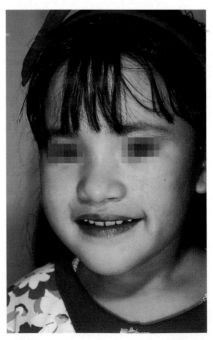

6-8D

CASE 3: Hypertrophic Port-wine Stain on Right Midface (Zone III)

History (Figure 6-9, *A*)

This 21-year-old patient had a 7 × 12 cm hypertrophic port-wine stain on the right midface (*Z-III*, zone III). An attempt to reduce the vascular malformation by argon laser was unsuccessful because of the resistant nature of the lesion's advanced stage. The patient requested removal of the entire lesion because of cosmetic concerns and occasional bleeding from the superficial vessels. The goals of surgery were (1) excision of the vascular malformation, (2) coverage with uninvolved adjacent skin, (3) preservation of facial structures and functions, and (4) creation of scars in aesthetic lines.

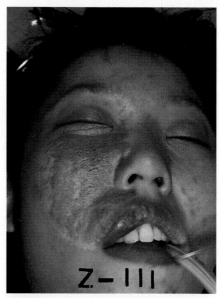

6-9A

Surgical Procedures (Figure 6-9, *B* to *E*)

A 320 cc rectangular expander (6 × 15 cm) was inserted partially under the lateral edge of the hemangioma and the uninvolved skin of the midface. The subcutaneous pocket was dissected from a 2.0 cm incision behind the right ear lobe. The remote valve system was positioned under the thicker postauricular skin. The expander was filled with 125 ml of saline at surgery to reduce hematoma formation and shorten the duration of expansion.

At surgery a 12 cm dome flap was created. Since the defect measured 7 cm across, a 14 cm flap would be pre-

ferred in order to advance the flap along preauricular and temporal lines, the subciliary line, nasomaxillary line, nasolabial fold, and eventual marionette fold. Therefore intraoperative expansion with 50 ml of saline more than the final expander volume of 300 cc produced an additional 2 cm of tissue. A 1 × 7 cm dermal strip of skin along the lateral edge of the hemangioma was raised in continuity with the lateral oral commissure. This strip would be sutured to the tissue over the zygoma to suspend the oral commissure in symmetry with the opposite side. In addition, a 0.5 × 6 cm free dermal graft, removed from the center

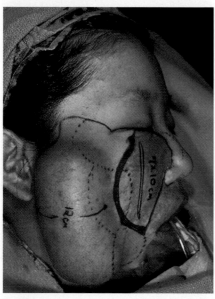

6-9B

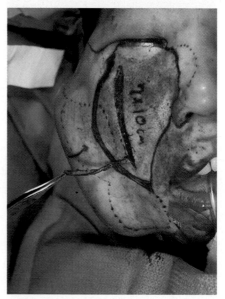

6-9C

of the malformation, would be used to support the lower lid by suspension from the medial canthal ligament across the lid margin to the temporoparietal fascia.

A total capsulectomy of the dome unfurled the expanded tissue for maximal use. Releasing capsulot-

omies around the base of expansion contributed to additional tissue for reconstruction. Creation of dermal fat mounds for the cheeks and nasolabial fold accentuated the dimensional results of the final reconstruction.

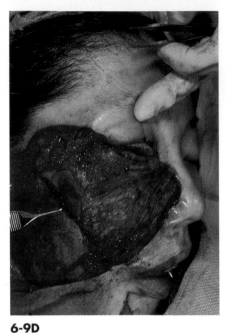

6-9D

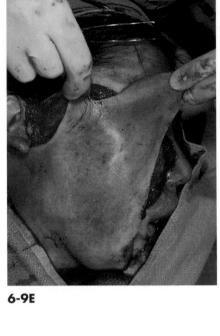

6-9E

Results (Figure 6-9, *F* and *G*)

Three years after her major reconstruction, the patient's replacement skin remains similar in quality to the opposite side and has normal sensation and color. The lower lid retains its supportive role without bowing or ectropion, but alar flare is absent. The oral commissure

is slightly lower than the opposite side with movement but at rest is symmetric to the contralateral side. The patient completed her reconstruction 5 years later with a reduction of the vascular component to the upper lip with a long-duration 532 nm Nd:YAG laser and a surgical removal of excess tissue along the marionette fold.

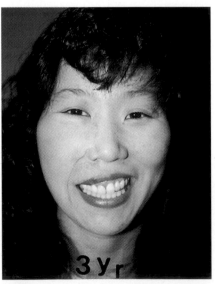

6-9F

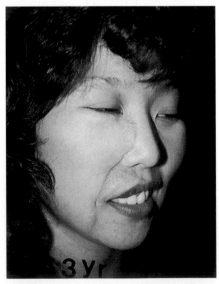

6-9G

CASE 4: Skin Graft Scar on Two Thirds of Right Midface (Zones II, III, and VI)

History (Figure 6-10, *A*)

This 34-year-old patient had a hemangiosarcoma resected from her right midface and covered with a skin graft. The patient received no other adjuvant treatment for her tumor. The 6 × 9 cm skin graft was located in the medial two thirds of her face. Vertical pleat lines (replaced fibrosis of hemangioma) were present along the right upper lip. Normal facial movement was present after her initial skin graft surgery. The goals of reconstruction were to (1) excise the skin graft scar, (2) resurface areas with normal adjacent skin, and (3) preserve all facial functions and anatomic relationships.

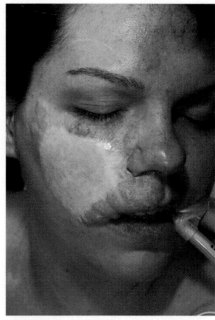

6-10A

Surgical Procedure (Figure 6-10, *B* to *D*)

Two 600 cc round expanders were inserted through a 2.5 cm retrolobular incision in the subcutaneous plane of the midface and neck. Each expander was filled to 300 cc at surgery to decrease hematoma formation. Serial expansions for 12 weeks (20 to 25 cc/expander/week) created a large 15 × 22 cm dome flap with temporary gravitational distortion to the oral commissure.

At the second stage, intraoperative expansion was performed with the addition of 100 ml of saline to the final expanded volume of 1200 cc to gain more tissue.

The large expanded cervicofacial flap was elevated, with excellent distal blood supply. A complete capsulectomy opened the domed flap. Base capsulotomies permitted more effective flap advancement. A dermal strip graft (1 × 7 cm) suspended the oral commissure to the zygoma. A narrower dermal strip graft (0.5 × 7 cm) was extended from the medial canthal ligament, under the lid margin, and to the temporoparietal fascia. These autogenous grafts resisted the downward forces on these mobile structures in the immediate postoperative period.

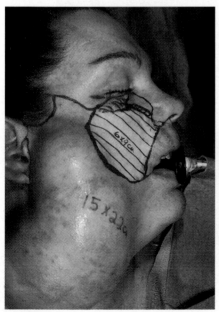

6-10B

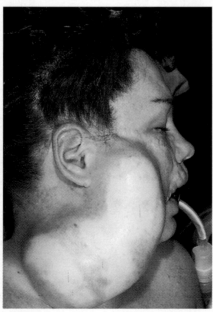

6-10C

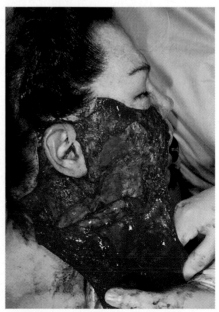

6-10D

Results (Figure 6-10, *E* and *F*)
Two years after reconstruction the patient has an aesthetic inset of the expanded flap along the preauricular temporal line, infraorbital crease, nasomaxillary line, perialar-to-nasal sill, philtral ridge, and upper lip line and down to the marionette fold. The incision was also extended along the postauricular sulcus and hairline. Facial symmetry and movement have been preserved with removal of the skin graft scar. Skin sensation has partially returned.

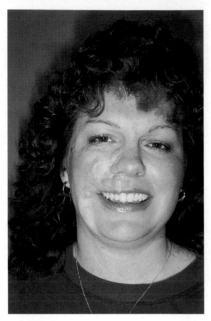

6-10E

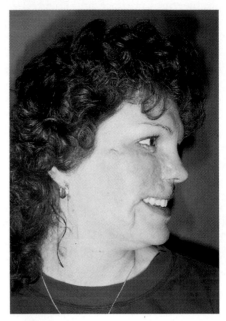

6-10F

CASE 5:   Hypertrophic Scar on Left Midface and Neck (Zones IV and V)

History (Figure 6-11, *A*)
This 16-year-old male had a hypertrophic scar on the lateral lower third of the midface and upper neck (*Z-IV & V*, zones IV and V). A recent attempt to expand the neck skin resulted in implant exposure and infection. Because the patient was referred from a distance, two separate expansion processes were planned to (1) expand first the noninfected midface skin and (2) delay expansion to the neck skin until complete resolution of infection.

The first expansion reconstruction was to remove the midfacial scar by stretching and advancing the midfacial skin toward the preauricular and mandibular lines. The second was to excise the neck scar component and advance the expanded neck skin to meet the scar along the mandibular outline. Thus the goals of surgery were to (1) remove the entire zone IV and V scar by two separate expansion processes, (2) preserve facial and neck functional and anatomic relationships, and (3) hide the incision scars along aesthetic lines.

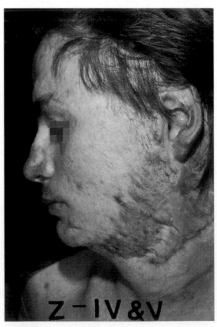

6-11A

First Surgical Procedure (Figure 6-11, *B*)

A 640 cc rectangular expander (8 × 15 cm) was inserted in the subcutaneous plane of the anterior two thirds of the midface through a 2.5 cm retrolobular incision. The expander was filled with 300 ml of saline at surgery to minimize hematoma formation and to reduce the duration of expansion. The patient's plastic surgeon performed weekly serial expansion. When sufficient tissue was produced with an expansion dome of 15 cm (5 cm width of facial scar component × 3 = 15 cm), the patient returned for scar excision.

At surgery, intraoperative expansion was performed by adding 50 to 75 ml of saline to gain more tissue. After excision of the facial scar the expanded tissue was advanced along the preauricular line and mandibular margin. Complete capsulectomy and base capsulotomies allowed efficient use of the flap.

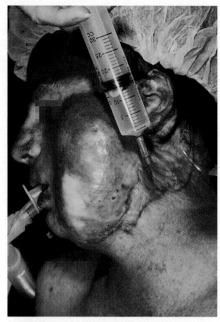

6-11B

Results (Figure 6-11, *C* and *D*)

Six months after surgery the patient demonstrates aesthetic facial reconstruction. Facial movement was preserved, and skin sensation partially returned.

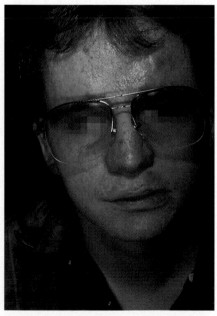

6-11C

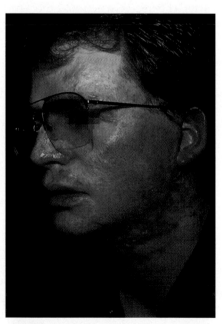

6-11D

Second Surgical Procedure (Figure 6-11, *E* and *F*)
A 640 cc rectangular expander was inserted in the subcutaneous plane of the neck through the same 2.5 cm retrolobular incision 1 year after resolution of the infection. Serial expansion was performed weekly until sufficient expanded dome tissue was produced to complete the reconstruction (7 cm scar width × 2.5 = 17 cm dome diameter). The remainder of the neck portion of the burn scar was excised, with advancement of the neck skin to the mandibular seam line.

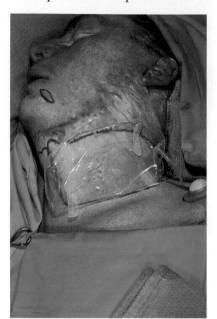

6-11E

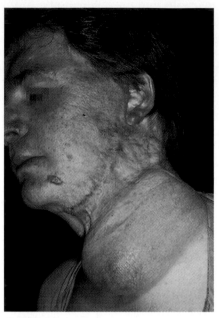

6-11F

Results (Figure 6-11, *G* and *H*)
Six years after the reconstructions, the entire hypertrophic burn scar has been replaced with normal skin from the midface and neck. The final scar lines are hidden in the lines of aesthetic closure. Facial movement and proportions have been preserved.

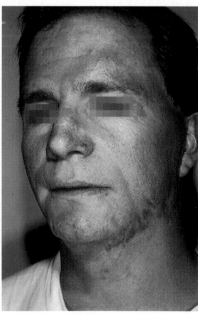

6-11G

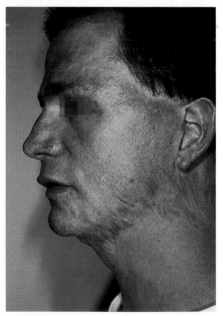

6-11H

CASE 6: Hypertrophic Lower Lip and Neck (Zones V and VII)

History (Figure 6-12, *A*)

This 21-year-old patient developed hypertrophic burn scars along her lower lip, chin, and midneck. Scar contractures tethered down the left oral commissure and restricted full neck extension. The patient also had minimal burn scars to the upper lip and left midface. The upper lip scar responded to 1 ml of intralesional betamethasone (Celestone) with reduction of erythema, itching, and prominence. The goals of surgery were to (1) remove the neck contractures, (2) release the scarred lower lip and left oral commissure, (3) restore cervicofacial relationships, and (4) resurface with normal skin along aesthetic lines of closure.

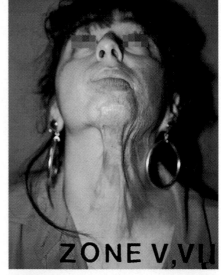

6-12A

First Surgical Procedure (Figure 6-12, *B* and *C*)

Two 600 cc round expanders were inserted in the preplatysmal plane along each side of the vertical neck contractures. A 2.5 cm retrolobular incision on each side permitted the large pocket dissections for each expander and allowed the placement of the remote valve systems under the postauricular scalp skin. Each expander was filled with 300 ml of saline at surgery to prevent hematoma formation. Serial expansions were performed weekly with the addition of 20 to 25 ml. When sufficient tissue was produced, the vertical scar contractures and underlying fibrotic platysmal bands were excised. The defect was replaced with the expanded skin, which was closed in a Z-plasty closure.

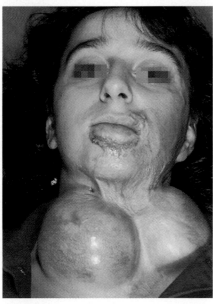

6-12B

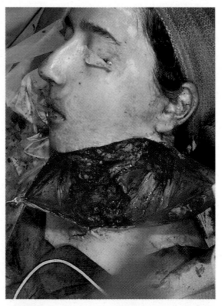

6-12C

Results (Figure 6-12, *D*)

Six months after neck reconstruction, the scar contracture has been broken effectively by the zigzag closure and platysmal resection. The lower lip and left commissure deformities are still present.

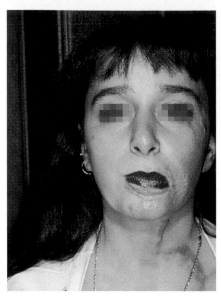

6-12D

Second Surgical Procedure (Figure 6-12, *E*)

A 25 cc round expander was inserted in the subcutaneous plane of right chin skin through a 2.5 cm retrolobular ear incision. The expander was positioned 1 cm within the chin scar. Serial expansion for 6 weeks produced sufficient tissue to advance the skin across three fourths of the lower lip and chin complex. The mucocutaneous border of the lip was reestablished. A left commissuroplasty redefined and partially released the corner of the mouth.

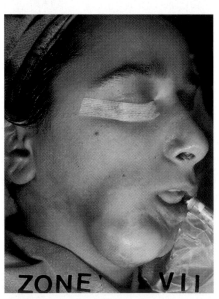

6-12E

Results (Figure 6-12, *F* and *G*)

One year after completion of the reconstructions, the vermilion border and left commissure have improved, with elevation of the corner of the mouth. Expanded tissue has partially resurfaced the scarred chin skin, with preservation of the mental sulcus.

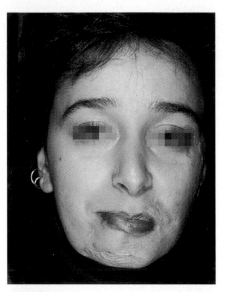

6-12F

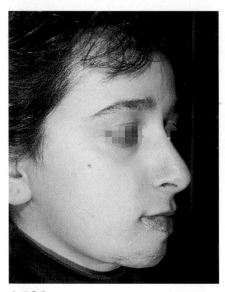

6-12G

CASE RESULTS: NECK EXPANSION

Cervical skin demonstrates elasticity and movement that can be advantageous to tissue expansion. Expansion of donor neck skin has allowed reconstruction of difficult problems such as burn scar contractures, congenital nevi, and traumatic scars (Table 6-4). In the past these entities were managed with relaxing incisions (Z-plasties), skin grafts, and local flaps. Implant insertion and expansion under the platysma muscle may cause it to bunch up under the mandible and lead to potential nerve injury.

Neck skin may be advanced in a transverse or vertical direction. Expanded tissue, moved in a cephalad or caudad direction, demonstrates an innate ability to contract and shorten, which may result in loss of acuity in the cervicomandibular angle. In contrast, expanded skin transposed in a horizontal direction, toward either the neck midline or the sides of the neck,

■ **Table 6-4** Types of Neck Defects in 74 Reconstructions

Type	Number
Trauma	
Scar	9
Skin graft	15
Burn contracture	23
Premalignancy	
Giant hairy nevus	27

tends to form hypertrophic scars. These shortcomings are related to the regional motor vectors of the neck exerted by flexion-extension and lateral rotary movements. The underlying platysma muscle also plays a significant role in scar hypertrophy, often observed after burn trauma.

Vertical Expanded-Skin Advancement

When a defect involves the upper portion of the neck below the mandible, donor skin in the lower aspect of the neck may be expanded. Cephalad advancement results in an acceptable reconstruction, with the scar located under or at the mandibular margin. The cervicomandibular angle may be recreated by the use of multiple permanent tacking sutures from the capsulodermal layer of the expanded neck flap to tissues along the neck angle.

Expansion of skin of the upper third of the neck to resurface a defect on the lower third of the midface above the mandible may lead to several postsurgical sequelae. The native cervicomandibular sulcus may be lost because of excessive skin tension during cephalad advancement of tissue. The lip commissures may also be pulled as a result of tethered skin. Thus reconstruction of the lower third of the midface at times is better managed by expanding any available cheek skin, which is then advanced down to the mandibular border.

Forty-seven patients in the author's series completed skin expansion of the neck with tissue advancement in a vertical direction (Table 6-5).

Horizontal Expanded-Skin Advancement

When a lesion is primarily located in the midneck, two laterocervical expanders may be used to advance tissue to the midline with Z-plasty closure. Compression on the mandibular branch of the facial nerve or on the jugular veins has never resulted in facial muscle paresis or venous hypertension. When a defect exists on the lateral aspect of the neck, expansion of the adjacent donor neck skin with a single balloon results in adequate tissue for replacement.

Twenty-seven patients underwent skin expansion of the neck with tissue advancement in a horizontal direction (Table 6-5).

■ **Table 6-5** Tissue Advancement of 74 Neck Reconstructions

Advancement	Number
Vertical	47
Horizontal	27

Complications

The major complication rate remained low (3%) with neck expansion (Table 6-6). Minor complications of flap ischemia and implant exposure did not result in termination of the process but required an additional corrective procedure. Major complications of infection aborted the process and occurred in burn scar contractures and in previously expanded tissue.

■ **Table 6-6** Complications in 74 Neck Reconstructions

Type	Number
Minor (16%)	
Flap ischemia	3
Exposure	
Implant	3
Valve	6
Major (3%)	
Infection	2

CASE REPORT AND ANALYSIS: Neck Reconstruction

Burn Scars and Contracture of Neck and Chest Wall

History (Figure 6-13, *A*)
This 42-year-old patient had hypertrophic burn scars and an anterior neck contracture. The goals of surgery were to (1) remove the hypertrophic scars to the anterior and lateral neck and keloidal scar over the sternum, (2) release the contracture to the midneck, (3) restore neck anatomy and function, and (4) ensure acceptable postsurgical scars.

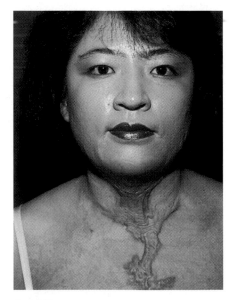

6-13A

Surgical Procedure (Figure 6-13, *B* to *D*)

Two 500 cc round expanders were inserted in the subcutaneous plane to each lateral neck. Two 500 cc rectangular expanders were placed in the subcutaneous plane on either side of the keloidal scar on the sternum. Each set of a round and a rectangular expander was placed into a single large pocket dissected from a 2.5 cm retrolobular incision. The valve systems for the round neck expanders were located under the postauricular scalp skin. The pockets for the valve system of each rectangular chest expander were dissected from 2.5 cm transaxillary incisions.

Intraoperative filling of the expanders to tissue tolerance prevented hematoma formation. Serial expansions began 3 weeks after insertion, with each expander filled with 15 to 20 ml of saline. After 12 weeks of expansion, sufficient tissue was produced to replace the excised scar formation. The fibrotic platysmal bands were removed to release the neck contracture. A Z-plasty skin closure of the chest and anterior neck scar was possible because of the amount of expanded tissue. The lateral neck closures paralleled the mandibular outlines.

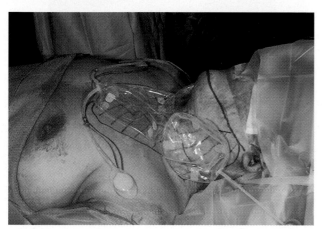

6-13B

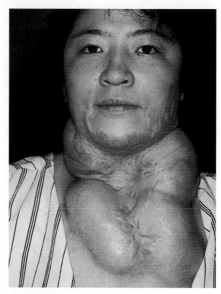

6-13C

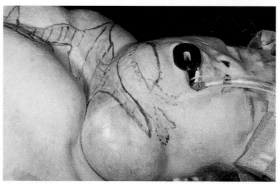

6-13D

Results (Figure 6-13, *E* and *F*)
Two years after surgery the patient has an acceptable chest and anterior neck scar. The new scar has not re-

sulted in a cervical contracture. The patient is able to wear open-neck clothing. Normal skin sensation has partially returned.

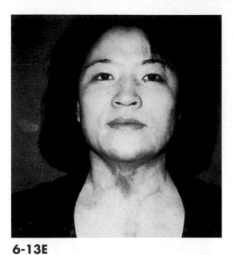

6-13E

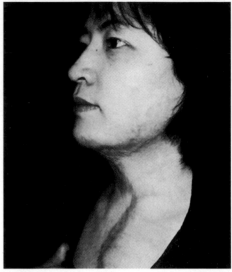

6-13F

CASE REPORTS AND ANALYSES: Complex Combined Procedures

CASE 1: **Skin Graft to Right Forehead for Giant Hairy Nevus of Right Temporoparieto-occipital Scalp**

History (Figure 6-14, *A* and *B*)
This infant had a giant hairy nevus of the right forehead and temporoparieto-occipital scalp. Because of the potential for malignant degeneration and aesthetic deformity, the forehead portion was excised and covered with a 5 × 8 cm split-thickness skin graft at 3 years of age. The right frontalis muscle did not func-

tion postoperatively and resulted in a 2 cm ptosis of the brow. The goals of surgery were to (1) remove the remaining portion of the congenital nevus, (2) replace the forehead skin graft with normal adjacent forehead skin and muscle, (3) resurface the scalp defect with normal adjacent scalp, and (4) elevate the right ptotic brow to match the opposite side.

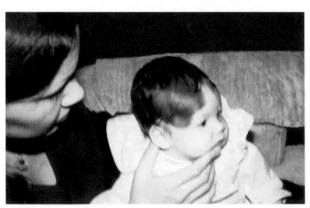

6-14A

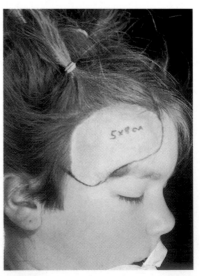

6-14B

Surgical Procedure (Figure 6-14, *C* and *D*)

At age 7, two 1000 cc rectangular expanders (10 × 20 cm) were inserted under the periosteum of the left forehead and frontal temporoparieto-occipital scalp. The expanders were located under a portion of the nevus to prevent their slippage from the defect's leading edge during serial expansion. The pocket for the expanders was developed from a 3.0 cm incision in the postauricular area of the left ear. The remote valves were positioned under the left neck skin.

Each expander was filled with 150 cc (ml) of saline at surgery to reduce hematoma formation and prevent the development of any soft tissue septum between the expanders. Serial expansions were begun 2 weeks later by filling each expander weekly with 25 ml. Once the galeal-periosteal resistance was overcome within 3 to 6 weeks, expansion proceeded more efficiently, with administration of larger volumes of saline into each balloon.

Serial expansions continued for 4 months until sufficient tissue was generated by measurement across the expansion domes. Since width of the nevus averaged 15 cm, expansion had to produce a mound at least 30 cm across (15 cm × 2 = 30 cm dome width). This amount of tissue was achieved by filling the anterior expander to 900 cc and the posterior expander to 1300 cc.

Intraoperative expansion to each balloon gained an additional 2 to 3 cm at surgery. After removal of expanders, a complete dome capsulectomy and base capsulotomy unfurled the flaps and permitted maximal advancement to cover the entire defect. The forehead was replaced with expanded frontalis muscle and skin. The right brow was elevated and fixed by sutures to match the opposite side.

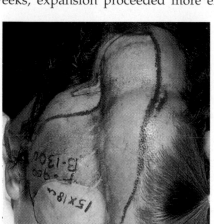

6-14C

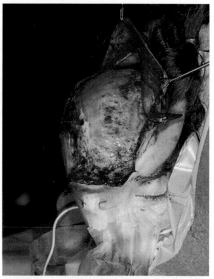

6-14D

Results (Figure 6-14, *E*)

Eight years after her surgeries the patient has functional and aesthetic reconstruction. The brow complex is symmetric to the opposite side at rest. Right frontalis muscle movement exhibits weakness compared with that on the left side. The entire nevus and skin graft have been removed, with replacement of hair-bearing tissue in the scalp and normal skin of the forehead. Hair density is less than before because of increased distance between hair shafts from expansion. Skin sensation has return to near-normal levels in most portions of the expanded flaps.

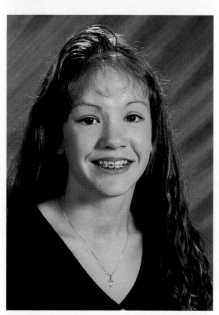

6-14E

CASE 2: Skin Graft for Burn Scar of Left Forehead and Temporoparietal Scalp

History (Figure 6-15, *A*)

This 7-year-old patient sustained a full-thickness burn to his left cheek, forehead, and scalp that was covered by a split-thickness skin graft. A previous expansion process to his left cheek resulted in an upward advancement of a lower cheek flap to replace the scarred tissue. Evaluation identified a 3 × 10 cm skin graft over his forehead and a 10 × 16 cm skin graft on the temporoparietal scalp. The goals of surgery were to (1) advance the cheek flap incision scars to the preauricular and temporal crease lines, (2) resurface the forehead scar tissue with normal skin, and (3) replace the area of alopecia with hair-bearing scalp.

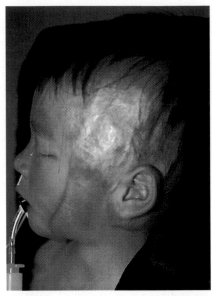

6-15A

Surgical Procedure (Figure 6-15, *B* to *D*)

A 100 cc round expander was inserted under the previously expanded cheek flap through a 2.5 retrolobular incision. Two 640 cc, 8 × 18 cm rectangular expanders were placed under the periosteum of the forehead and adjacent scalp tissues through a 2.5-cm incision in the right postauricular sulcus. The remote valve systems of the two scalp expanders were buried under the periosteum of the right temporal scalp. The valve for the cheek expander was placed under the postauricular scalp. Serial expansions were done weekly for 3 months to obtain sufficient skin to cover the scalp, forehead, and cheek. The dome of the scalp flaps measured 20 cm across.

At surgery, intraoperative expansion was performed on the three expanders to gain additional tissue. After the forehead and scalp expanders were removed, capsulectomies and base capsulotomies released and unfurled the hemispheric flaps. The forehead flap was advanced laterally to resurface the 3 × 10 cm scarred remnant of the forehead and to define the anterior and temporal seam lines. The expanded scalp flap replaced the entire skin graft over the temporoparietal area. The expanded cheek flap was advanced in a cephalad and posterior direction to replace scar tissue between the eyebrow and ear and thus to position the new scar along the ear's normal crease lines.

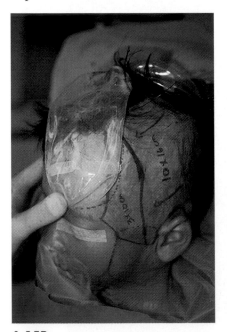

6-15B

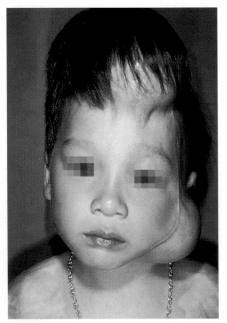

6-15C

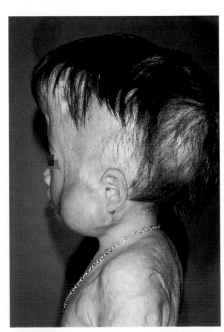

6-15D

Results (Figure 6-15, *E* and *F*)
One year after the major reconstructive procedures, hair density and distribution in the former areas of scalp alopecia have provided a stable, aesthetic cover. The brow and lateral commissure of the eyelids have regained symmetry with the opposite side. The fore-

head aesthetic unit has been reestablished with a functioning frontalis muscle. Maturation of the vertical midface scar should improve, with less erythema and thickness. The redundant submental skin is scheduled for later resection.

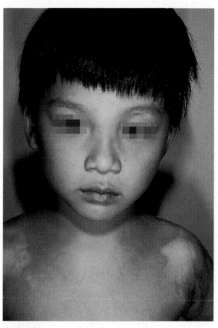

6-15E

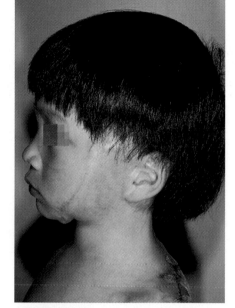

6-15F

CASE 3: Giant Hairy Nevus of Right Forehead-Hemiscalp and Cheek

History (Figure 6-16, *A*)
This 4-year-old patient had a congenital giant nevus on the lateral aspect of her right forehead, half of the brow, the cheek, and half of her entire scalp. Because of the potential for malignant degeneration and cosmetic deformity, tissue expansion was indicated. The lesion's size and location required two expansion procedures 6 months apart to complete the major portion of her reconstruction. The goals of surgery were to (1) remove the entire nevus; (2) establish the aesthetic and functional units of the forehead, eyebrow, eyelid commissure, and scalp; and (3) minimize visible scars.

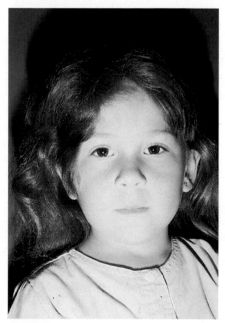

6-16A

First Surgical Procedure (Figure 6-16, *B* and *C*)

At the first surgery, three expanders were inserted in the subperiosteal plane under the forehead and adjacent normal scalp tissue. Two 400 cc round expanders were positioned under normal forehead and occipital scalp tissue. An 800 cc rectangular expander was placed between the round expanders. All expanders were inserted through a 3.0 cm left postauricular incision that created a single large pocket. The expanders were filled to maximal tissue tolerance to reduce hematoma formation.

Serial expansion continued weekly. After 3 months, each expander generated a 20 cm–wide hemispheric flap. Further flap expansion was not possible because of tissue thinning. A 20 cm flap was expected to result in about 10 cm of advancement. Since the nevus measured at least 20 cm across, an additional expansion procedure was anticipated.

Intraoperative expansion was performed to gain extra tissue. Dome capsulectomies of the flaps maximized their potential areas for coverage. Capsulotomies permitted greater mobilization of the flaps. The thickened capsules on the base of the skull were removed to allow more efficient flap advancements and to reduce contour irregularities.

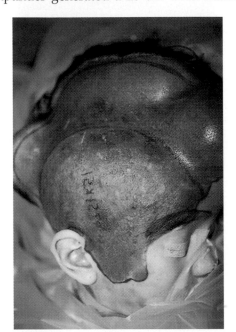

6-16B

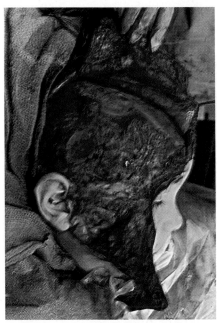

6-16C

Second Surgical Procedure (Figure 6-16, *D*)

The second surgical procedure 6 months later involved insertion of a 400 cc round expander under the forehead and frontal scalp tissues, an 800 cc rectangular expander under the parieto-occipital scalp, and a 400 cc round expander under the cheek tissue. The cheek expander was inserted through a 2.5 cm retrolobular incision and positioned in the subcutaneous layer. The scalp expanders were inserted through the previous left postauricular incision scar in the subperiosteal plane.

Reexpansion of the scalp and forehead complex was completed in 8 weeks to obtain sufficient tissue to resurface the remaining 10 × 10 cm remnant. In general, reexpansion of tissue proceeded more rapidly than during the first expansion process and achieved the same flap dimensions. Serial expansion of the cheek tissue was done weekly for 12 weeks.

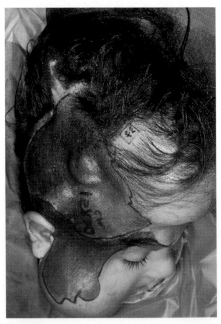

6-16D

Results (Figure 6-16, *E*)

Two years after her complex expansion procedures, the patient has a small remnant of nevus on the cheek and lateral tail of the brow. A scattered growth of nevoid cells is seen in the temporal portion of the advanced flap. All the scalp nevus has been successfully removed. Facial aesthetics and function have been restored. The frontalis muscle is active with brow symmetry. Scalp resurfacing of the entire hemiscalp remains stable, with adequate hair density and distribution. Sensation has slowly returned to the reexpanded tissue. Scars are hidden along aesthetic crease lines.

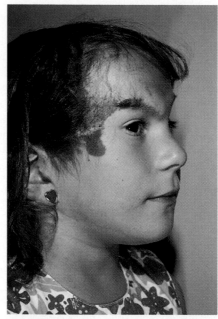

6-16E

CASE 4: Burn Deformity of Ear and Skin Grafts to Right Lower Cheek and Neck

History (Figure 6-17, *A*)

This 21-year-old patient sustained a burn injury that destroyed the helical rim and antehelical crura of her right ear and resulted in full-thickness skin loss to the lower third of her midface and most of her right neck. Secondary scar contracture deformed the ear remnant. The skin graft developed areas of hyperpigmentation and contractures. The goals of surgery were to (1) reconstruct the right pinna, (2) resurface the midface and neck graft sites, (3) reestablish facial aesthetics and function, and (4) minimize incision scars along aesthetic lines.

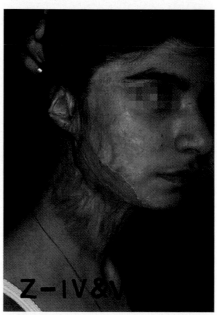

6-17A

Surgical Procedure (Figure 6-17, *B* and *C*)

A 100 cc rectangular expander was inserted in the subperiosteal plane above and behind the right ear remnant through a 2.5 cm incision of the temporal scalp. The same incision permitted the insertion of a 300 cc round expander in the subcutaneous plane of the cheek. An 800 cc rectangular expander was positioned in the subcutaneous plane under neck and adjacent chest skin through a 2.5 cm incision along the deltopectoral crease line. All expanders were filled to tissue tolerance to decrease hematoma formation.

Serial expansions of the expanders continued weekly for 4 months until sufficient tissue was generated (cheek: 13 × 14 cm; supraauricular area: 8 × 12 cm; neck-chest: 14 × 28 cm). The expanded cheek flap was expected to be advanced at least 6 cm to lie beneath the mandibular margin. The expanded neck-chest flap was anticipated to resurface the 7 cm–wide neck scar, meeting the mandibular seam line. The expanded tissue above and behind the ear remnant was expected to provide sufficient thin, hairless cover over both the cartilaginous framework and the postauricular sulcus.

Intraoperative expansion was performed on all expanders to gain additional tissue. Capsules were removed from the domes of all flaps to unfurl them for more efficient coverage. The cartilaginous framework (6-17, *C*), created from contributions of the seventh, eighth, and ninth ribs, was spliced onto the existing remnants of the antehelix and concha.

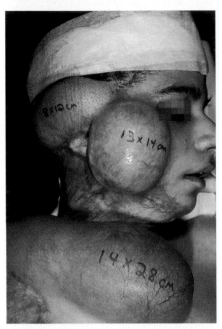

6-17B

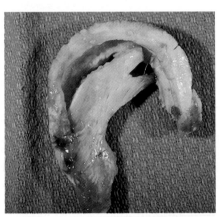

6-17C

Results (Figure 6-17, *D* and *E*)

Three years after reconstruction the ear's projection and delicate outline match the opposite ear's dimensions. The mandibular margin is defined by the seam line of opposing flaps. The scar tissue has been resur-

faced by soft pliable skin, with preservation of normal facial and neck aesthetics. Although the lower lid exhibits a 1 mm scleral show, the patient does not complain of dryness or tearing.

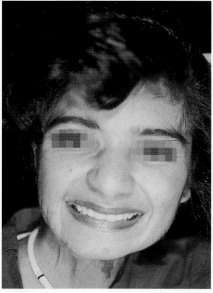

6-17D

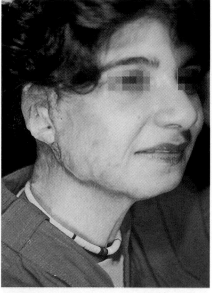

6-17E

CASE 5: Full-face Grafting

History (Figure 6-18, *A* and *B*)

This 14-year-old patient sustained burns to 40% of his body from a gasoline explosion. Split-thickness grafts were placed in aesthetic units. The patient wanted resurfacing with more supple skin for a more natural, mat masklike, facial appearance. Since replacement

tissue would be derived from limited donor sites, multiple expansion procedures were planned. The goals of reconstruction were to (1) resurface the graft sites with supple neck skin; (2) establish facial function and aesthetics without distortions to the oral commissure, nasal flare, and eyelids; and (3) minimize incisional scars.

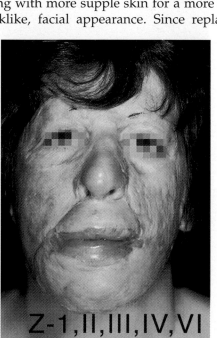

Z-1,II,III,IV,VI

6-18A

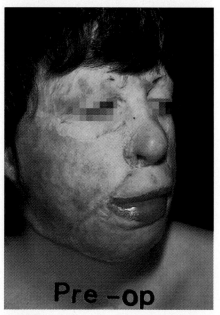

Pre -op

6-18B

First Surgical Procedure (Figure 6-18, *C* and *D*)
Two 1000 cc rectangular expanders were inserted in the subcutaneous plane of the neck in a single pocket through a 2.5 cm incision behind both ear lobes. Each expander was filled to 500 cc to maximal tissue toler- ance at surgery. Serial expansion was performed weekly for 4 months until the overlying tissue became too thin. A total dome capsulectomy released and un- furled the flaps for efficient advancement up to the level of the oral commissure.

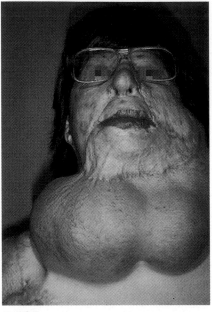

6-18C

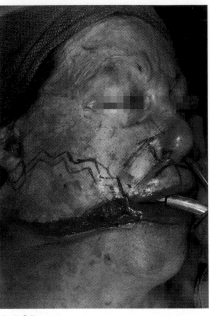

6-18D

Second Surgical Procedure (Figure 6-18, *E* and *F*)
After 6 months a 400 cc rectangular expander was in- serted in the subcutaneous plane under the advanced skin above each mandibular margin. Expansion of the supramandibular skin preserved the mandibular out- line and sulcus by avoidance of a tented appearance. Serial expansion for 3 months created a 12 cm-wide hemispheric flap. The released flap was able to be mo- bilized upward to the level of the nasal sill.

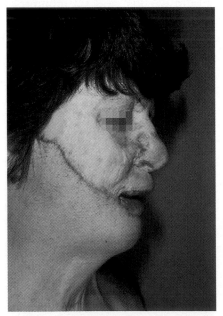

6-18E

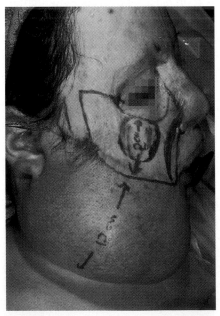

6-18F

Third Surgical Procedure (Figure 6-18, *G*)

Six months later a 300 cc rectangular expander was inserted in the subcutaneous plane under each of the larger donor midfacial skin sites through the same retrolobular incision scars. Serial expansion for 3 months produced a hemispheric dome flap that was advanced to the infraorbital sulcus and above the level of the eyelid commissures. Static suspension of the lower lid was performed with a dermal strip graft that extended from the medial caudal ligament to the lateral temporoparietalis fascia.

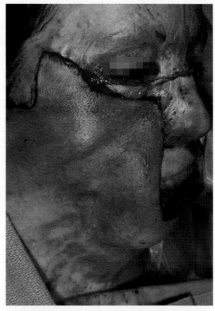

6-18G

Fourth Surgical Procedure (Figure 6-18, *H*)

After another 6 months the excess portions of the medial flaps were advanced to the nasomaxillary line, toward the philtral columns, along the upper lip lines, around the commissures, across the lower lip vermilion borders, and down the mental prominence.

Secondary procedures, including lower lip reduction, eyebrow grafting, and cheek augmentation with silicone implants, were also performed to enhance the major reconstructive procedures.

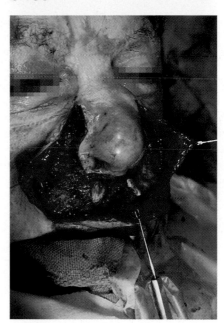

6-18H

Results (Figure 6-18, *I*)

Three years after his major reconstructions, the patient demonstrates dimensional effect created by supple skin over underlying autogenous and alloplastic facial mounds. Sensation to the stretched skin has partially returned. The major aspects of facial aesthetics have been realized. Although a degree of lower lid bowing still exists, the patient does not complain of dryness or tearing.

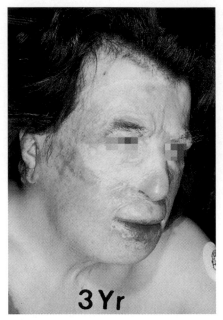

6-18I

SUMMARY

Reconstruction of the scalp, forehead, midface, and neck presents a challenge for expansion surgery. Functional and aesthetic concerns are paramount during and after tissue expansion, which offers the optimal tissue replacement for many patients. The surgeon should attempt small and distant incisions to reduce early complications from exposure and infection. A dimensional reconstructive approach is required for symmetry and function with preservation of facial muscles and their nerves. Complications can be significantly reduced with attention to detail in surgical approach and technique, sterility during filling, and preservation of structures.

CHAPTER

7

Nasal Reconstruction

Tissue expansion for small and isolated nasal defects ideally involves expansion of direct nasal skin. In this way, optimal conditions are provided to match skin texture, thickness, and color. However, the preexpanded median forehead flap remains the method of choice for nasal defects too large to be repaired by expanded nasal skin or adjacent cheek skin. The expansion process is necessary not only to provide sufficient skin (10 to 12 cm wide) to reconstruct the entire nasal tip, alar rims, and columella, but also to permit direct closure of the forehead donor site. Whenever expansion is not employed, the standard-designed median forehead flap (5 to 6 cm wide) frequently falls short both in supplying adequate skin and in permitting primary closure of the forehead site.

Although expansion of adjacent cheek skin and distal sites, (e.g., scalp, arm, deltopectoral region) are possible, the disadvantages of such surgeries far outweigh their benefits. Since the introduction of tissue expansion of the forehead flap, the prepared flaps possess an increased vascular supply and have greater dimensions, leaving sufficient tissue to close the donor area with an acceptable scar. For smaller nasal defects, long-term expansion or intraoperative expansion with miniexpanders provides optimal tissue replacement.

ANATOMIC CONSIDERATIONS

The nasal skin is thin and lax over the root and dorsum but becomes more adherent over the nasal tip, alae, and columella. The number of sebaceous and sweat glands increases in the lobular skin, which covers the support provided by the upper lateral and alar cartilages.

The skin over the nasal root, dorsum, and alae is innervated by the nasal branch of the ophthalmic division of the fifth cranial nerve (Figure 7-1). The greater part of the sides of the nose is supplied by the second division of the trigeminal nerve.

The arteries to the nasal skin are derived from the facial artery, which supplies the skin of the side of the nose and alar rims. The septal branches travel to the septum and the alae. The ophthalmic artery provides blood to the skin of the root and dorsum. The major veins follow the course of the arteries.

The primary blood supply to the nasal skin is abundant and permits safe expansion for coverage of smaller defects.

Forehead Flaps

The vascular network of the forehead is based on significant axial vessels that define skin territories on which various flaps are designed. The median forehead skin is abundantly supplied by the supratrochlear, supraorbital, and frontalis branches from the internal carotid artery. The lateral portion of the forehead skin derives its blood supply from the superficial temporal artery and the zygomatico-orbital branches of the external carotid artery.

Tissue expansion of the median or paramedian forehead area for nasal reconstruction incorporates the supratrochlear neurovascular bundles located at the midpoint between the inner canthus and the inner eyebrow border. This deep axial vessel predictably becomes a vertical dermal plexus nourishing the adjacent skin and contributing small vessels to the underlying frontalis, procerus, and depressor corrugator muscles. From these anatomic relationships, the surgeon may insert an expander under the periosteal, subgaleal, or epigaleal plane as long as the vascular territory supplied by the supratrochlear vessels is preserved. Within this expanded territory, a reliable median or paramedian flap, incorporating this axial vessel, may be elevated from the expanded tissues with or without the underlying muscle complexes (procerus, corrugator, frontalis).

The advantages of a subperiosteal or subgaleal expander pocket include rapid and safe dissection, a bloodless field, and protection of the axial blood supply. The disadvantages of such a deeper expander pocket relate to transposing a thicker and unnatural flap because of muscle inclusion. Secondary

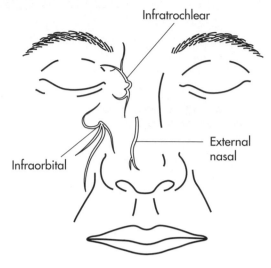

Figure 7-1 Cutaneous nerves of the nose.

debulking procedures may be required to thin the transposed flap.

The advantage of an epigaleal expander pocket is the expansion of skin from which a thin, pliable, arterially based median or paramedian forehead flap is raised and transferred to the nasal defect. The initial disadvantage of an epigaleal pocket is the special care needed to preserve the supratrochlear vascular bundle as it enters the dermal layer. Intraoperative Doppler tracing of the supratrochlear artery is mandatory during both pocket dissection and flap elevation.

Flap Design
A subtotal or total nasal reconstruction, including tissue for infolding and columellar development, requires a flap measuring about 8 cm in vertical and horizontal dimensions. The meridian measurement of the expanded dome flap should be about twice the width of the designed flap. In the forehead the final measurement of the dome flap therefore should be about 16 to 18 cm across to permit tension-free closure of the donor site. The adult forehead provides an area of about 5 to 7 cm in vertical height and 12 to 16 cm width.

Expander Insertion
The expander's shape and size are selected on the basis of the amount of forehead skin available and the dimensions of the actual or anticipated nasal defect. Usually a 100 to 160 cc round or rectangular expander will fit into the donor site and, after expansion, provide sufficient tissue for a subtotal or total nasal reconstruction. A remote minivalve or incorporated valve system may be advocated, because both types possess certain advantages that offset their drawbacks. For example, the remote valve system obviates the

possibility of inadvertent balloon puncture during filling, which can occur with an incorporated valve expander. However, a remote valve requires creation of an additional pocket and time to remove it and increases the risk for valve exposure and infection.

Surgical Considerations

The requirements and priorities for nasal reconstruction must be determined on the basis of existing or anticipated deficiencies.

Limited Nasal Defects
Insertion of an expander under available nasal skin may be indicated before surgical resection of a lesion or after a defect has been established. At the second stage the expanded skin replaces the affected nasal skin containing the defect (e.g., congenital nevus, scar). Cartilage or bone grafts may be inserted under the expanded skin. Lining may be provided at the second stage by turning down adjacent skin or mucosal flaps or by using them as grafts (partial thickness, full thickness, or composite).

In contrast, an expander should not be inserted under nasal skin at resection or when unstable tissue conditions exist after a resection has been completed. The chances for implant exposure and infection along the closure line are higher under these circumstances. Expanded nasal skin is more easily advanced in a horizontal direction across the nose. Vertical advancement is more difficult because of immediate tissue stretchback. Expansion of remaining nasal skin provides the ideal replacement because of like tissue and avoidance of more complicated incision scars associated with local transposition of nasal flaps.

Larger Nasal Defects
Nasal skin expansion may not be possible when minimal nasal donor skin exists or is anticipated after resection. In these cases, median forehead skin is the donor tissue of choice. When the nasal tip, alar folds, and columella are to be reconstructed, expanded median forehead skin provides ample tissue to create them by infolding techniques. In addition, the donor forehead defect may be approximated by primary skin closure. Provision of structure (cartilage and bone grafts) and lining may be included at the second stage.

SURGICAL TECHNIQUE

Nasal Expansion

For limited nasal defects, a small nasal expander may be inserted with the patient under local or general

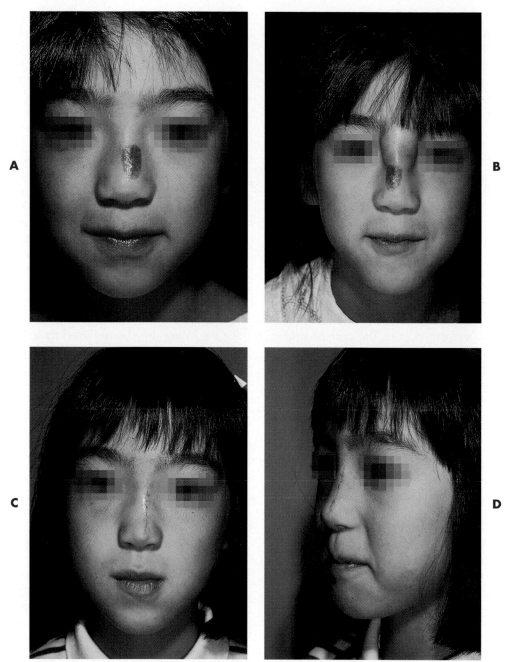

Figure 7-2 **A,** This 7-year-old patient had a 1 × 2 cm congenital nevus on the dorsum of her nose. Because of the slight risk for malignant degeneration and the cosmetic deformity, tissue expansion was chosen to remove the lesion. **B,** Vertical 2.0 cm incision was made in the midforehead behind the precapillary line. A subperiosteal dissection in the midforehead was converted to a subcutaneous plane at the level of the nasal root. The dissection was carried down to the distal end of the nevus. Balloon retraction required surgical repositioning of the expander toward the nasal tip. Thereafter, serial expansion of a 5 cc rectangular expander was performed weekly for 4 weeks. This produced sufficient tissue to permit primary closure of the defect after surgical excision of the nevus. **C** and **D,** The patient 1 year after her reconstruction. The defect has been approximated in a single vertical line closure. No deformity to the bony or cartilaginous structures resulted from the expansion forces.

anesthesia (Figure 7-2, *A*). A 2.0 cm vertical incision is made behind the precapillary line in the midforehead. A subgaleal or subperiosteal tunnel is dissected from the scalp incision, past the nasal root, and downward to the farthest extent of the donor nasal skin. The use of long scissors facilitates the nasal dissection from a distant site.

A 1.5 to 5.0 cc round or rectangular expander is pushed down with the aid of a plastic suction cannula. The remote valve is inserted into its own subperiosteal pocket under the scalp away from the incision. The selection of the expander's size and shape is determined by the dimensions of available donor tissue. The expander is filled to tissue tolerance to maintain the pocket size and to reduce the incidence of hematoma formation. Serial expansion may begin within a few weeks and continues weekly until sufficient tissue has been produced (Figure 7-2, *B*).

At the second stage, intraoperative expansion may provide additional tissue before expander removal. After the lesion has been excised, the expanded tissue is advanced to resurface the defect with a single line closure (Figure 7-2, *C* and *D*). Additional tissues, such as cartilaginous grafts and turn-down lining flaps, may be included to complete the reconstructive effort.

Forehead Expansion

For larger and more complex defects, expander insertion for development of a median or paramedian forehead flap may be performed with the patient under local or general anesthesia (Figure 7-3, *A* and *B*). The round (100 cc) or rectangular expander (160 cc) is outlined on the forehead skin in a median or paramedian location. The location of the supratrochlear vessels is determined by Doppler recording. A vertical incision is made about 2.5 cm posterior to the frontal hairline and measures less than 3 cm in length. The downward dissection may be performed either in an epigaleal plane or at the subperiosteal level. If an epigaleal plane is developed, care must be taken to reduce injury to the supratrochlear vessels when they penetrate into the dermal layer. With a subperiosteal approach the dissection is quicker, safer, and less bloody than with elevation in the subgaleal plane.

The surgical pocket should exceed the expander base by 1 cm to flatten the expander. The remote valve is inserted in the same incision under the epigaleal or subperiosteal plane away from the balloon. The expander is filled with saline containing bacitracin through the buried remote valve to tissue tolerance. Implant and valve integrity is tested with a small amount of methylene blue–stained saline to determine leakage. Suction drainage is rarely used because the expanded implant tamponades any significant bleeding.

Serial expansion usually begins 1 to 2 weeks after insertion to permit early capsule formation and decrease postoperative pain. Saline filling is performed weekly or every other week to patient tolerance. When a hemispheric dome flap 16 to 18 cm across is achieved, an 8 cm–wide flap transposition can be designed to reconstruct the alar folds, nasal tip, and columella and permit primary closure of the donor site (Figure 7-3, *C*).

An intraoperative Doppler study can identify the ipsilateral dominant supratrochlear vessels. The dermal, epigaleal, or subperiosteal designed flap with an intact supratrochlear vessel is elevated over the expander without problems (Figure 7-3, *D*). The flap is rotated about 175 degrees into the nasal defect. The flap's distal end is thinned to permit infolding for the delicate alar and columellar structures. Capsulectomy or multiple capsulotomies may unfurl the domed flap, adding both length and width to the original shape.

Dermal flaps have the advantages of being thin and supple, which reduces the need for secondary debulking procedures. Epigaleal flaps contain a sturdier blood supply and provide more bulk for the nasal reconstruction. Subperiosteal flaps are the most reliable and contribute a portion of the corrugator and procerus muscle-skin bulk to the reconstructive site, but secondary debulking procedures of the inlayed flap may be required to contour the nasal profile.

Simultaneous incorporation of autogenous cartilage grafts from the ribs or concha and tissue provision for the lining may be required to reconstruct the nasal defect. The donor site is closed by primary intention (Figure 7-3, *E* and *F*).

After 3 months the remaining dog-ear defect at the nasal root may be divided and inset. Minor secondary procedures such as flap defattening may be done at later stages to define the nasal shape.

CASE RESULTS

Since 1979 the author has reconstructed 69 nasal defects produced by congenital nevi, neoplasia, and trauma (Table 7-1). Expansion reconstruction was begun when wound healing was completed. Seven patients sustained scar contractures with degrees of choanal atresia but demonstrated minimal cartilaginous deformities or losses. Eleven patients had varying sizes of skin grafts that presented cosmetic problems. Eight patients had subtotal nasal deformities

■ **Table 7-1**   Types of Nasal Defects in 69 Reconstructions

Type	Number
Trauma	
Scar contracture	7
Skin graft	11
Subtotal loss	8
Total loss	5
Malignancy	
Superficial multifocal basal cell cancers	12
Mohs' chemosurgical defect	15
Benign lesions	
Congenital nevus	11

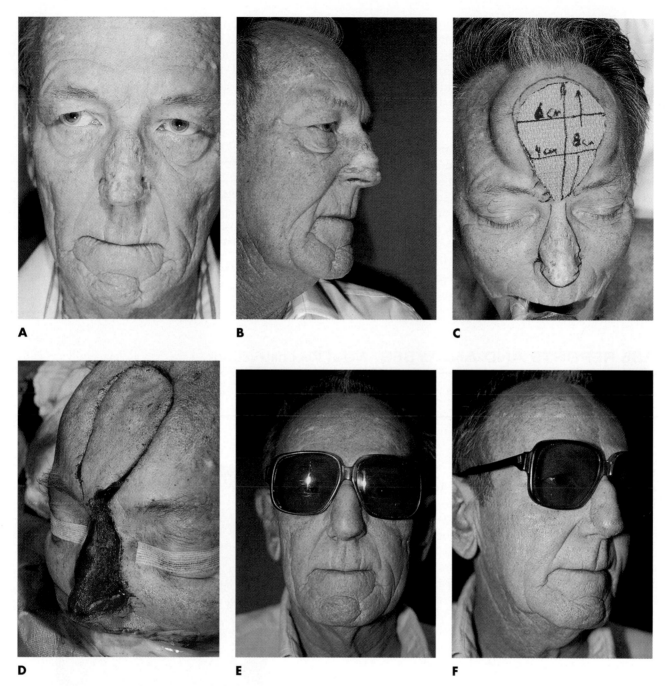

Figure 7-3 **A** and **B,** This 57-year-old patient had multifocal basal cell cancers on the skin of the nasal dorsum. The patient had undergone four previous excisions on the actinically damaged skin. The surgical plan was to expand the midforehead at the site of an intended glabellar flap to resurface the entire nasal skin and permit primary closure of the forehead donor tissue. The forehead skin was spared significant actinic changes and could serve as a useful donor site. **C,** Round 100 cc expander was inserted under the periosteum of midforehead tissue through a 3 cm sagittal scalp incision about 2 cm behind the hairline. The remote valve system was positioned under the periosteum of the right parietal scalp. Serial expansion was begun 2 weeks after balloon insertion, with 10 to 20 ml of saline weekly. After a 16 to 18 cm hemispheric flap was generated by the expander, the patient was considered for the second stage of reconstruction. An 8 cm–wide glabellar flap was required to cover the nasal dorsum after skin excision (the template measures 6 cm across). This left behind at least 8 cm of forehead skin to permit a vertical line closure. **D,** At surgery a Doppler tracing identified the dominant supratrochlear vascular bundle on which the flap was based. The expanded glabellar flap was raised from the periosteal level and rotated on its left supratrochlear vascular bundle. Maximal thinning of the expanded flap was performed to retain a thin layer of subcutaneous fat and the expanded skin. Subdermal blood flow should be excellent because of increased flow in a delayed flap. **E** and **F,** The patient 2 years after his surgery. Minor secondary procedures included flap division and inset and a few debulking procedures to contour the nasal profile. No columellar skin coverage was required. The donor vertical forehead scar has matured and is barely visible. Brow elevation by the frontalis muscles was preserved after expansion.

from trauma, with partial loss of skin, bone and/or cartilage, and inner lining. Five patients had total loss of nasal cover, structures, and lining from trauma. Twelve patients had multifocal superficial basal cell cancers over the entire nasal skin, and 15 underwent Mohs' surgery for basal cell cancer that resulted in subtotal nasal deformities. Eleven patients had significant congenital nevi on their noses.

All patients underwent long-term tissue expansion for 4 to 16 weeks, depending on the amount of skin required to complete the reconstruction. For smaller defects on the nasal skin, expansion of either nasal skin or the forehead median flap ranged from 4 to 8 weeks. For subtotal or total nasal deformities, forehead tissue expansion required up to 16 weeks because of the complex reconstructive processes. Minor secondary procedures were common and consisted of dog-ear revisions, insettings, bulk reductions, and structural alterations.

Complication rates were lower than in other areas of facial expansion (Table 7-2). Minor complications occurred with malposition of expanders, ineffective expansion, and delayed exposure of cartilage or bone. The two major complications were infection and partial flap loss.

■ **Table 7-2** Complications in 69 Nasal Reconstructions

Type	Number
Minor (11.6%)	
Malposition of expander	2
Ineffective expansion	5
Bone/cartilage exposure	1
Major (2.9%)	
Infection	1
Flap loss	1

CASE REPORTS AND ANALYSES: Nasal Reconstruction

CASE 1: Multifocal Basal Cell Cancers with Premalignant Skin Lesions

History (Figure 7-4, *A*)

This 58-year-old patient underwent numerous nasal skin biopsies for premalignant changes and multifocal basal cell cancers. The patient requested complete resurfacing of his nose to eliminate the cancers. Mid-forehead skin was selected for expansion because of the absence of degenerative skin changes and abundance of available donor tissue. The goals of reconstruction were to (1) excise the entire diseased dorsal nasal skin, (2) resurface with expanded thin, supple forehead skin, (3) approximate the forehead donor site with a vertical midline closure, and (4) minimize the nasal scars along aesthetic lines of closure.

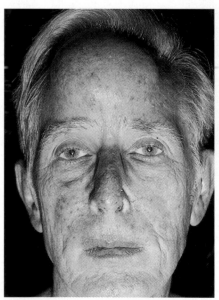

7-4A

Surgical Procedure (Figure 7-4, *B* to *D*)

A 200 cc round expander was inserted under the forehead skin above the midforehead muscles in the thin subcutaneous fatty layer through a 2.5 cm sagittal scalp incision 5 cm from the precapillary line. The remote valve was positioned in the subperiosteal space of the right parietal scalp. Intraoperative saline filling reduced the incidence of hematoma formation. Serial expansion was begun 3 weeks later, with the addition of 10 to 15 ml of saline weekly.

After 3 months of expansion the hemispheric flap measured 18 cm across. Intraoperative expansion gained additional skin at surgery. The median flap was designed to be 8 cm across to permit full coverage from ala to ala and along the nasomaxillary lines. The forehead flap was based on the right supratrochlear neurovascular bundle, which was located by preoperative Doppler examination. The flap's distal half was maximally debulked of capsule and subcutaneous tissue in order to present thin, supple skin on the nasal tip. The entire dorsal nasal skin was excised down to the perichondral and periosteal layers. Since the columella and nasal alae were not included in the resection, internal nasal lining was preserved. The excess remaining forehead tissue was approximated for a vertical midline closure.

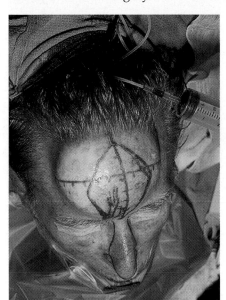

7-4B

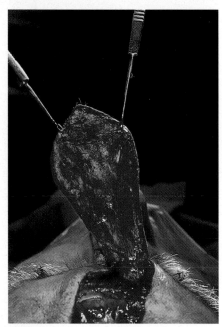

7-4C

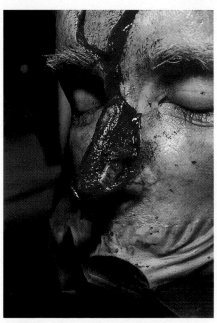

7-4D

Results (Figure 7-4, *E* and *F*)

Two years after his nasal reconstruction by skin coverage alone, the patient's nasal profile and transposed skin present an aesthetic and functional reconstruction. The frontalis, corrugator, and procerus muscles continue to function under the aesthetic midline skin closure. Brow symmetry is balanced. The seam line closures follow the aesthetic lines on and along the nose. The patient's transposed forehead skin remains free of basal cell cancers.

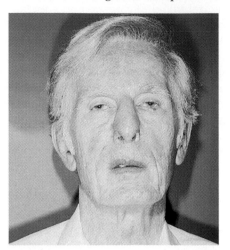

7-4E

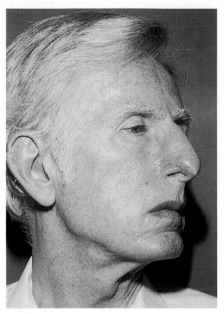

7-4F

CASE 2: Subtotal Nasal Tip Loss after Mohs' Surgery

History (Figure 7-5, *A*)

This 70-year-old patient underwent Mohs' surgery for an invasive, sclerosing basal cell cancer to her nasal tip. The final defect included full-thickness loss of her entire nasal tip skin, cartilage support, and lining. The septal, upper lateral, and alar cartilages were treated in an open manner until scar contracture produced the secondary defect. At that time the patient requested reconstruction. The goals of surgery were to (1) provide a projecting contoured nasal tip with skin, support, and lining and (2) minimize the surgical procedures and scars.

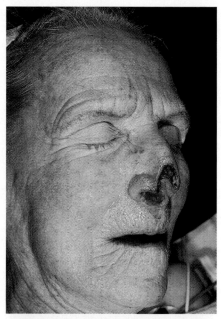

7-5A

Surgical Procedure (Figure 7-5, *B*)

A 200 cc round expander was inserted in the subperiosteal space in the forehead's midline through a 2.5 cm sagittal incision about 5 cm behind the frontal hairline. The remote valve was positioned in a subperiosteal location on the right parietal scalp. Intraoperative filling with 50 ml of saline reduced hematoma formation. Serial expansion continued weekly for 3 months until an 18 cm hemispheric median forehead flap was generated.

At surgery, intraoperative expansion gained 1 to 2 cm of tissue. An 8 cm–wide flap was elevated based on the right supratrochlear vascular bundle. Its distal half was debulked to create a supple flap that could be infolded to resemble the alar rims and columella. Adjacent skin flaps were turned down for inner lining. Conchal cartilage grafts were spliced on the remnants of the septal, upper lateral, and alar cartilages. The expanded contoured flap was placed over the supportive and lined tissues. Secondary procedures, such as division and inset of the flap base, debulking, and contouring, were performed 3 to 6 months after the major stages of reconstruction were completed.

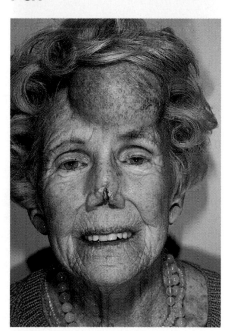

7-5B

Results (Figure 7-5, *C* and *D*)

One year after her final revision surgery the patient has a stable, aesthetic nasal tip symmetric to the cephalic portion of her nose. Minimal secondary tissue contracture has occurred. The midline forehead scar is camouflaged by her hair but continues to be less apparent with maturation. The brow complexes have not widened and possess frontalis and depressor corrugator muscle activity.

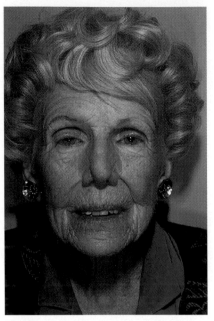

7-5C

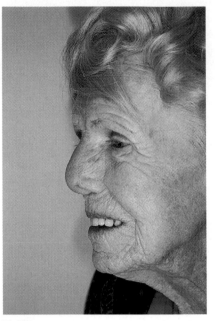

7-5D

CASE 3: Subtotal Nasal Deformity with Forehead and Cheek Burn Scar Contractures

History (Figure 7-6, *A*)

This 7-year-old patient sustained flame burn injuries to the right forehead, nasal, and cheek skin. A complete right choanal contracture existed, with partial atresia to the left choana. The patient requested resurfacing of his right forehead, interbrow area, nose, and medial cheeks with supple thin skin. Because of the complex injuries, two expansion periods were scheduled to complete the reconstruction. The goals of surgery were to (1) expand the left forehead skin and advance it over the functioning right frontalis muscle, (2) expand and advance both cheek skins to the nasomaxillary lines, (3) reexpand the median forehead skin for nasal skin cover, (4) reinforce the nasal cartilaginous structures of the alae and columella, and (5) minimize scar lines.

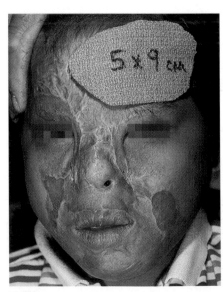

7-6A

Surgical Procedure (Figure 7-6, *B* to *L*)

A 100 cc round expander was inserted under the mid-forehead skin in the subcutaneous fat through a 2.5 cm sagittal incision 5 cm behind the precapillary line (Figure 7-6, *B*) A 200 cc round expander was inserted in the medial aspect of each cheek in the subcutaneous fat through 2.0 cm retrolobular incisions. The valve for the forehead expander was positioned in the subperiosteal plane under the right parietal scalp, and the valves for the cheek expanders were located under postauricular scalp skin. Intraoperative saline filling prevented hematoma formation. Serial expansions continued weekly until sufficient tissue was generated for advancement coverage.

At surgery, intraoperative expansion gained additional tissue. After the forehead expander was removed, dome capsulectomy and base capsulotomies effectively advanced the skin over the excised scar. After forehead flap advancement the same expander was reinserted under the flap in the forehead's midline. Bilateral cheek flap advancements to the naso-maxillary and nasolabial lines effectively resurfaced the scarred areas.

The forehead exander was slowly filled with saline about 4 weeks after flap inset to create a median flap. Axial blood flow through branches of the previously transected supratrochlear arteries was reestablished by Doppler examinations. Forehead expansions continued for 12 weeks until an 18 cm hemispheric flap was created.

At surgery, intraoperative expansion again gained tissue. An 8 cm–wide median forehead flap was elevated, debulked at its distal half, and transposed to the nose based on the right supratrochlear pedicle. After the entire scarred nasal skin was excised, an iliac bone graft was secured to the nasal bone by interosseous fixation to provide nasal projection. Conchal grafts were carved to reinforce the deformed alar-columellar cartilages. The thin, supple forehead flap was infolded to create the alar rims and columella and insetted onto the newly created structures. Final flap division and inset were performed 3 months later.

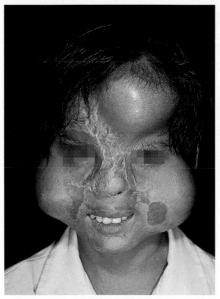

7-6B

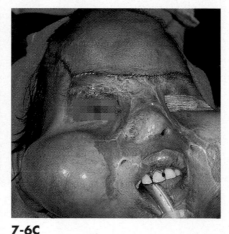

7-6C

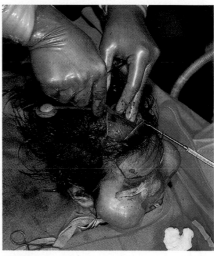

7-6D

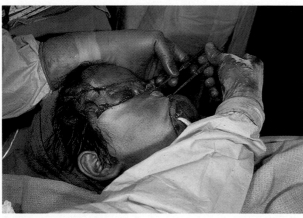

7-6E

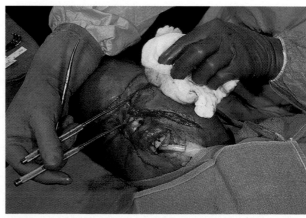

7-6F

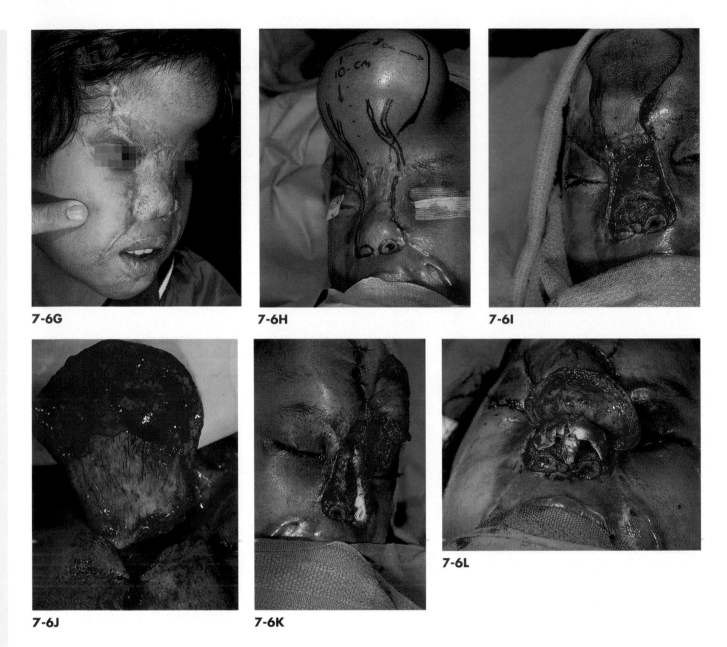

7-6G

7-6H

7-6I

7-6J

7-6K

7-6L

Results (Figure 7-6, *M* and *N*)

Five years after his reconstructions the patient's visible scars are fading. The forehead muscles are functional under the twice-expanded skin flap. The nasal profile, projection, and definition remain acceptable as a functional and aesthetic unit. The patient has not requested further debulking procedures to thin out the nasal dorsum.

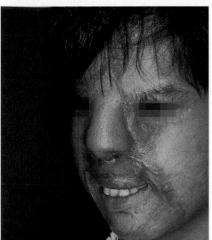

7-6M

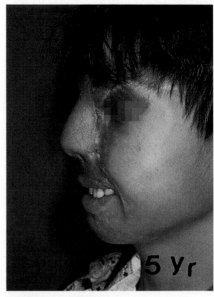

7-6N

CASE 4:   Total Nasal Loss

History (Figure 7-7, *A* and *B*)

This 37-year-old patient sustained a gunshot wound through his mentum and nose that resulted in a central mandibular bone loss of 5 cm and total nasal ablation. The patient requested reconstruction of his mandible and lip elements for oral continence and stability, as well as a total nasal reconstruction. The goals of surgery were to (1) reestablish mandibular continuity for oral continence and stability; (2) provide soft tissue replacement for the chin and lower lip; (3) provide skin, bone/cartilage structures, and inner lining for a functional, aesthetic nasal reconstruction; and (4) minimize visible scars.

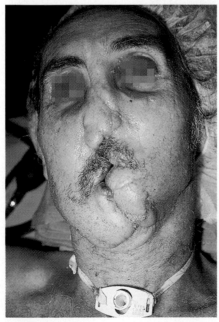

7-7A

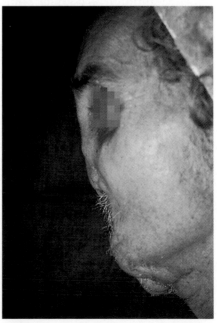

7-7B

First Surgical Procedure (Figure 7-7, *C* and *D*)

A free tissue transfer, based on the deep circumflex iliac vessels, established mandibular continuity with a vascularized 5 cm iliac bone graft. The transferred soft tissue also provided sufficient bulk to augment the chin. A 200 cc round expander was inserted in the sub-periosteal plane of the midforehead through a 2.5 cm sagittal incision 5 cm behind the frontal hairline. The expander was filled to tissue tolerance to reduce hematoma formation. Serial expansion continued for 3 months to generate an 18 cm hemispheric flap.

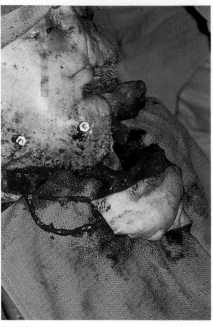

7-7C

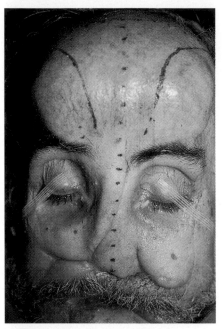

7-7D

Second Surgical Procedure (Figure 7-7, *E* to *I*)

At surgery, intraoperative expansion provided additional tissue for the reconstruction. A 10 cm–wide median forehead flap was elevated and based on the right supratrochlear vessels. The flap's distal half was debulked to produce a thin, supple skin cover. The nasal skin was opened through a midline approach and used as turn-down flaps for lining. A cantilever iliac bone graft provided nasal bone replacement. Conchal cartilages were used to reconstruct the alar rims and replace the upper lateral cartilages. The median forehead flap was infolded to create soft tissue replacement of the columella, alar folds, and dorsal skin. The flap provided the cover over the structural arrangements.

Secondary surgeries involved division and inset of the forehead flap, nasal debulking and contouring procedures, and chin and lower lip revisions.

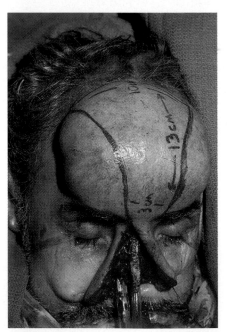

7-7E

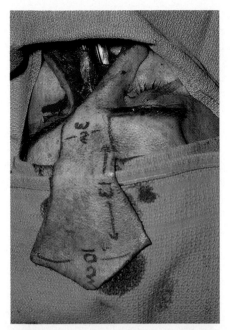

7-7F

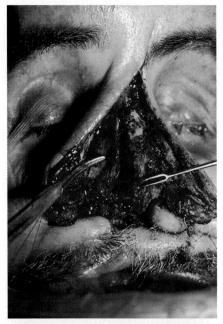

7-7G

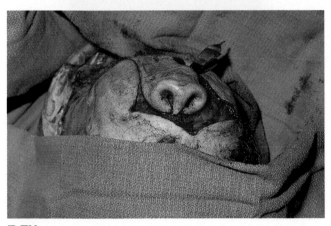

7-7H

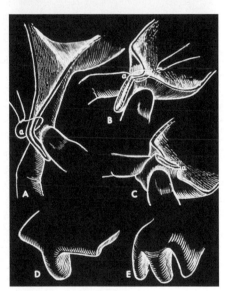

7-7I

Results (Figure 7-7, *J* and *K*)

The patient is shown 6 months after completion of the major reconstructive procedures. The vertical midline forehead scar should improve with further maturation. Frontalis muscle function has partially returned.

The nasal complex remains a dimensional, aesthetic, and functional reconstruction. Mandibular stability has provided oral continence and an aesthetic chin and lower lip complex.

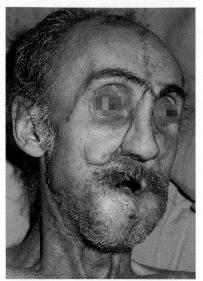

7-7J

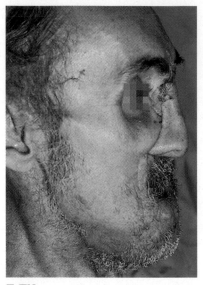

7-7K

SUMMARY

The use of tissue expansion for nasal reconstruction has provided ideal coverage of like skin from either the nose or the median forehead, with minimal donor site scars. Intraoperative expansion may be useful for small nasal defects. Long-term expansion of residual nasal skin or glabellar skin is required for larger defects. The addition of cartiligenous or bone grafts creates a dimensional reconstruction, along with provision of lining from turn-down flaps. Secondary procedures, such as division and inset of dog-ear defects and debulking of fat, may be required to complete the final nasal profile.

8 Reconstruction of Acquired and Congenital Auricular Defects

Several authors have reported their experience with tissue expansion in the reconstruction of traumatic auricular defects[1-6] and congenital microtia.[7-11] Tissue expansion has proved to be particularly applicable in these deformities because of the extent of skin deficiency or loss, including scarring.

The concept of expanding local tissue cannot be overemphasized in the reconstruction of a three-dimensional auricle. Tissue expansion can create donor tissue that is virtually the same color, thickness, texture, and sensation as the recipient site. Expanded skin from the postauricular area is thin, pliable, well vascularized, and non–hair bearing. The wide expanse of postauricular skin usually produced will comfortably drape over the autogenous cartilaginous framework, eliminating distortions of the hairline and the need for skin grafts in the postauricular sulcus. Secondary elevation of the reconstructed auricle with a skin graft may be considered at the patient's request.

Direct trauma can cause major auricular deformities that require partial or total reconstruction of the helical or antihelical complex. Major defects may also result from tumor resection or burns. In such patients the amount of remaining cartilage and skin is often insufficient for reconstruction of a three-dimensional structure. In congenital microtia the limiting factor for an aesthetic reconstruction is skin availability. Tissue expansion produces pliable, vascularized, non-hairbearing skin. This skin will adapt to the contours of the new auricular framework, creating a posterior sulcus and reducing the encroachment of hair on the reconstructed site.

ANATOMIC CONSIDERATIONS

The external ear consists of the auricle (pinna) and the external auditory meatus. Its purpose is to collect and convey sound waves to the tympanic membrane.

The skin of the auricle is thin, hairless, and tightly adherent to the underlying cartilaginous structures. The skin of the lateral auricular surface is supplied by the great auricular nerve over its lower third and the auriculotemporal nerve over its upper two thirds (Figure 8-1). The medial surface is supplied over its lower half by the great auricular nerve and over its upper half by the lesser occipital nerves.

Intrinsic auricular ligaments maintain the cartilage in position, and extrinsic ligaments attach the auricle to the temporal bone.

The six intrinsic auricular muscles are rudimentary and supplied by the facial nerve. The auricle receives its arterial supply from the external carotid through the posterior auricular artery in back and the superficial temporal artery in front. Its venous drainage involves the superficial temporal veins in front and the external jugular vein below. The lymph vessels of the ear eventually drain into the deep cervical chain.

The cartilaginous framework consists of the helix, antihelix, and concha. The *helix* forms the auricle's outer margin and includes the crus helicis, which enters into the conchal floor and continues into the lobule's fibrofatty tissue. On the posterosuperior helical aspect is the small darwinian (auricular) tubercle. The *antihelix* (anthelix) runs parallel with the helix and ends inferiorly in a small tubercle called the antitragus. Superiorly, the antihelix divides into the superior and inferior crura, which form the boundary of a shallow depression known as the fossa triangularis. The *concha* cartilage forms the auricle's central deep cavity and is divided into upper and lower parts by the ridge known as the crus helicis. The lower part of the concha leads into the external auditory meatus and is bounded by the tragus, which forms a backward projection partially obscuring the external auditory meatus.

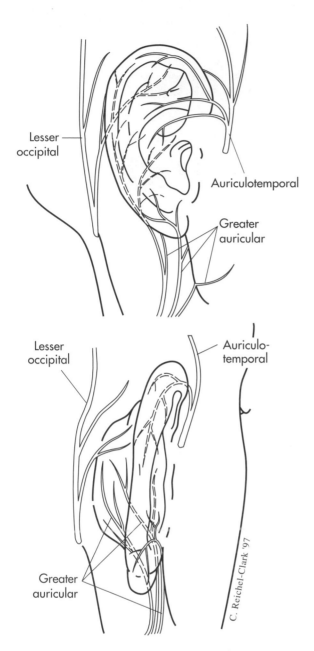

Figure 8-1 Cutaneous nerves of the ear.

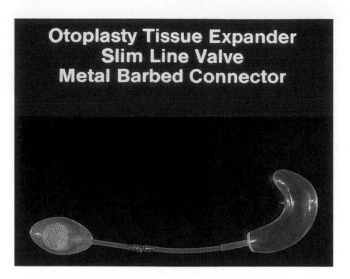

Figure 8-2 Customized otoplasty expander is designed with a commalike curve. The expander measures about 2.5 cm in width and 6.5 cm in length. This shape follows the curvature of a normal ear and utilizes as much of the non-hair-bearing skin as possible for expansion. The slim, low-profile valve reduces the chance of a skin erosion, as may occur with a prominent valve under thin donor skin.

EXPANDER SYSTEM

The tissue expander is designed with a gently curving shape, measuring about 6.5 cm long and 2.5 cm wide (Figure 8-2). This shape seems to be optimal for simulating the configuration of the ear, for limiting the expansion of non-hair-bearing skin, and for minimizing the tendency to migrate inferiorly. The expander may be used for either the right or the left ear. Although the mandrel volume is about 35 cc, more than 100 cc can be safely inflated into the expander. A suture tab should be placed on the expander's forward end to fix the unit and prevent inferior migration. A low-profile valve permits easy insertion and reduces the risk for erosion of the overlying skin.

SURGICAL TECHNIQUE

Ear deformities have unique variations (Figure 8-3, *A*). Detailed preoperative assessment and meticulous surgical technique are critical to success. If possible, comparison of templates from the normal and deformed ears is useful in identifying the auricular defects (Figure 8-3, *B*). When both external pinnae are destroyed or deformed, a reliable template may be obtained from a parent or sibling.

Long-term expansion techniques may not be indicated in patients who cannot psychologically tolerate the large bulge on the side of their head or whose donor site is unacceptable for expansion. Expansion of unstable tissue (scarred, contaminated, infected, or irradiated) can result in implant exposure or unsuitable skin.

Incision(s)

Incisions may be placed in the adjacent scalp or along the hairless border of the postauricular scalp. These locations represent distant sites that eliminate any potential weak spots near the expander unit. The author's preferred incision site is the border of the postauricular hairline, caudad to the ear level (Figure 8-3, *C*). The remote incision is about 2.5 to 3.0 cm long and is designed to reduce implant exposure, contamination, and infection. Any scalp incision can result in scar alopecia or may compromise blood supply to the expanded ear flap.

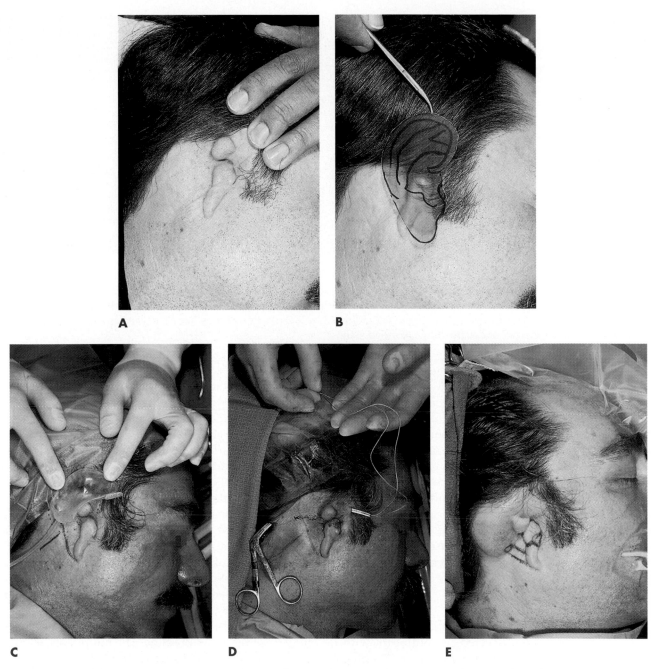

Figure 8-3 **A,** This 47-year-old patient demonstrated signs of congenital microtia, with retained cartilaginous remnants and a displaced lobule. **B,** Template of the normal ear has been superimposed on the defective site to identify the reconstructive needs and deformed remnants. **C,** Radial 2.5 cm incision along the border of the postauricular hairline is planned to eliminate the risk of implant exposure with a distant location. Incisions within the scalp can lead to scar alopecia, adding to the problems of reconstruction. **D,** Deep subcutaneous dissection along the expander's proposed location under the non-hair-bearing skin is performed from the postauricular incision site. The distal end of the pocket should be to the level of the helical root to position the balloon in an optimal location. An absorbable suture from the expander's anterior tab to the anticipated helical root keeps the expander in its dissected pocket. The remote valve may be positioned under the skin of the lateral middle to lower neck. **E,** Serial expansion with saline is performed weekly, with 5 to 10 cc (ml) per filling. When the final saline volume of 90 to 120 cc has been attained, the second stage of reconstruction may be scheduled. This amount of tissue provides the thin anterior cover as well as tissue to create the posterior sulcus. *Continued*

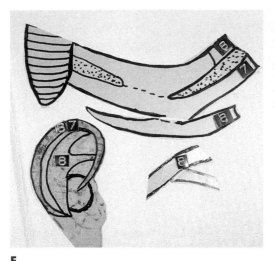
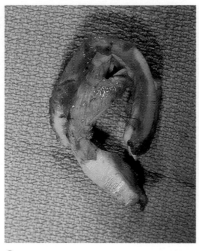
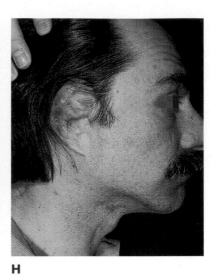

F   **G**   **H**

Figure 8-3, cont'd   F and G, Templates of the cartilaginous ear framework are designed on radiographic film and outlined on the exposed synchondrosis of the sixth to eighth ribs. The ninth rib contributes to the formation of the helical strut. **H,** The patient 1 year after his reconstruction. The lobule was adjusted by a Z-plasty transposition. The cartilaginous framework has gradually been unveiled from under the thin expanded skin.

Pocket Location

The skin pocket is located in the non-hair-bearing area behind and in front of the ear remnants. The plane of dissection lies in the deep subcutaneous tissue above the posterior and superior auricular muscles. Dissection is extended above the apex of the helical rim and anterior to the helical root. The pocket is continued behind the ear to the level of the antihelical-conchal complex. Unless a lobular defect exists, the pocket should be confined to the area above the lobule. The pocket is slightly larger than the base dimension of the curved expander and may extend slightly into the hairline.

Insertion of Expander Unit

From the posterior hairline incision, the tunnel for the valve and its pocket is dissected in continuity with the expander pocket. The pocket for the low-profile valve may be placed in the middle to lower neck, posterior to the sternocleidomastoid muscle. The valve is positioned deep in the subcutaneous plane to prevent erosion and to allow for easy palpation and injection. The exit site of the spinal accessory nerve at the posterior border of the sternocleidomastoid muscle must be preserved during dissection.

The tubing length is adjusted, and the tissue expander, remote valve, and tubing are assembled before insertion. The unit's watertight seal is tested by injecting 5 to 10 ml of saline colored with methylene blue, which helps detect leakage during surgery and confirm accurate needle placement during expansion.

To fix the expander in its optimal position, a small nick is made in the skin anterior to the helical root for passage of a percutaneous absorbable 4-0 suture (Figure 8-3, *D*). The needle is first passed through the skin nick at the helical root, into the expander pocket, and then out of the skin opening at the hair-bearing border of the postauricular scalp. The needle is passed through the suture tab in front of the expander and returned into the pocket and out through the skin nick. The suture ends are gently pulled through the skin, fixing the expander in its final position and preventing implant descent. After the suture is tied, a fine nonabsorbable 7-0 suture closes the stab wound, burying the absorbable suture and reducing risk of suture tract infection to the expander.

When the remote valve is inserted, the tubing should be taut to prevent curling, which can lead to skin erosion. The injection valve is tested in situ for filling and withdrawal of saline. The inferior aspect of the expander pocket is closed with a few absorbable sutures to prevent implant descent. The tubing is displaced from the incision and buried under local tissue with absorbable sutures. The primary incision is approximated in layers with 5-0 absorbable subdermal sutures and 6-0 nonabsorbable skin sutures.

Expansion Technique

Serial expansion is begun 1 to 2 weeks after surgery. The final volume should be 90 to 120 cc of saline to provide enough tissue for anterior draping and formation of a posterior sulcus (Figure 8-3, *E*). About 5 to 10 ml of saline is added to the expander each week. If expansion failed to produce enough tissue during 3 to 4 months of expansion, intraoperative expansion at the second stage can gain 1 to 2 cm of tissue.

Second Stage of Reconstruction

At the second stage the expander is removed by either incising along the borders of the congenital auricular remnants in a microtic ear or cutting through the scar lines of a traumatized ear. Sufficient exposure of the operative site permits precise shaping and positioning of the cartilage framework in situ. The cartilaginous base of the antihelix is constructed from the contralateral costal synchondrosis of the sixth to eighth ribs (Figure 8-3, *F* and *G*). The ninth rib can be attached to the antihelical frame to form the helical strut.

Conchal depth and creation of a normal angle of auricular deviation are achieved by adding shaped cartilage blocks under the spliced framework. After insertion of the graft into its pocket, the incision is closed under a suction catheter. The posterior sulcus may be defined with bolster sutures tied over small cotton pledgets. The degree of sulcus depth and framework detail depends on the amount of skin available, pliability and thinness of the skin, and character of the delicate three-dimensional framework. Additional minor surgeries may be required to deepen the base of the concha, construct the tragus, and deepen the sulcus. The lobule's position is adjusted by a Z-plasty transposition (Figure 8-3, *H*).

CASE RESULTS

The curved expander was inserted in 52 of the 60 patients in the author's series for various degrees of helical and antihelical loss produced by burns, trauma, or cancer (Table 8-1). In 23 of these patients the defects involved primarily a major portion of the helical rim, and in 20 patients the defects involved both helical and antihelical complexes. Nine patients had reconstruction for total ear loss. Reconstruction was begun when wound healing was complete.

Seven patients underwent reconstruction for congenital microtia and one for a defect resulting from an arteriovenous malformation. In general, expansion volumes greater than 70 cc of saline are recommended to produce sufficient skin laxity to profile the contour details of the ear, to form a posterior sulcus, and to maintain a normal hairline. Secondary procedures, such as conchal deepening, postauricular skin grafts, or repositioning, were performed in 35 patients, who demonstrated significant tissue deformity or loss.

■ **Table 8-1** Types of Ear Defects in 60 Reconstructions

Type	Number
Trauma/malignancy	
Helical rim	23
Helical rim/antihelix	20
Total loss	9
Congenital	
Microtia	7
Arteriovenous malformation	1

■ **Table 8-2** Complications in 60 Ear Reconstructions

Type	Number
Minor (30%)	
Implant malposition	3
Skin contraction	15
Major (20%)	
Open infection	
Exposed balloon	5
Exposed tubing	2
Exposed valve	2
Closed infection	
Cellulitis	3

The reconstructed ears were satisfactory in terms of color, texture matching, and sensation. Appropriate return of sensation to touch and temperature required more than a year in some patients.

Complication rates were significantly higher than in other facial areas of expansion (Table 8-2). Minor complications were defined as malposition of the expander and delayed skin contraction. The most common minor complications were attributed to contraction of the expanded skin on the firm cartilaginous framework. Although the skin contraction did not deform the graft, depth of the postauricular sulcus was decreased. To minimize this distracting effect, expansions were maintained for a longer period (3 to 4 months) and stretched to larger volumes (more than 100 cc). The superior and inferior auricular muscles were excluded from the flaps. It is hoped these maneuvers will reduce the incidence of postoperative skin shrinkage.

Major complications primarily involved implant exposure with open infections or closed infections from a break in sterile technique. Contamination of the implant and thin skin required removal of the implant and a delay of at least 4 months for tissue healing before another expansion attempt.

CASE REPORTS AND ANALYSES

CASE 1:   Traumatic Loss of Helical Rim

History (Figure 8-4, *A*)
This 7-year-old boy sustained loss of the right helical rim after a dog bite. The injury was managed by direct closure of tissue. About 1 year later the patient underwent auricular reconstruction of his helical rim. The goals of surgery were to (1) provide sufficient non-hair-bearing skin for coverage of the cartilaginous framework, (2) create a posterior sulcus for auricular projection, and (3) minimize visible scars.

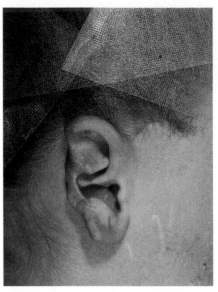

8-4A

Surgical Procedure (Figure 8-4, *B* and *C*)
A 2.5 cm incision was made along the border of the postauricular scalp. A subcutaneous pocket was dissected adjacent to the posterior ear remnant under hairless skin. The remote valve was placed under skin of the lower neck. The expander was filled with 5 cc (ml) of saline to tissue tolerance. A final volume of 130 cc of saline was achieved over 10 weeks.

At surgery, intraoperative expansion with an additional 10 cc gained more tissue for the reconstruction.

After the expander was removed from an extended postauricular incision, the edges of the cartilaginous remnants were exposed through an incision along the posterior ear scar. A framework was fabricated from rib cartilages and spliced onto the antihelical and conchal portions of the ear. The thin, supple expanded skin covered the dimensional framework on its anterior and posterior surfaces. Cotton bolsters accentuated the posterior sulcus.

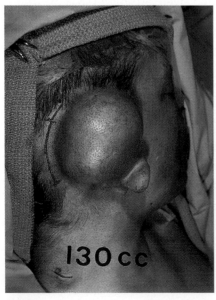

8-4B

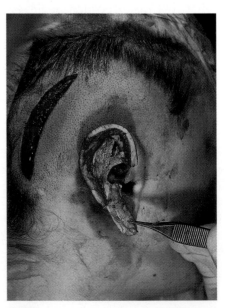

8-4C

Results (Figure 8-4, *D*)

One year after reconstruction the dimensions of the patient's auricle closely match those of the opposite side. The cartilaginous framework provides a delicate profile of the helical rim symmetric to the antihelix. The ear is projected away from the skull with an adequate sulcus and angle.

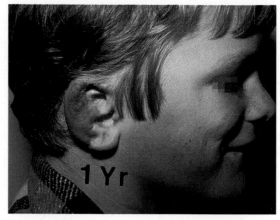

8-4D

CASE 2: Traumatic Loss of Helical-Antihelical Rims, Scar to Midface, and Alopecia on Parietal Scalp

History (Figure 8-5, *A*)

This 15-year-old patient lost a portion of his right parietal scalp and ear and sustained hypertrophic scars to his midface from a motor vehicle accident (*Z-IV & V*, zones IV and V). A skin graft was placed over the scalp injury, with primary closure for the injured ear. The facial lacerations developed into hypertrophic scars. The goals of surgery were to (1) resurface the area of scar alopecia with normal hair-bearing scalp tissue, (2) replace the scarred midface skin with supple adjacent skin, (3) reconstruct the ear framework, and (4) minimize the surgical scars.

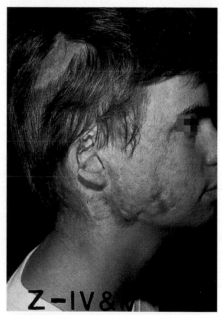

8-5A

First Surgical Procedure (Figure 8-5, *B* and *C*)
A 200 cc round expander was inserted in the subcutaneous plane of the midface through a 2.5 cm incision along the border of the postauricular hairline. A 400 cc rectangular expander was positioned within the subcutaneous tissue of the midneck through the same incision. Intraoperative filling was performed in both implants to reduce hematoma formation. Serial expansions continued for 3 months until sufficient skin was obtained.

Intraoperative expansion was done with both expanders to gain additional tissue. After the expanders were removed, dome capsulectomies and base capsulotomies permitted inferior and posterior advancement of the cheek flap below the mandibular margin and cephalad advancement of the neck flap to the mandibular seam line.

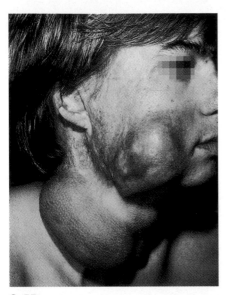

8-5B

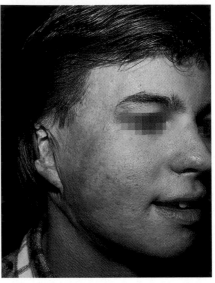

8-5C

Second Surgical Procedure (Figure 8-5, *D* and *E*)
About 8 months later a second expansion procedure was begun to replace skin and cover a helical and antihelical framework. A 2.5 × 6.5 cm curved ear expander was inserted under the postauricular skin through the same borderline scar used for the first procedure. Serial expansions continued for 3 months until the expander volume exceeded 100 cc.

At surgery, intraoperative expansion gained extra tissue before implant removal. The scar line along the ear's posterior aspect was reopened to expose the edges of the cartilaginous remnants. An ear framework constructed from rib cartilages was inset and spliced to the main frame of the helical and antihelical remnants. The thin, supple expanded skin covered the additional structures and provided enough skin for a posterior sulcus.

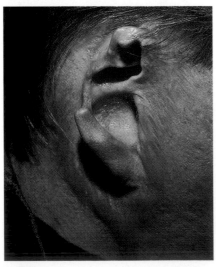

8-5D

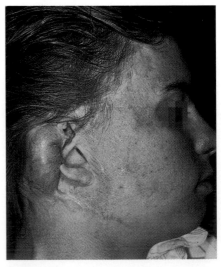

8-5E

Results (Figure 8-5, *F* and *G*)
Three years after the reconstructions the aesthetic and functional aspects of expansion have been realized, with normal skin coverage of the midcheek and neck, a dimensional autogenous ear reconstruction, and hidden scar seam lines. The outline of the mandibular margin is symmetric to the opposite side.

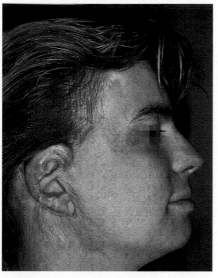

8-5F

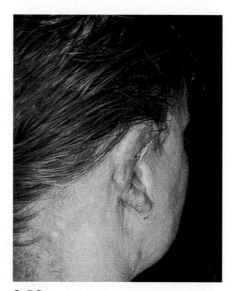

8-5G

CASE 3: Microtia of Right Ear

History (Figure 8-6, *A*)
This 5-year-old patient demonstrated the classic signs of microtia of the right ear. The lobule was malpositioned, with an unusable hillock of cartilaginous remnants. The patient had no hearing loss in the opposite ear. The goals of reconstruction were to (1) construct a framework symmetric to the opposite side, (2) provide sufficient projection of the ear with a posterior sulcus, and (3) minimize visible scars.

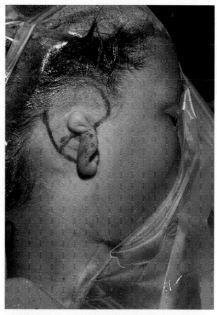

8-6A

Surgical Procedure (Figure 8-6, *B* to *F*)

A 2.5 × 6.5 cm otoplasty expander was inserted under the thin hairless skin above and behind the ear remnants through a 2.5 cm incision at the borderline of the postauricular scalp. A template of the ear frame was traced from the opposite side. The remote valve was positioned in the lower neck. After the subcutaneous pocket was created, the expander was filled with methylene blue-colored saline to detect any leakage during insertion. A percutaneous absorbable suture was passed from a stab wound at the helical root through the implant's anterior tab and back out through the skin to guide and fix the expander tip in its proper po-sition. The expander was filled to tissue tolerance to reduce hematoma formation. Serial expansion continued for 3 months until 100 cc (ml) of saline filled the implant.

At surgery, intraoperative expansion was used to gain additional tissue. After expander removal, a skin incision was made along the anticipated posteroinferior edge of the sulcus to hide the scar position. A cartilaginous framework was carved from sixth to eighth ribs and inserted under the thin, supple expanded skin. Sufficient tissue was present to infold the framework into the scaffolding of the ear graft and to provide a postauricular sulcus.

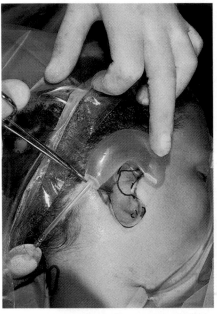

8-6B

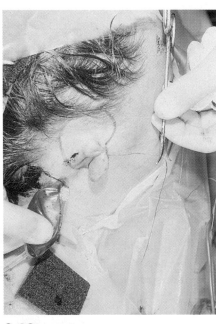

8-6C

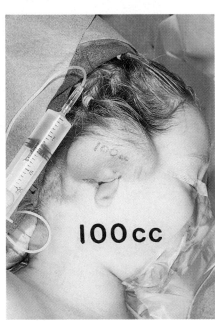

8-6D

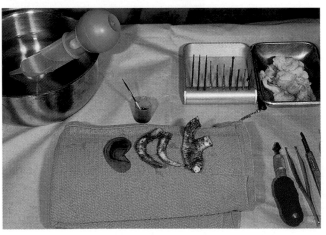

8-6E

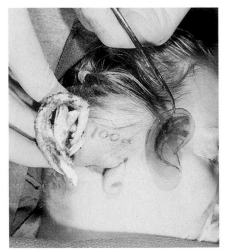

8-6F

Results (Figure 8-6, *G*)

One year after lobular transposition to complete the reconstruction, the patient's corrected ear closely resembles the opposite side, with an acceptable configuration, adequate projection, a defined posterior sulcus, and the absence of transposed hair on the external pinna.

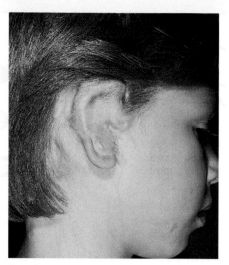

8-6G

SUMMARY

Over the past 15 years, tissue expansion has gradually become accepted as a useful adjunct to ear reconstruction with an autologous framework. The advantage of expanded tissue in these patients is the addition of more tissue with similar color, texture, and sensation. In patients with traumatic injuries the creation of well-vascularized tissue allows improved anterior draping of skin over the cartilaginous framework and production of a well-defined posterior sulcus. Encroachment of hair on the reconstructed ear is minimized because of the extra tissue produced by expansion. Under favorable conditions, tissue expansion is an acceptable and reliable method for partial or total ear reconstruction. The use of expansion technique in congenital ear reconstruction is still under investigation.

REFERENCES

1. Brent B: Ear reconstruction with an expandable framework of autogenous rib cartilage, *Plast Reconstr Surg* 53:619, 1974.

2. Mutimer KL, Mulliken JB: Case report: correction of cryptotia using tissue expansion, *Plast Reconstr Surg* 82:601, 1988.

3. Neumann CG: The expansion of an area of skin by progressive distention of a subcutaneous balloon, *Plast Reconst Surg* 19:124, 1957.

4. O'Neal RM, Rorich RJ, Izenberg PH: Skin expander as an adjunct to reconstruction of the external ear, *Br J Plast Surg* 37:517, 1984.

5. Quaba A: Case report: reconstruction of a post traumatic ear defect using tissue expansion, *Plast Reconstr Surg* 80:266, 1987.

6. Sasaki GH: *Ear reconstruction: guidelines and case analyses,* Tissue expansion booklet, Midland, 1987, Dow Corning Wright.

7. Brent B: The acquired auricular deformity: systematic approach to its analysis and reconstruction, *Plast Reconstr Surg* 59:475, 1977.

8. Bauer B: Reconstruction of the microtic ear, *J Pediatr Surg* 19:440, 1984.

9. Brent B: The correction of microtia with autogenous cartilage grafts. II. Atypical and complex deformities, *Plast Reconstr Surg* 66: 1980.

10. Tanzer RC: Total reconstruction of the auricle, *Plast Reconstr Surg* 47:523, 1971.

11. Brent B: The correction of microtia with autogenous cartilage grafts. I. The classic deformity, *Plast Reconstr Surg* 66:1, 1980.

continuation of the musculocutaneous nerve, pierces the lacertus fibrosus, travels under the median cephalic vein, and then takes a superficial course, dividing into anterior and posterior branches that supply the skin over the anterolateral and posterolateral aspects of the forearm (see Figure 9-1). In addition, the medial antebrachial cutaneous nerve, a branch of the medial cord of the brachial plexus, divides at the middle of the brachium into volar and ulnar branches. These branches assume a superficial position above the lacertus fibrosus as they pass through the elbow to innervate the skin of the ulnar half of the forearm down to the wrist.

During development of a surgical pocket in the subcutaneous tissue within the antecubital fossa, the dissection should remain in the superficial plane to avoid injury to these important sensory nerves and to avoid needless venous bleeding. The brachial artery and median and radial nerves are below the lacertus fibrosus and should not be injured during expansion surgery.

In the olecranon region the only important structure that may be injured during expansion is the ulnar nerve (Figure 9-2). This mixed nerve reaches the elbows behind the medial intermuscular septum within the medial olecranon groove in contact with the periosteum under the triceps tendon. The nerve exits this area between the heads of the flexor carpi ulnaris muscle but still remains under the deep fascia. Therefore dissection in a plane superficial to the investing fascia should prevent any nerve injury.

Forearm

The skin on the dorsal surface is thicker and has more hair follicles than skin on the volar surface of the forearm. Skin from both areas is mobile and rests on a moderate amount of subcutaneous fat.

The antebrachial fascia covers the forearm as a strong aponeurotic sheet, closely adherent to the underlying surface of the volar and dorsal muscles. The fascia is strengthened around the olecranon process and incorporated anteriorly by the laceratus fibrosus. The distal portion of the fascia at the wrist level extends to the transverse and dorsal carpal ligaments of the hand. The radius, ulna, and interosseous membrane form a septum that divides the forearm into volar flexor or dorsal extensor compartments.

As previously mentioned, the lateral posterior aspect of the forearm skin is supplied by the lateral cutaneous nerve of the forearm, a terminal branch of the musculocutaneous nerve, which becomes cutaneous at the lateral border of the biceps, 2.5 cm above the elbow (see Figure 9-2). Its anterior and posterior branches descend on the dorsal and volar aspects of the radial side of the forearm and wrist skin. The medial cutaneous nerve of the forearm is a direct branch of the medial cord of the brachial plexus. Its anterior and posterior branches supply the front and back of the ulnar side of the forearm to the wrist. The large central strip of skin on the dorsal surface of the forearm is supplied by the posterior cutaneous nerve of the forearm, a branch of the radial nerve, which becomes cutaneous about 5 cm above the lateral epicondyle.

Four other important sensory nerves become superficial in the forearm and provide cutaneous sensation in the hand (Figure 9-3), as follows:

1. The superficial (sensory) branch of the radial nerve divides at the lateral epicondyle into superficial and deep branches. The superficial branch pierces the deep fascia in the middle of the forearm and supplies the skin of the dorsum of the hand and wrist.
2. The palmar cutaneous branch of the median nerve arises 2.5 cm above the wrist, passes obliquely downward under the flexor carpi radialis tendon, and then pierces the deep antebrachial fascia between that tendon and the tendon of the palmaris longus muscle. The cutaneous distribution of this nerve supplies sensation to the thenar eminence and the hollow of the palm.

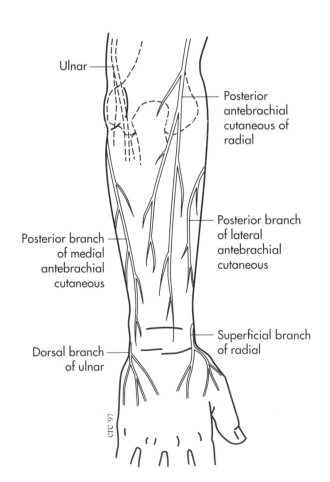

Ulnar

Posterior antebrachial cutaneous of radial

Posterior branch of medial antebrachial cutaneous

Posterior branch of lateral antebrachial cutaneous

Superficial branch of radial

Dorsal branch of ulnar

Figure 9-2 Cutaneous nerves of the dorsal forearm and hand.

3. The palmar cutaneous branch of the ulnar nerve arises from the ulnar nerve about 10 cm above the wrist crease in the middle of the forearm. This nerve branch pierces the antebrachial fascia just above the wrist crease and distributes itself over the hypothenar eminence in the palm.
4. A terminal branch of the radial nerve pierces the antebrachial fascia about 5 cm above the styloid process of the radius and crosses over the underlying tendons to supply the skin over the radial aspect of the thenar eminence.

The expander unit is placed above the deep fascia in the middle layer of the subcutaneous fatty plane. Inadvertent injury to any of these four cutaneous nerves of the forearm may result in prolonged neuromatous formation in the forearm or hand.

Hand

The hand can be conveniently divided into the palmar region, dorsal aspect, and the phalanges. The palmar region consists of a triangular central concave part bounded on the radial side by the thenar eminence and on the ulnar side by the hypothenar eminence. The skin of the central palm is thick and coarse, is thin-ner over the thenar and hypothenar eminences, and then becomes especially firm and subject to callus formation over the metacarpal heads. The volar skin has no hairs or sebaceous glands but contains abundant sweat glands. The skin is bounded tightly to the deep investing palmar fascia and palmar aponeurosis, which is continuous with the antebrachial fascia in the forearm, represented at the wrist by the transverse and volar carpal ligaments. The adipose layer, between the skin and the deep palmar fascia, is divided by multiple fibrous bands and septa, which create a tough cushion in the palm. When skin creases are present, intervening subcutaneous fat is minimal.

In contrast to the tightly bound palmar skin, the dorsal skin is thinner and pliable, containing numerous sebaceous glands and short hairs. The dorsal skin owes its mobility to the underlying dorsal subcutaneous space of loose areolar tissue and fat. Several superficial veins travel within this defined space, along with the cutaneous nerve supply derived from the sensory branches of the ulnar and radial nerves (Figure 9-4).

Tissue expansion is accomplished most favorably on the dorsum of the hand by expander placement within the dorsal subcutaneous space. Neuromatous formation in the sensory nerves may inadvertently occur from the expansion procedures. Tissue expansion of the palmar skin is most difficult to execute because of the firm attachments of the bands and septa from thick skin to the palmar aponeurosis and deep

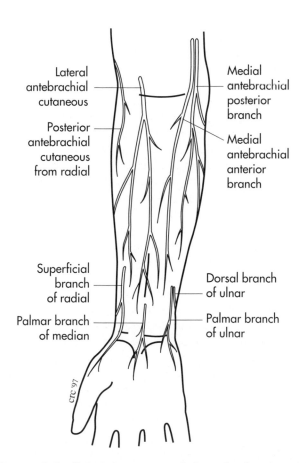

Figure 9-3 Cutaneous nerves of the volar forearm and hand.

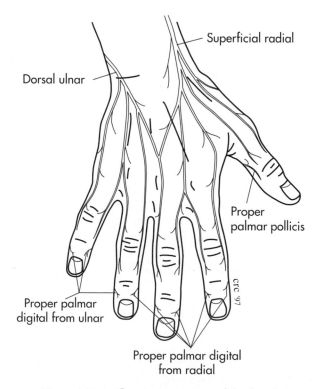

Figure 9-4 Cutaneous nerves of the hand.

fascia. Significant pain can be expected during expansion of palmar skin.

Strategic Considerations

Tissue expansion at the shoulder, brachium, antebrachium, and dorsum of the hand may be done safely and effectively within the subcutaneous fatty plane. In general, however, the complication rate increases as the expansion process descends down the upper extremity, possibly because of the lesser amount of subcutaneous fat and thinner skin in the distal forearm and dorsal hand. In addition, the number of musculocutaneous perforators from the muscles to the overlying skin is expected to be significantly reduced in the distal portions of the upper extremity because of absence of muscles in favor of their tendons. Thus the deleterious effects of any nonyielding part of the expander system, such as the backing, silicone reinforcements around entry points on the expander, implant corners and edges, and high-profile valves, are magnified with thin skin and reduced adipose tissue.

Expanded flaps are more effectively advanced from side to side rather than in a cephalad-to-caudad direction on the extremity. If the flap is expected to be advanced in an up or down direction, the addition of a second expander to the defect's opposite end may be advisable. A second expansion process should be discussed initially with the patient whenever an inadequate amount of coverage is anticipated from the first procedure, depending on the defect's size.

Excess tissue at the incision closure may not positively influence the scar's outcome. Any incision that crosses joint lines can be expected to develop into a hypertrophic, widened and thickened scar, whether or not expansion is done. A significant number of extremity scars tend to become widened even when they do not intrude into the joint spaces.

Injury to the cutaneous sensory nerves to the hands is inevitable during skin expansion in the forearm or dorsum. Nerve injury may occur during expander insertion or stretching and certainly is expected during the second stage of flap advancement. Numbness, paresthesias, or pain can be annoying sequelae after the surgeries are completed.

Expander Selection

In the upper extremity, expander size and shape are determined not only by the defect's configuration but also by the donor site dimensions. Useful available tissue is restricted by the extremities' cylindric nature. In addition, the number of the donor sites is progressively reduced proceeding from the brachium to the hand. If possible, the expander should be as long as

the length of the defect. Because of their larger base diameters, round expanders usually produce more tissue than rectangular ones. The use of one expander on either side of the defect frequently is required because of the paucity of donor tissue from a single side.

Textured-wall expanders offer no significant advantages over smooth-wall expanders during the expansion process. Larger incisions are required for the insertion of textured expanders. As previously mentioned, implants that possess unyielding backers, edges, or silicone reinforcements should be avoided because of the potential for skin erosion and implant exposure.

Surgical Technique

After the defect's size and location have been outlined, the available donor skin adjacent to the defect should be assessed (Figure 9-5, *A*). Expanded donor tissue may be advanced either from side to side (ulnar to radial) or in a caudad-to-cephalad direction. Whenever possible, expanded tissue should be advanced from a radial-to-ulnar direction so that the final vertical scar seam is positioned on the hidden side of the upper extremity. When expanded tissues are moved in a cephalad or caudad direction, a highly visible scar line across the extremity is anticipated.

After a local or general anesthetic is administered, the extremity is prepared with Betadine paint. The expander and its remote valve are outlined on the donor skin adjacent to the defect. A 2 to 4 cm incision may be made within the defect, along its border, or distant from it (Figure 9-5, *B*). Remote incisions permit earlier balloon expansion because of absence of weak points over the expansion site(s). Potential sites for remote incisions include the axillary, elbow, or wrist crease lines. Paralesional incisions, however, are placed on the side of the defect opposite the location of the pocket that will accommodate the expander balloon. In these cases, dissection of a tunnel under the defect permits access for creation of the balloon pocket. The balloon may be inflated early, with less risk for incisional dehiscence. Intralesional incisions possess the greatest potential for incisional dehiscence, implant exposure, and periprosthetic infection.

The balloons are inflated with saline to tissue tolerance to reduce the occurrence of hematomas; smooth out implant folds, which can penetrate new incision closures; and maintain the pocket size. Serial expansion may begin 2 or 3 weeks after surgery. Expansion is completed when the dome width from a single expander is 2.5 to 3 times the defect width (Figure 9-5, *C*).

At the second stage a capsulectomy or capsulotomy is performed to unfurl the domed flap. Any subcutaneous fatty tissue under a benign defect should be saved to act as autogenous filler material (Figure 9-5, *D*). The

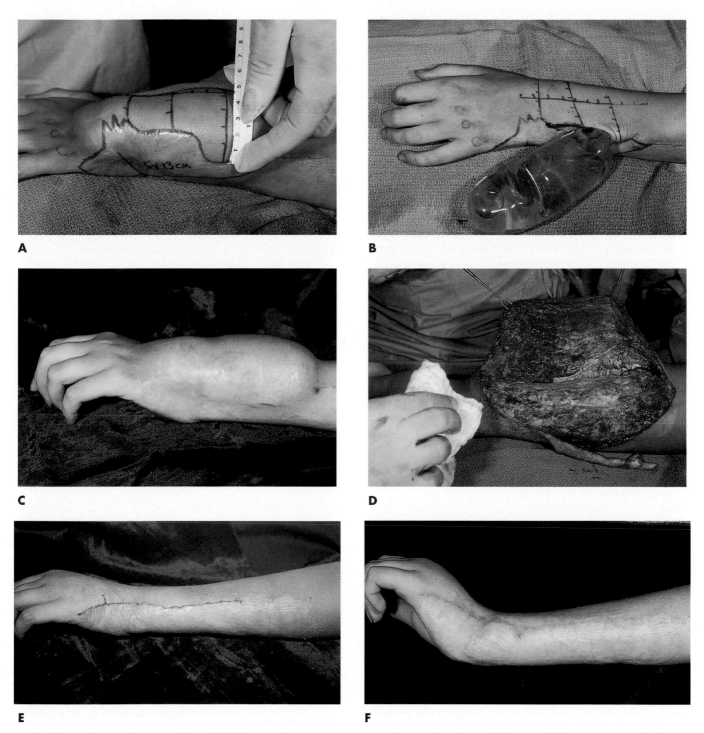

Figure 9-5 A, This 15-year-old patient had a 5 × 13 cm burn scar contracture on the ulnar aspect of her left distal forearm. The available donor skin was adjacent to the defect on the dorsum of the forearm. **B,** Paralesional 3 cm incision was made along the border of the defect and donor site. A pocket in the subcutaneous fat under the donor skin was dissected to accommodate the expander. A separate pocket in the proximal dorsal forearm distal to the antecubital fossa was created for the remote valve. **C,** Serial filling of the tissue expander with saline was performed weekly until the dome width measured three times the defect width. **D,** Expanded flap was elevated along the length of the scar defect after expander removal. A capsulectomy and base capsulotomy unfurled the domed flap. Any subcutaneous fat or de-epithelialized scar bed was preserved to act as filler material under the thinned expanded flap. **E,** Expanded flap was advanced in a lateral direction to replace the excised scar bed. The sutures were removed after 2 weeks. The new scar was treated to prevent hypertrophy. **F,** Six months after surgery the patient has supple skin coverage and near-normal return of sensation. Full wrist and finger extension is not restricted. Scar maturation has not resulted in scar hypertrophy across the wrist joint.

expanded flap is then drawn over the area of the excised defect by advancing it in a lateral or vertical direction (Figure 9-5, *E*). The patient receives a systemic antibiotic during the first and second stages of expansion surgery. Oral postoperative antibiotics are continued for 5 to 7 days.

Case Results

Since 1979 the author has performed 260 upper extremity reconstructions for removal of nevis, scars, and skin grafts (Table 9-1). More than 50% of reconstructions required three or more expansion periods when large lesions were encountered or flap advancement was primarily in an axial direction. Multiple expansions of previously stretched tissue always resulted in a higher morbidity to the reconstructive site. Repeat expansion created thinner skin flaps with more fat loss, which produced a concavity or depression at the reconstructed site. Sensory changes in the expanded skin increased with serial expansions, ranging from pares-

thesias, dysesthesias, painful neuromas, and sympathalgias to complete loss of feeling.

Immediate complications were classified as minor (5.4%) or major (0.8%) (Table 9-2). Depending on severity, the problem was corrected to ensure continuation of the expansion process or the procedure was terminated, primarily because of infection. Deleterious side effects were also observed after an extended postoperative recovery. These involved sensory changes, as previously described, and development of wider hypertrophic scars and concave deformities. Intraoperative expansion facilitated secondary scar revisions. Limited lipoinjections improved significant tissue depressions. Localized liposuction techniques or corticosteroid injections flattened elevated tissue.

■ **Table 9-1** Sites of 260 Shoulder and Upper Extremity Reconstructions

Site	Number
Shoulder	44
Brachium	85
Forearm	91
Dorsum of hand	35
Finger	5

■ **Table 9-2** Complications in 260 Shoulder and Upper Extremity Reconstructions

Type	Number
Minor (5.4%)	
Malposition	1
Implant failure	3
Exposure	
Silicone implant	3
Tubing	1
Valve	1
Wound dehiscence	5
Major (0.8%)	
Infection	1
Flap necrosis	1

CASE REPORTS AND ANALYSES: Shoulder and Upper Extremity Reconstruction

CASE 1:   Unstable Hypertrophic Scar on Right Back, Shoulder, Brachium, and Elbow

History (Figure 9-6, *A*)

This 23-year-old patient had an unstable burn scar contracture to the right back, shoulder, brachium, and elbow. Scar irritation and breakdown occurred from the pressure and movement of her brassiere strap. In addition, shoulder movement was restricted because of the underlying scar bed along the scapula and posterior axillary fold. The goals of surgery were to (1) excise the entire scar and release the underlying fibrosis along the medial border of the scapula and axilla, (2) resurface with supple adjacent skin, and (3) minimize the development of a hypertrophic scar.

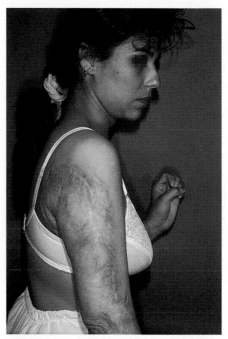

9-6A

Surgical Procedure (Figure 9-6, *B* to *D*)

A 500 cc rectangular expander and a 600 cc round expander were placed in the back through a 3 cm horizontal incision on the lateral aspect of the brachium within the burn scar. These expanders were positioned in the subcutaneous plane above the subjacent trapezius and latissimus dorsi muscles. The remote valves for these expanders were located posterior to the clavicular fossa along the upper border of the trapezius muscle.

A 1000 cc rectangular expander was placed in the subcutaneous plane under the uninvolved skin of the anteromedial aspect of the brachium through the same incision on the lateral brachium. Its valve was also positioned above the clavicular fossa.

A 400 cc round expander was inserted in the subcutaneous fat in the proximal aspect of the lateral forearm through a 2.5 cm incision within the lateral scar of the elbow. Its valve was located in the midforearm. Intraoperative filling of the four expanders reduced the chances for hematoma formation.

Serial expansion of the expanders was performed weekly until sufficient tissue was generated to cover the anticipated defect. Intraoperative expansion at

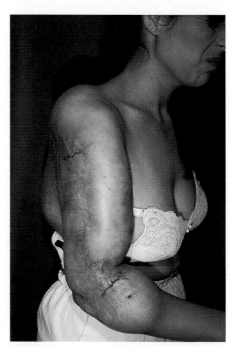

9-6B

surgery gained 2 cm of skin. Capsulectomies and base capsulotomies unfurled the flaps for the most efficient advancement of tissue. The underlying subcutaneous fat and the dermal portions of the scars were retained for filling purposes. The areas of deep fibrosis along the scapula and posterior axilla were excised.

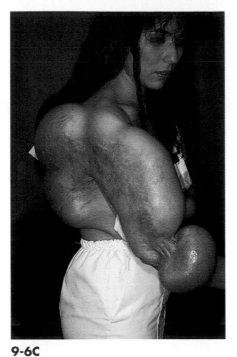

9-6C

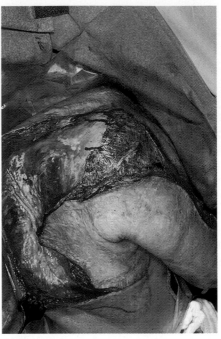

9-6D

Results (Figure 9-6, *E*)

Six months after surgery the patient has minimal scar hypertrophy. The shoulder and elbow exhibit full range of motion. The resurfaced skin is soft and supple, with return of normal sensation.

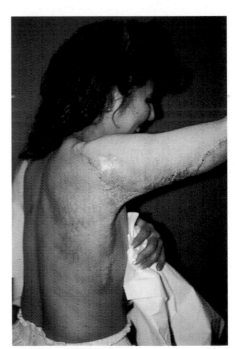

9-6E

CASE 2: Keloidal Burn Scar on Right Shoulder

History (Figure 9-7, *A*)

This 19-year-old patient had a mature burn scar over her right shoulder. The scar underwent episodic breakdown and fissure formation after movements of the shoulder girdle. The patient also experienced restricted full motion of this ball-and-socket joint because of underlying fibrosis along the superomedial aspect of the scapula. The goals of surgery were to (1) excise the keloidal burn scar and subjacent fibrosis, (2) regain full range of joint movement, and (3) produce minimal scarring.

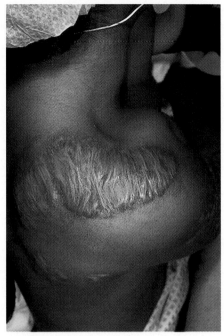

9-7A

Surgical Procedure (Figure 9-7, *B* and *C*)

A 400 cc rectangular expander was inserted in the deep subcutaneous plane of normal neck and back skin. A 500 cc rectangular expander was positioned on the scar's opposite side, extending from the lateral clavicle down to the lateral aspect of the scapula. Both expanders were inserted through a single 2.5 cm vertical incision into a burn scar below the inferior angle of the scapula. The remote valves were positioned in the midback away from the incision. Intraoperative filling with 300 to 400 ml of saline into each expander prevented hematoma formation.

Serial expansions continued for 3 months until a 15 × 30 cm medial flap and a 17 × 30 cm lateral flap were generated. Each flap was expected to contribute 7 to 8 cm of inward advancement to replace the 10 cm–wide scar. More tissue was expanded than needed to account for tissue contraction with full range of shoulder movement. Capsulectomies and base capsulotomies permitted efficient use of the flaps. The areas of deep tissue fibrosis were resected and released the shoulder girdle. The flaps were advanced inward with triangulated permanent sutures in dermal-to-deep tissue to reduce tension on the line of closure.

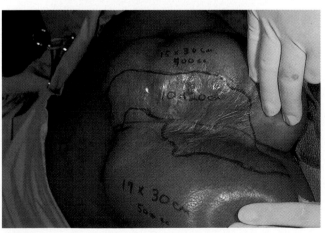

9-7B

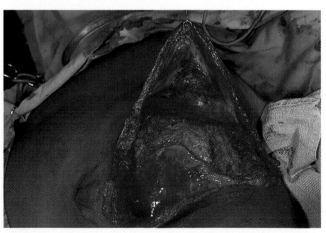

9-7C

Results (Figure 9-7, *D*)

One year after surgery the patient has minimal scar hypertrophy, scar widening, and neuromatous pain. The shoulder exhibits unrestricted movement. The burn scar contractures have been successfully removed and replaced with supple skin.

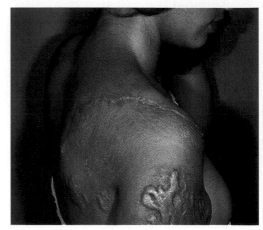

9-7D

CASE 3:   Giant Hairy Nevus on Deltoid Area of Left Shoulder

History (Figure 9-8, *A*)

This 5-year-old patient had an 11 × 15 cm giant hairy nevus on her left shoulder. A previous attempt at reduction surgery at age 4 resulted in an intralesional hypertrophic scar and did not significantly reduce the lesion's original dimensions. The patient was referred for expansion surgery to (1) eliminate the chance for malignant degeneration, (2) preserve range of motion to the shoulder joint, (3) minimize the visible scar, and (4) prevent scar hypertrophy.

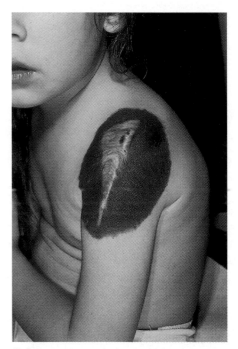

9-8A

Surgical Procedure (Figure 9-8, *B*)

A 400 cc rectangular tissue expander was inserted in the subcutaneous plane under clavicular and neck skin. A 600 cc rectangular expander was positioned lateral to the lesion, extending from the back, posterior axillary fold, and lateral aspect of the brachium. Each of the remote valves was located under back skin. Both expander systems were placed into their respective pockets through a 3.0 cm incision within the central intralesional hypertrophic scar. Intraoperative filling with 200 to 300 ml of saline into each expander reduced hematoma formation.

Serial expansions continued for 3 months until more than the calculated amount of flap was achieved. The extra tissue was provided to reduce the chances of tissue contraction, hypertrophic scar formation, and restricted shoulder motion. At surgery, capsulectomies and base capsulotomies unfurled the flaps for efficient coverage. Permanent sutures from the dermis to the deep bed advanced the flaps to relieve tension along the line of closure.

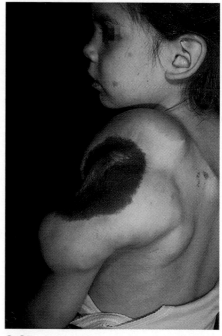

9-8B

Results (Figure 9-8, *C* and *D*)

Three years after surgery the patient shows a 2 to 3 cm widening of the deltoid scar, which has remained free of thickening and pain. The patient has minimal concerns because this scar blends with the surrounding skin. The shoulder girdle has unrestricted movement. There is an absence of nevoid cells along the scar line.

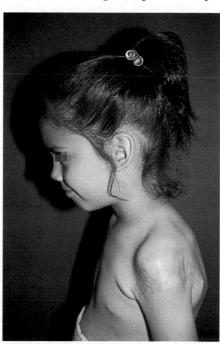

9-8C

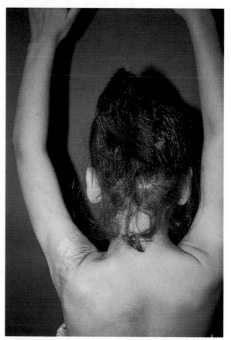

9-8D

CASE 4: Tattoo on Left Midbrachium

History (Figure 9-9, *A*)

A 23-year-old patient had an 8 × 8 cm tattoo on the lateral aspect of his midbrachium. Salubrasion of the tattoo had resulted in scarification and residual pigmentation. The goals of surgery were to (1) excise the scarred pigmentation of the tattoo and (2) minimize the visible scar.

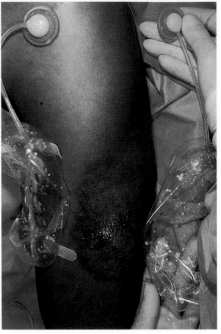

9-9A

Surgical Procedure (Figure 9-9, *B* and *C*)

Two 600 cc rectangular expanders were inserted in the subcutaneous plane of the adjacent uninvolved skin through a 3.0 cm intralesional incision. The anterior expander was positioned lower than the distal end of the tattoo and the posterior expander above the proximal end. These staggered locations were selected to ensure adequate skin for the closure of the ends of the square-shaped tattoo. Intraoperative filling with 200 ml of saline into each expander prevented hematoma formation.

Serial expansion continued until sufficient skin was generated from each expander to cover the defect. At surgery, intraoperative expansion was used to gain 2 to 3 cm of tissue. Capsulectomies and base capsulotomies opened the expanded flaps. An attempt was made to retain the subcutaneous fat beneath the scarred tattooed lesion for additional filling. Skin closure was performed by advancing flaps with absorbing sutures in a triangulated pattern from the dermis into deeper tissue.

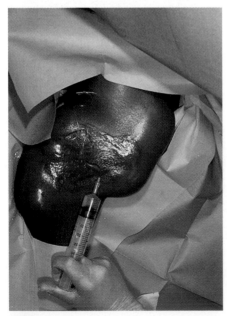

9-9B

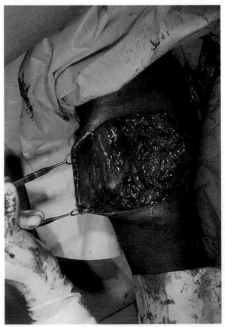

9-9C

Results (Figure 9-9, *D*)

Two years after his procedures the patient's scar remains soft without hypertrophy but exhibits 1 cm of widening. The soft tissue contour did not become depressed and therefore did not require autogenous filling by lipoinjections.

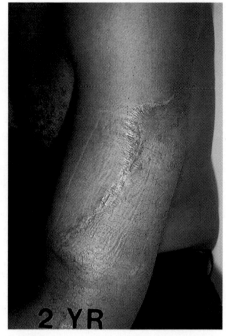

9-9D

CASE 5: Large Congenital Nevus on Distal Right Brachium

History (Figure 9-10, *A*)

This 8-year-old patient had a 3.5 × 10 cm congenital nevus on the posterior aspect of the distal right brachium. Because of its malignant potential, the lesion was removed by expansion technique. The goals of surgery were to (1) excise the nevus and (2) minimize the surgical scar.

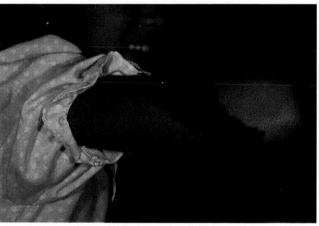

9-10A

Surgical Procedure (Figure 9-10, *B*)

A 200 cc rectangular expander was inserted in the subcutaneous layer of brachial skin from a 2.5 cm incision in the axilla. The remote valve was located under skin of the lateral brachium. Intraoperative filling with 150 ml of saline prevented hematoma formation.

Serial expansion continued weekly for 2 months until sufficient skin was generated. At surgery, intraoperative expansion was performed to gain tissue. Capsulectomies and releasing capsulotomies maximized use of the expanded flap. An attempt was made to salvage the deep subcutaneous fat under the nevus for filling material. Skin approximation was performed by advancing the flaps with absorbable sutures placed from the dermis into the deep tissue in a triangulated pattern.

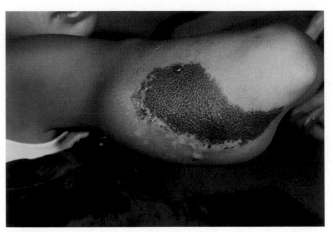

9-10B

Results (Figure 9-10, *C*)

Six months after surgery the patient shows eradication of the nevus and acceptable contouring of the expanded area. The nonhypertrophic scar has begun to blend with the surrounding skin.

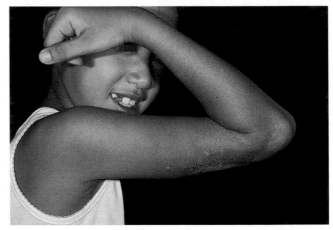

9-10C

CASE 6:   Tattoo on Left Forearm

History (Figure 9-11, *A*)

A 26-year-old patient had an 8 × 12 cm tattoo to the dorsum of his left forearm. The goals of surgery were to (1) remove the tattoo, (2) resurface the area with normal tissue without a contour deformity, and (3) minimize the visible scar.

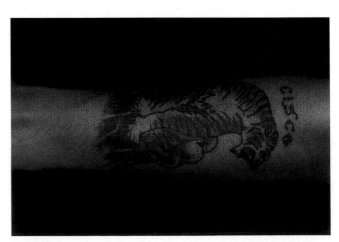

9-11A

Surgical Procedure (Figure 9-11, *B* and *C*)

A 300 cc rectangular expander was inserted in the subcutaneous plane of adjacent volar skin through a 2.5-cm intralesional incision. The expander's valve was incorporated into the implant's dome. Intraoperative filling with saline prevented hematoma formation and brought the valve toward the skin for ease of palpation.

Serial expansion continued for 3 months to obtain an 18 cm hemispheric flap for 9 cm of advancement. Intraoperative expansion was done to gain 2 cm of tissue. A long paralesional incision permitted expander removal. A complete capsulectomy and releasing capsulotomies maximized use of the expanded flap. A zigzag skin closure was performed by advancing the flaps with dermal-to-deep sutures.

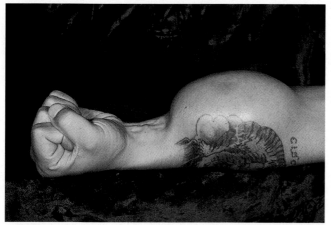

9-11B

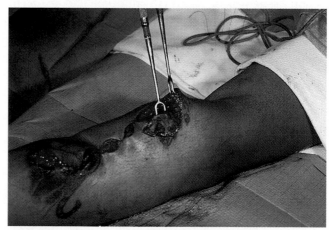

9-11C

Results (Figure 9-11, *D*)

Two years after his procedures the patient has a slightly widened scar, but it has matured without hypertrophy or neuromatous pain. The contour of the reconstructed site is flat without a depression, as may occur from fat atrophy.

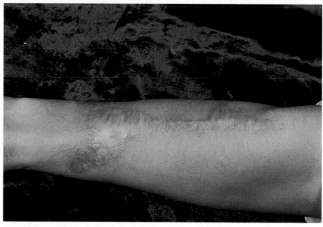

9-11D

CASE 7:   Hypertrophic Burn Scar to Dorsum of Distal Left Forearm and Hand

History (Figure 9-12, *A*)

A 14-year-old patient sustained a scald burn to the dorsum of her distal left forearm and hand. The 5 × 13 cm scar was thickened and caused itching and pain. The goals of surgery were to (1) excise the scar bed, (2) preserve distal skin sensation and extensor tendon glide, and (3) limit the visible scar.

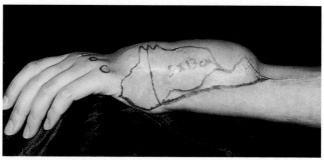

9-12A

Surgical Procedure (Figure 9-12, *B*)

A 200 cc rectangular expander was inserted in the subcutaneous space of the dorsal hand and forearm skin through a 2.5 cm incision into a proximal forearm burn scar. The remote valve was positioned in the proximal forearm. Intraoperative filling with 100 ml of saline prevented hematoma formation.

Serial expansions continued for 3 months until sufficient tissue was obtained (15 cm dome flap = 7.5 cm of advancement). At surgery, intraoperative expansion gained 2 cm of tissue. A capsulectomy and base capsulotomies unfurled the expanded flap. The expanded skin was advanced in an ulnar direction to provide stable coverage.

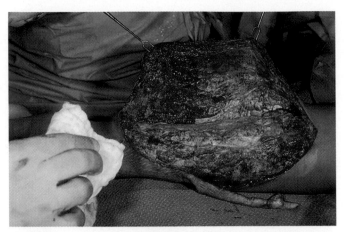

9-12B

Results (Figure 9-12, *C*)

Six months after surgery the patient has supple skin coverage and near-normal return of sensation. Full wrist and finger extension is not restricted. Scar maturation has not resulted in scar hypertrophy across the wrist joint.

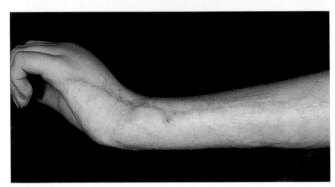

9-12C

HIP AND LOWER EXTREMITY

Anatomic Considerations

Hip

The skin of the hip region is of moderate thickness. The subcutaneous fat layer may be thick over the lateral portions of the hip and gluteal buttock regions, forming an efficient cushion.

The cutaneous nerves of the hip and adjacent thighs are numerous and threaded throughout the fatty layer (Figure 9-13). Sensation to the superior aspect of the gluteal region is served by cutaneous branches from the posterior rami of the first, second, and third lumbar nerves. The lateral cutaneous branch of the iliohypogastric nerve provides sensation to the superolateral hip skin. The cutaneous branches from the posterior rami of the first, second, and third sacral nerves supply the posterior hip skin adjacent to the intergluteal fold. Twigs from the posterior branch of the lateral cutaneous nerve of the thigh terminate over the greater trochanter, and cephalic branches from the posterior cutaneous nerve provide sensation over the inferior half of the buttocks.

The deep fascia is strongly attached to the iliac crest and forms a dense white sheet over the superior origins of the gluteus medius muscle to the posterior iliac crest. However, when this fascia approaches the upper border of the gluteus maximus, it changes to a thin, transparent cover over the entire muscle.

Tissue expanders are placed within the subcutaneous fatty layer overlying the deep fascia. The numerous sensory branches may be damaged during the insertion phase or after the expanded flaps are elevated and advanced. Abnormal cutaneous sensory changes range from numbness to dysesthesias. After reconstruction, fat atrophy from expansion ischemia or traumatic necrosis of fatty tissue may cause soft tissue depressions.

Thigh

The thigh extends from the hip to the knee. The inguinal ligament stretches between the pubic spine and the anterosuperior iliac spine and forms the boundary between the abdomen and thigh. The inferior gluteal crease line defines the posterosuperior extent of the

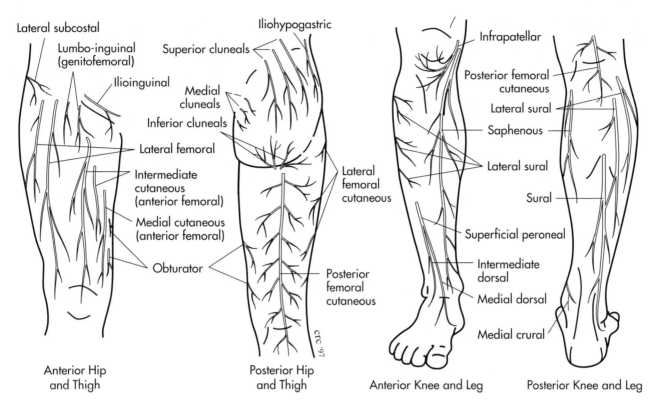

Figure 9-13 Cutaneous nerves of the hip and lower extremity.

thigh. The superior border of the patella forms the lower thigh boundary.

The skin of the thigh is thicker over its anterolateral aspect but thinner on its posteromedial side. The subcutaneous fat forms a prominent layer that varies in thickness throughout the thigh. Between the superficial and deep layers of adipose tissue reside the cutaneous nerves of the thigh, internal saphenous vein and its numerous draining branches, and the lymphatic vessels and lymph nodes clustered below the inguinal ligament, around the fossa ovalis (hiatus saphenus) and saphenous vein, and below the deep fascia within the femoral canal.

Cutaneous Nerves.   The ilioinguinal nerve (branch of first lumbar nerve, L1) provides sensation to the scrotal and penile skin and the upper medial adjacent thigh skin (see Figure 9-13). The lumboinguinal nerve, the femoral component of the genitofemoral nerve (from L1-L2), pierces the deep fascia lateral to the fossa ovalis and supplies a small area below the middle of the inguinal ligament. The posterior branch of the lateral cutaneous nerve (from L2-L3) exits from the deep fascia at the lateral end of the inguinal ligament and divides into anterior and posterior branches. These branches travel down the lateral thigh skin to the knee.

The intermediate cutaneous nerve of the thigh (branch of femoral nerve from L2-L3) divides into two or three branches that innervate the anterior thigh skin

down to the knee. The anterior branch of the medial cutaneous nerve of the thigh (branch of femoral nerve) provides sensation over the inner thigh skin down to the knee. The third cutaneous branch of the femoral nerve, the saphenous nerve, exits from the deep fascia at the medial knee and provides sensation to the anteromedial aspect of the leg.

The posterior thigh skin derives its sensory branches medially from the anterior cutaneous rami of the femoral nerve, posteriorly from the posterior femoral cutaneous nerve, and laterally from the lateral femoral cutaneous nerve.

Long Saphenous Vein.   This vein originates from the dorsal venous plexus in the foot, passes in front of the medial malleolus, ascends upward on the medial thigh, and empties into the femoral vein within the fossa ovalis. Numerous tributaries enter the long saphenous vein in the midthigh and around its entry at the saphenofemoral junction.

Lymph Glands and Vessels.   A superficial horizontal cluster of lymph nodes resides along the inguinal ligament and receives drainage from the genitoperineal areas. Another superficial but longitudinal group of nodes parallels the route of the long saphenous vein and accepts drainage from the lower extremity. Drainage from the lateral side of the foot and the posterolateral lower extremity usually enters the popliteal lymph glands, which eventually enters the deep inguinal lymph stations along the femoral canal.

Deep Fascia (Fascia Lata). The deep fascia of the thigh completely surrounds the conical thigh as a tight-fitting sleeve over the muscle groups. The fascia lata attaches itself to the anterosuperior iliac spine, inguinal ligament, pubic arch, ischial tuberosity, and sacro-tuberous ligament. Posteriorly the fascia lata merges into the gluteal fascia and iliac crest. At the knee level the fascia lata inserts into the patella, femoral condyles, and fibular head. In the posterior knee it continues as the popliteal fascia. In the lateral thigh the fascia lata thickens from its fusion with the conjoined tendon (iliotibial tract) for the gluteus maximus and tensor fasciae latae muscles.

Tissue expanders may be safely positioned in the midlevel of the thigh's subcutaneous fat. Because of the thickness of fat and the rigidity of anterior thigh skin, the surgeon should place expanders in the superficial or midlevel of fat to maximize the effects of balloon stretching. Many cutaneous nerves traverse the subdermal planes in the thigh and provide sensation below the knee and to the upper leg. Inadvertent injury to them during the insertion, expansion, and reconstruction phases may produce complete numbness or dysesthesias in the lower extremity skin.

Knee

The knee region is anatomically defined by a horizontal circumferential line 7.5 cm (3 inches) above the base of the patella and below at the level of the tibial tuberosity. The anterior knee is dominated by the patellar-femoral-tibial hinge joint. The corrugated skin and thin layer of subcutaneous fat in the anterior knee is partly separated from the patella by the prepatellar bursa.

The posterior knee is defined primarily by the popliteal fossa, which contains the lateral (common peroneal) and medial (tibial) popliteal nerves, popliteal artery and vein, the posterior cutaneous nerve, and lymph nodes (Figure 9-14). Within the popliteal fossa the tibial nerve gives off a cutaneous branch (sural nerve) that provides sensation to the posterior calf. The common peroneal nerve also provides a lateral cutaneous nerve to the calf (lateral sural) and a sural communicating branch that joins the main sural nerve in the lower third of the calf (see Figure 9-13). The common peroneal nerve ends by dividing into the superficial (musculocutaneous) and the deep (anterior tibial) peroneal nerve. The musculocutaneous branches of the common peroneal nerve provide sensation to the lower lateral leg. The deep structures within the depths of the popliteal fossa are protected by the deep fascia, composed primarily of circular fibers. The popliteal fascia is pierced by the small saphenous vein and the sural nerve, which travel within the subcutaneous fatty layer.

Expansion must be judiciously performed around the knee joint because of the thin subcutaneous fat and tight skin. Full flexion and extension of this joint may be restricted by the physical restraints of the large balloons as expansion proceeds. Injury to the important cutaneous branches that pass through the popliteal fossa may produce irreversible numbness or dysesthesias to the terminal fibers as they course to the skin of the leg, ankle, and foot.

Leg

The skin of the leg to the ankle is thinner than that of the thigh. The subcutaneous layer of fat on the anterior leg surface is generally less thick than that found on the posterior calf. The deep fascia does not form a complete investment around the leg because it fuses with the periosteum on the medial surface of the tibia. The deep fascia originates on the anterior border of the tibia and sweeps laterally and posteriorly to reach the tibia again at its posteromedial border. The deep fascia gradually becomes thinner in the distal leg but regains its thickness at the ankle as the inferior extensor retinaculum. A number of cutaneous nerves within the subcutaneous fat distribute their sensory fibers to the anterior and posterior leg (see Figure 9-13).

The anterior skin surface receives sensation from the medial branch of the saphenous nerve (femoral nerve) and the lateral sural nerve (lateral cutaneous branch from common peroneal nerve). The lower lateral aspect of the leg, dorsal ankle, and dorsum of the foot derive their cutaneous sensation from the superficial (musculocutaneous) branch of the common peroneal nerve. The posterior leg receives cutaneous sensation from the terminal fibers of the thigh's posterior cutaneous nerve, posterior branch of the medial cutaneous nerve, cutaneous branches of the common peroneal (lateral sural and sural communicating branches), and the sural nerve (tibial nerve).

Skin expansion on the posterior leg is easier and safer to perform than on the anterior surface. The

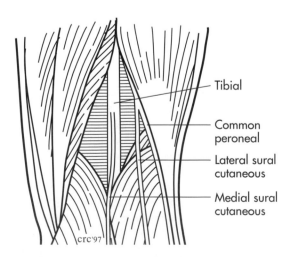

Tibial

Common peroneal

Lateral sural cutaneous

Medial sural cutaneous

crc'97

Figure 9-14 Cutaneous nerves of the popliteal fossa.

skin overlying the tibial tuberosity and anterior tibia is taut, thin, and supported by a thin layer of subcutaneous fat. Injury to cutaneous leg nerves can produce numbness and dysesthesias of the ankle and foot.

Ankle

The ankle is defined by the ankle joint and is bounded superiorly by the distal tibia and fibula and inferiorly by the talus. The dorsal ankle skin is thin and lax with minimal subcutaneous fat, and the plantar skin is thick and firm. The deep fascia is tough and continuous with the leg fascia. The ankle fascia forms five restricting bands that keep the tendons in contact with the bones and assist in the formation of osteoaponeurotic tunnels, through which tendons and their synovial sheaths pass. The structures over the deep fascia on the dorsal ankle include the long saphenous vein, saphenous nerve, and superficial peroneal (musculocutaneous) nerve (Figure 9-15).

Skin expansion around the ankle may be painful and limited by the paucity and thinness of the donor sites. Ankle flexion and extension are restricted by the enlarging balloons.

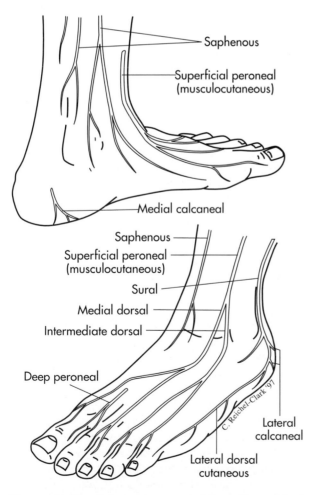

Figure 9-15 Cutaneous nerves of the ankle and foot.

Foot

The dorsal foot skin is thin, less sensitive, and pliable with a minimal layer of subcutaneous fat. The deep fascia in the dorsum is a thin membranous layer continuous with the transverse and cruciate crural ligaments. The significant structures under the dorsal skin include the dorsal venous plexus, which drains into the saphenous vein; lateral musculocutaneous branch of the peroneal nerve; medial terminal branches of the saphenous nerve; and terminal branches of the anterior tibial (deep peroneal) nerve between the large and second toes (see Figure 9-7).

Expansion of the dorsal foot tissue may be compromised by the thinner skin and negligible subcutaneous fat. Donor skin may be limited, without sufficient stretch to cover an adjacent defect.

The skin on the sole is thicker, unyielding, and highly sensitive with numerous sweat glands. A layer of entrapped fatty tissue is subdivided into lobules by septal bands that connect the skin to the deep plantar fascia. The deep fascia lies above the deeper vessels, muscles, and tendons and is referred to as the *plantar aponeurosis.* This tough, glistening white sheet is dense and protective of the more delicate underlying structures. The cutaneous nerves consist of the medial plantar nerve (three and one-half digits on the large toe side of the foot), lateral plantar nerve (remaining one and a half digits), and the medial calcaneal branches of the posterior tibial nerve to the heel skin.

Plantar skin expansion is extremely difficult because of pain, nonpliable skin, and balloon location. Infection rates increase with expansion of ankle and foot skin.

Strategic Considerations

Tissue expansion in the hip, thigh, and posterolateral calf can be safely and effectively accomplished. Expansion around the knee and ankle may be compromised by the minimal donor tissue and restricted joint motion. The plantar surface is the only area where tissue expansion may not be applicable, because the skin is too thick and nonpliable, similar to the palmar skin, and significant pain occurs during expansion of this unyielding tissue.

Tissue expanders may be positioned within the subcutaneous fatty plane above the deep investing fascia in the hip, thigh, knee, leg, ankle, and dorsum of the foot. The surgeon should consider the deleterious effects of expansion on the fatty layer, especially in the hip and thigh. Expansion often results in a significant concave depression or irregularities in these areas, primarily because of fat necrosis. These contour changes are accentuated by the natural round curvatures of the hip and the conical shape of the thigh.

Expansion of anterior thigh tissue may be problematic because of the thick, unyielding skin and fat. If the subcutaneous fat layer is extremely thick, as from obesity, the expander should not be placed directly over the deep fascia, but rather in the midlevel of the subcutaneous fatty tissue. This superficial position, about 1 to 2 cm below the skin surface, permits more effective expansion of the overlying skin.

Cutaneous sensory nerves can be traumatized during expander insertion, injured during tissue stretching from ischemia, and irreversibly transected during the second stage of excision and flap advancement. Sensory alterations include numbness, paresthesias, and neuromatous pain. Permanent injury to proximal nerves with terminal branches around the ankle and foot may keep patients from recognizing skin trauma caused by poorly fitting shoes, improper ambulation, or accidents. Sensory alterations in the skin of the buttocks, thighs, knees, and leg are disturbing to the patient but do not lead to more serious consequences as they can in the ankle and foot.

Expansion under the inguinal ligament may injure the superficial lymph nodes and vessels and the greater saphenous vein. No adverse effects have resulted from permanently removing these structures during the reconstructive phase. No limb lymphedema from multiple expansion has occurred during the author's 17 years of clinical experience.

Advancement of expanded skin in a transverse direction is always more effective than in a cephalad-to-caudad direction. More than one expansion process may be required to reconstruct a large defect completely, especially when the expanded flap is advanced in a vertical direction.

The incidence of implant exposure and closed cellulitis increases as the surgical procedures progress down to the lower leg, ankle, and foot. The exact causes for these morbidities are unknown but may be related to thinner skin and fat, opportunities for local trauma, and dependent swelling and edema that encourages streptococcal cellulitis. Intraoperative expansion may be beneficial in reconstructing small defects in the lower extremity to obviate the problems caused by long-term presence of a foreign body.

Expander Selection

In the hip and lower extremity, rectangular expanders are useful because of their length and the lack of available donor tissues. An expander on each side of the defect permits more tissue to be advanced. The pocket may be dissected in an encompassing manner to surround the defect with two expanders. Round or crescent-shaped expanders may be required, depending on the defect's size and shape and amount of donor tissue.

Surgical Technique

After selection of the size, shape, and location(s) of a single balloon or multiple expanders, the skin is prepped with an antibiotic solution. The patient receives systemic antibiotics just before the incision is made. The anticipated field of dissection is injected with 0.5% lidocaine (Xylocaine) with epinephrine (1:400,000). The incision site must be selected on the basis of minimizing visible scars and maximizing prevention of premature dehiscence or suture line infections.

If a convenient crease line (e.g., axillary fold, nape of neck, intergluteal fold, umbilicus, infragluteal fold, inguinal line, knee fold, ankle crease) or previous scar is available and distant from the problem site, the surgeon may select it to camouflage the incision scar. If the defect (e.g., scar, skin graft, nevus) is wide enough, an incision may be made within the defect's center. In either case the dissection is done straight down to the mid–fatty plane or the deep fascia. Tunneling by finger or instrument dissection creates a pathway from the distant incision or under the lesion to the outlined expander pocket. Tissue elevation continues along the side(s) of the defect, creating a slightly larger cavity in the shape of the expander(s).

The smooth-wall expander(s) is inserted and positioned within the pocket along with its pretested remote valve system. The expander is filled with saline containing methylene blue (0.5 ml) and bacitracin (100,000 U/500 ml saline) to tissue tolerance to reduce hematoma formation and implant folds and maintain the surgical pockets. Methylene blue may reveal any leakage points within the implant system during the first stage of implant insertion. The need for surgical drains to remove fluid is unlikely at the insertion phase. The prolonged presence of drains also can cause retrograde infection of the implant.

Two to 3 weeks after implant insertion the expander(s) may be filled with saline in the office to tolerance, as determined by patient comfort and ischemic skin changes. Serial expansion continues weekly or every 2 weeks until dome measurements (2.5 to 3 × defect width) are sufficient for the second reconstructive surgery. During lesion excision, every effort must be made to preserve the subcutaneous fat layer under the defect. By conserving adipose tissue, more cutaneous nerves may be left intact to provide as much sensation as possible to the expanded skin. In addition, the retained adipose layer can reduce the degree of concavity at the reconstructed site.

Capsulotomies and capsulectomies may be required to unfurl the domed expanded flaps to maximize tissue coverage. Surgical drains may be necessary during the second stage of reconstruction because of copious oozing after capsule removal. After tissue healing, secondary procedures such as lipoinjection of fat under deficient areas may be considered. Scar revisions may also be needed later.

Case Results

Since 1979 the author has performed 173 hip and lower extremity expansions, primarily for scars, unstable skin, skin grafts, and nevi (Table 9-3). More than 50% of the reconstructions required two or more expansions to complete the coverage. About half the cases were performed with distant incisions and the other half with incisions in the defect's center.

Immediate minor (7.5%) and major (4%) complication rates involved expander problems, incision dehiscence, infection, and skin ischemia (Table 9-4). Minor complications often required correction of the problem, after which the expansion process could continue. Major complications resulted in termination of the procedure. In general the incidence of major complications increased as expansion occurred lower in the extremity. Cellulitis was often observed during expansion in the lower third of the leg, the ankle, and the foot. Flap necrosis occurred during expansion in the ankle and foot.

Delayed side effects were noted months after the reconstructions, including contour depressions from fat necrosis that developed either during expansion or at flap reconstruction. Serial lipoinjections were performed about 6 months to a year after the final surgery to diminish the acquired concavities. About 50% of patients reported abnormal cutaneous sensations in the lower leg, ankle, and dorsum of the foot. These neural changes included permanent numbness, paresthesias, dysesthesias, and neuromatous pain.

■ **Table 9-3** Sites of 173 Hip and Lower Extremity Reconstructions

Site	Number
Hip/buttock	41
Thigh	48
Knee	15
Leg	43
Ankle	8
Dorsum of foot	18

■ **Table 9-4** Complications in 173 Hip and Lower Extremity Reconstructions

Type	Number
Minor (7.5%)	
Malposition	1
Implant failure	2
Valve turnover	1
Implant exposure	
Envelope	2
Tubing	1
Valve	1
Wound dehiscence	5
Major (4%)	
Infection	4
Flap necrosis	3

CASE REPORTS AND ANALYSES: Hip and Lower Extremity Reconstruction

CASE 1: Giant Nevus on Right Hip, Buttock, and Thigh

History (Figure 9-16, *A* and *B*)

This 12-year-old patient had a 15 × 25 cm giant nevus on her right hip, buttock, and thigh. Two previous attempts at surgical reductions produced no significant change in the lesion's dimensions. This referred patient wanted the nevus removed because of its appearance and possible malignant degeneration. The goals of surgery were to (1) excise the entire pigmented lesion, (2) match the involved buttock skin to the opposite side, (3) provide a feminine hip contour without concavities, and (4) minimize visibility of the scars. Because of the lesion's size, multiple expansion periods were planned.

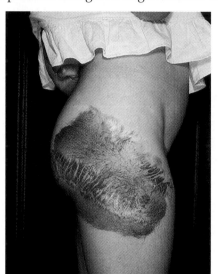

9-16A

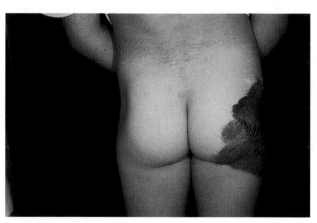

9-16B

First Surgical Procedure (Figure 9-16, *C* and *D*)

Two 1500 cc custom-made crescent expanders were inserted in the subcutaneous plane under adjacent skin through a 3.0 cm intralesional incision at the buttock crease line. The expanders encircled the lesion in a continuous pocket. The remote valves were located under the lateral trunk skin. Intraoperative filling with 500 ml of saline reduced hematoma formation and maintained the continuous pocket.

Serial expansions continued for 4 months to tissue tolerance of thinning and fat atrophy. Intraoperative expansion, capsulectomies, and capsulotomies maximized the expanded flaps for advancement. About 75% of the lesion could be removed.

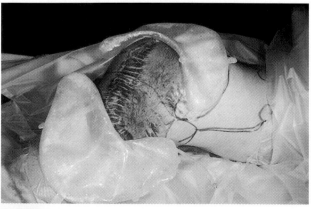

9-16C

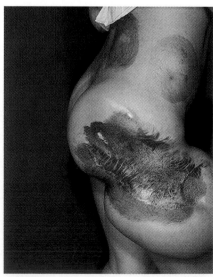

9-16D

Second Surgical Procedure (Figure 9-16, *E*)
After 6 months, two 1000 cc expanders were inserted above and below the residual nevus. The tissues were reexpanded over 3 months until calculation showed sufficient available tissue for the final coverage. Intraoperative expansion gained 2 cm of tissue. The remainder of the nevus was excised and covered with expanded tissue. A buttock lift and repositioning were also performed to match the opposite side.

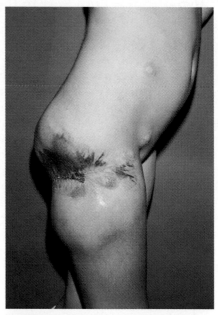

9-16E

Results (Figure 9-16, *F*)
Two years after her reconstructive procedures the patient shows complete nevus removal without persistent pigmentation along the scar line. The buttocks are in close symmetry to each other. The trunk, hip, and lateral thigh curvatures have been reconstructed with preservation of subcutaneous fat for autogenous filling.

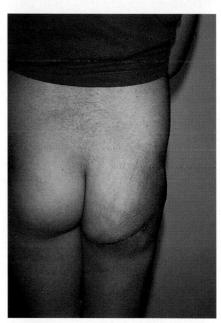

9-16F

CASE 2: Hypertrophic Burn Scar to Right Lateral Thigh and Knee

History (Figure 9-17, *A*)

This 20-year-old patient sustained a scald burn injury to her right lateral thigh and knee at an early age. Much of the burned area received skin grafts, and other sites were allowed to heal by secondary intent. An expansion procedure 6 months before consultation resulted in necrosis of the expanded flap, which required skin grafting. The patient wanted the residual scar contracture and recent skin graft removed and thigh contour improved. The goals of surgery were to (1) excise the remaining hypertrophic scar and skin graft, (2) resurface the area with normal supple skin, (3) reduce contour defects from fat atrophy, and (4) minimize the scar appearance.

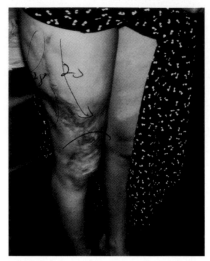

9-17A

Surgical Procedure (Figure 9-17, *B* to *D*)

Two 1000 cc rectangular expanders were inserted in the subcutaneous plane through a 3.0 cm incision within the proximal upper thigh scar. The expanders were positioned around the upper half of the patellar scar and along each side of the residual lateral thigh scar and graft. The valves were located under the uninvolved thigh skin of the upper lateral and medial thigh. Intraoperative filling with 500 ml of saline in each expander reduced hematoma formation.

Serial expansion continued weekly for 3 months until sufficient tissue was created. The scar was widest above the patella and measured about 15 cm. Therefore each expanded flap had to contribute at least 7.5 cm of tissue. Expansion proceeded until the diam-

eter of each hemispheric flap measured at least 15 cm. Intraoperative expansion to maximal tissue tolerance gained 1 to 2 cm for flap advancement.

At surgery the scar tissue was de-epithelialized and used as filler material to minimize depressions caused by expansion. Each flap underwent excision of its capsule to open the constricted domed flap. Base capsulotomies aided in further tissue advancement.

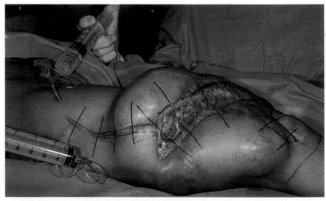

9-17C

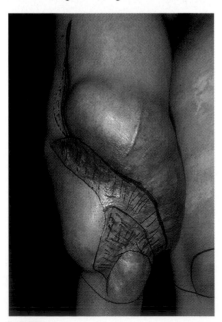

9-17B

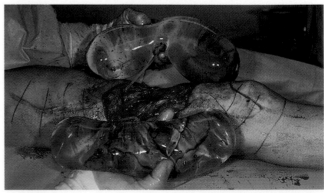

9-17D

Results (Figure 9-17, *E*)
One year after the major surgical procedure, most burn scar contractures and grafts have been replaced with softer unaffected skin. The visible scar is slowly maturing and less obvious. Areas of depression may be filled later with lipoinjected fat.

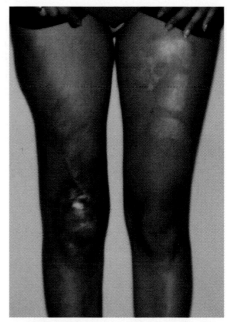

9-17E

CASE 3:   Unstable Scar Over Left Knee

History (Figure 9-18, *A*)
This 17-year-old male developed a hypertrophic scar over his left knee from a basketball injury. The patient received two intralesional steroid injections over 3 months. The overlying skin became atrophic, with bleeding and subsequent fat atrophy. Because of frequent cracking, bleeding, and breakdown on knee flexion, the patient was unable to play school sports. The goals of surgery were to (1) excise the injured tissue, (2) create stable skin coverage, and (3) minimize hypertrophic scarring.

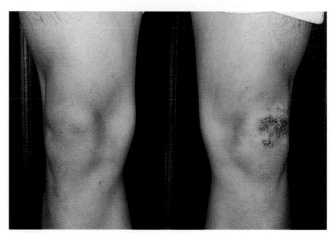

9-18A

Surgical Procedure (Figure 9-18, *B* and *C*)
Two crescent-shaped expanders were inserted around the 8 × 8 cm atrophic scar tissue in the subcutaneous plane through two 2 cm incisions in the flexion crease lines on either side of the knee. The remote valves were positioned under the skin of the lower medial thigh and the upper medial leg. Intraoperative filling with saline reduced hematoma formation and maintained a continuous single pocket.

Serial expansion continued for 3 months until sufficient skin was generated, as determined by the flaps' diameters. Intraoperative expansion was performed at surgery to gain more tissue. The expanded supple flaps were advanced over the de-epithelialized atrophic site in a horizontal closure.

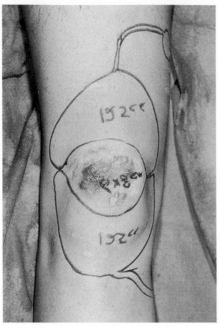

9-18B

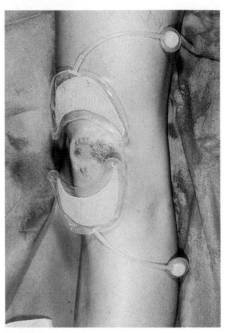

9-18C

Results (Figure 9-18, *D*)
One year after his reconstruction, the patient's tissues are stable with minimal scar hypertrophy. The contour of the reconstructed site is symmetric to the opposite side. The patient was able to resume his athletic career.

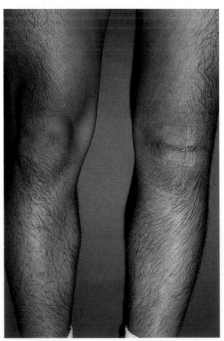

9-18D

CASE 4: Exposed Tibial Fracture Site

History (Figure 9-19, *A*)
This 17-year-old male sustained a complex open fracture and dislocation of the knee joint in a motor vehicle accident. After the initial vascular spasm subsided, foot sensation gradually returned. The gastrocnemius and soleus muscles, however, were significantly crushed and devitalized.

After several evaluations in the operating room, the proximal muscle portions were débrided. A split-thickness skin graft covered the exposed tissue. External fixation reduced and stabilized the femoral and tibial fractures. Although no significant bone loss was evident after fixation, two sites of tibial exposure were observed close to the fracture line. The exposed tibial cortices were treated with frequent silver sulfadiazine (Silvadene) dressings.

After 8 weeks of wound healing with no evidence of osteomyelitis, the patient was examined for coverage of his exposed tibia. The patient refused any free tissue transfers. A split-thickness skin graft for bone coverage was discarded as an option because of its proximity to the fracture line. Tissue expansion of the medial calf skin was chosen for more stable coverage.

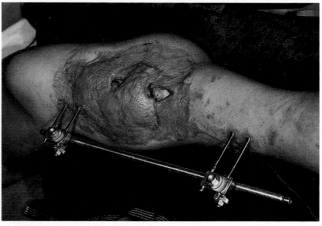

9-19A

Surgical Procedure (Figure 9-19, *B* and *C*)
A 600 cc rectangular expander was inserted in the deep subcutaneous plane of adjacent upper medial calf skin through a 3.0 cm midposterior calf incision. The valve was incorporated into the expander's anterior dome.

Serial expansions continued for 8 weeks until sufficient tissue was generated for flap coverage of the two exposed bone sites. Intraoperative expansion was performed to acquire more tissue. The exposed cortices were reduced down to bleeding cortical bone, and the unstable intervening tissue over the fracture site was removed. The expanded tissue was then elevated as a rotation-advancement flap to cover the fracture line and the adjacent portions of exposed bone.

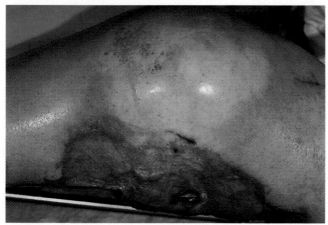

9-19B

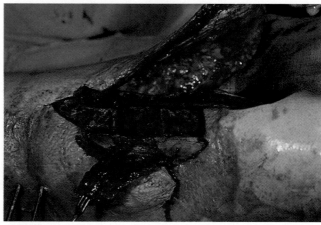

9-19C

Results (Figure 9-19, *D*)

The patient's reconstructive site is shown immediately after flap coverage. The "delayed" flap survived and provided stable tissue over the tibia. The external fixation was removed 8 weeks after flap coverage. The extremity was placed in a long-leg cast for 4 months. Primary bone healing at the fracture line was seen radiographically at 6 months.

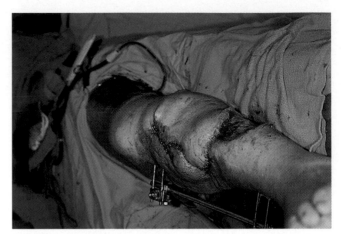

9-19D

SUMMARY

Tissue expansion may be performed safely and effectively for a variety of lesions of the upper and lower extremities, including the hip region. The rate of major complications, however, increases as surgery involves the distal aspects of the arm and leg. Signs of fat atrophy can be expected around and below the reconstructed site(s).

10 Abdominal and Back Reconstruction

ABDOMEN

The anterior abdominal wall is defined superiorly and inferiorly by bony margins and laterally by arbitrary lines. This large area consists of a platform of muscles rather than a bony floor. The abdomen is bounded above by the xiphoid process of the sternum and the costal margins of the seventh through tenth ribs. The lower boundary consists of the iliac crests, inguinal ligaments, and the pubis. The lateral borders are arbitrarily assigned as the midlevel of the lateral abdominal walls.

The abdominal skin is loosely attached to the subcutaneous layer and capable of stretching during pregnancy and obesity. Vertical fibers and septae hold the skin firmly adherent around the umbilicus and divide the subcutaneous fat into compartments. The *linea alba* extends from the xiphoid process to the pubis symphysis and is divided by the umbilicus into a supraumbilical portion (1.25 cm ½ inch) wide and an infraumbilical portion so narrow that it blends into the underlying rectus muscle fascia. The linea alba is a fibrous raphe formed by a meeting of the three lateral abdominal muscles.

The subcutaneous adipose layer of the anterior abdominal wall is soft, movable, and continuous with layers in the thorax, hip and external genitalia, and back. In the infraumbilical area the adipose layer can be separated into two distinct layers. The superficial layer, above *Camper's fascia*, is the *panniculus adiposus*, which may be several centimeters thick in obese people. The deeper layer, below *Scarpa's fascia*, contains no fat and consists of a yellow fibrous membrane. Scarpa's fascia forms a continuous sheet across the abdomen but attaches to the linea alba as it passes under it.

The abdominal skin is abundantly supplied by the lower six thoracic and first lumbar nerves (Figure 10-1). Each thoracic nerve distributes in a dermatomal pattern, with an anterior branch along the paramedian line and a lateral branch on the side. The lateral branch of the twelfth thoracic nerve is longer and crosses the iliac crest to provide sensation to the buttock. The first lumbar nerve divides into two large branches, the iliohypogastric and ilioinguinal nerves, which provide sensation to the groin and inguinal areas.

The abdominal skin is profusely supplied with corresponding superficial arterial branches from the posterior intercostal arteries and the superior and inferior epigastric arteries. In addition, the superficial external pudendal, the superficial epigastric, and the superficial circumflex iliac branches from the femoral artery supply the abdomen.

The deep fascia of the abdomen lies over the muscular portions of the external oblique muscle and its aponeurosis. The deep fascia continues medially over the rectus muscle sheath, which is formed by fusion of the separate aponeuroses of the external oblique, internal oblique, and transversus abdominis muscles. The deep abdominal fascia is a continuation of the fasciae of the latissimus dorsi and pectoralis major muscles.

Strategic Considerations

Tissue expansions may be safely and effectively performed within the subcutaneous fat layer of the anterior abdominal wall. The linear alba is important in tissue expansion because it must be elevated from its adherent underlying structures to create a subcutaneous pocket for tissue expansion across the midline. In the supraumbilical and infraumbilical areas the linea alba can expand with the adjacent skin during the expansion process. In addition, expansion can proceed efficiently even when its base is soft tissue only, such as muscles and fasciae, rather than bone. Expansion around the umbilicus is somewhat compromised because of its tethering nature.

Expanders are positioned in the adipose layer about 1 to 2 cm beneath the skin surface. Expanders in this superficial level permit more effective expansion of tissue than those in the deep level of the panniculus adiposus. The preferred incision site may be a 2 to 3 cm exposure within the suprapubic hair or in one of the lateral groin creases.

The consequences of adverse changes in cutaneous sensation are negligible in the abdomen and are not

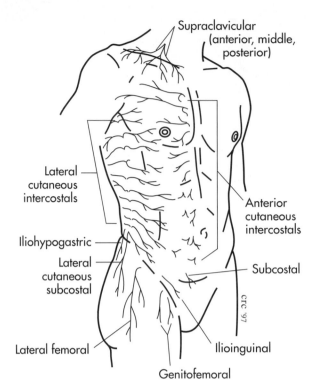

Figure 10-1 Cutaneous nerves of the abdomen.

likely to occur because of the segmental nature of its innervation.

Expander Selection

Conventional rectangular or round tissue expanders may be selected, depending on the defect's size and configuration. The expanders' length should be equal to or longer than the defect's length. The number of expanders inserted around the defect depends on its width, availability of donor skin sites, and effciency of expansion and anticipated coverage. Smooth-wall expanders without firm backers and edges are recommended.

Surgical Technique

After the defect's size and shape and available donor tissues are evaluated, the outlines of the selected expanders are marked on the skin. The surgical site is prepared with an antibiotic solution and injected by insufflation technique with lidocaine (Xylocaine, 0.5%) and epinephrine (1:400,000) to aid in hemostasis, dissection, and pain control.

Access incisions 2 to 3 cm long may be camouflaged within the pubic hair or along one of the inguinal crease lines. A 2 cm transverse incision inside the umbilicus is another reliable site for dissection of the surgical pockets. If the defect has stable skin cover, an intralesional incision may be used to avoid an additional scar. In this case the dissection is taken straight down to the superficial subcutaneous fat layer, tunneled under the defect, and then continued alongside the defect in the outline of the expander pocket.

For small lesions, a round expander may be placed directly under the defect's center through a remote incision. The remote valve is located away from the balloon in its own pocket. The balloon is filled to tissue tolerance by injecting methylene blue–colored bacitracin solution into its remote valve system.

Serial expansion is begun 2 to 3 weeks after insertion on a weekly or every-other-week basis until sufficient tissue has been developed (expander dome = 3 × defect width). At the second stage, intraoperative expansion for 5 to 10 minutes may gain 1 or 2 cm of tissue. After removal of the entire expander system, capsulotomies and capsulectomy unfurl the domed flap to provide optimal use of tissue.

Tissue flaps may be advanced either toward the vertical midline or to the groin crease line to reduce visibility of scars. However, vertical scars tend to hypertrophy and widen over time. In most cases the surgeon positions the final scar in the direction of the defect's longest axis. Any subcutaneous fat under the defect should be used as autogenous filling material, which may minimize formation of concavities within the reconstructed site. Surgical drains may be required after extensive tissue dissection and repositioning. Delayed revision of hypertrophic scars and lipoinjection for depressions may be performed in selected patients.

Case Results

Since 1979 the author has performed 11 reconstructions in the supraumbilical anterior abdomen and 23 expansion cases in the infraumbilical area. These surgeries were indicated for removal of scars, skin grafts, and nevi (Table 10-1). Ten percent of cases re-

■ **Table 10-1** Types of Defects in 34 Abdominal Reconstructions

Area/type	Number
Supraumbilical	
Scar	5
Skin graft	2
Nevus	4
Infraumbilical	
Scar	11
Skin graft	7
Nevus	5

quired two or more expansions to resurface the defect completely.

Two minor (5%) and two major (5%) immediate complications during abdominal expansion involved implant failure, exposure of expander balloon, and infections (Table 10-2). One year from the last surgery, no significant changes in sensation had developed. No patient requested filling of fat-deficient concavities.

■ **Table 10-2** Complications in 34 Abdominal Reconstructions

Type	Number
Minor (5%)	
Implant failure	1
Envelope exposure	1
Major (5%)	
Infection	2

CASE REPORT AND ANALYSIS: Abdominal Reconstruction

Congenital Giant Nevus on Anterior Chest Wall and Upper Abdomen

History (Figure 10-2, *A*)

This 3-year-old patient had a giant nevus across the lower half of her chest wall with adjacent abdominal involvement. Because of potential malignant development, the defect was assessed for removal by expansion technique. The goals of surgery were to (1) excise the nevus in stages because of its size and location, (2) preserve future development of the breast buds into normal mammary mounds, and (3) minimize scar formation under the anticipated inframammary fold lines.

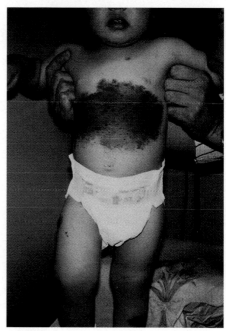

10-2A

First Surgical Procedure (Figure 10-2, *B* and *C*)

A 1000 cc rectangular expander was inserted in the subcutaneous plane under the nevus through a 3 cm incision within the right lateral extension of the lesion. The expander was located away from the anticipated inframammary folds but under uninvolved skin of the upper abdomen. The remote valve was positioned under skin of the right posterior axillary fold. Intraoperative filling with 400 ml of saline reduced the incidence of hematoma formation.

Serial expansion began 3 weeks after surgery and continued every 2 weeks for 4 months. Expansion was terminated because of tissue thinning above one of the expander's corners.

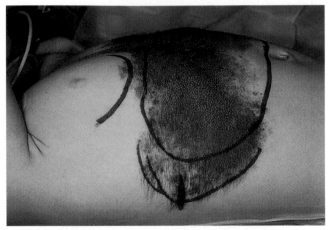

10-2B

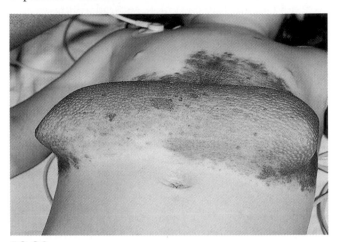

10-2C

Results (Figure 10-2, *D*)

The first expansion procedure resected 50% of the nevus without injury to the breast buds. After healing occurred, a second expansion process was begun 6 months later.

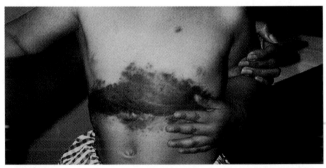

10-2D

Second Surgical Procedure (Figure 10-2, *E*)

Another 1000 cc rectangular expander was inserted in the same pocket through the previous incision scar. Intraoperative filling with 300 ml of saline reduced hematoma formation. Serial expansion of the previously stretched tissue continued for 8 weeks until tissue thinness at the expander edges terminated the expansion phase. The nevus was reduced further without violation of the breast buds.

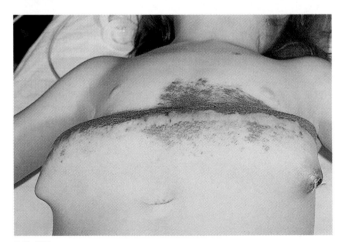

10-2E

Results (Figure 10-2, *F*)

Six months later the patient shows initial scar maturation. Further surgical procedures to remove the remnant are delayed until growth and development of the patient's breast mounds.

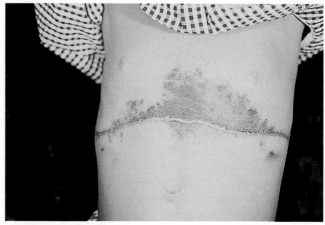

10-2F

BACK

The back extends from the nuchal ridge of the posterior skull to the posterior shoulders and thorax and down to the low back and posterior pelvis. The skin of the back is thick and firm, moving more easily in a transverse than in a cephalad-to-caudad direction. The subcutaneous fat is thick and fibrous, extending from the posterior skull down to the pelvis. The skin and fat are bound to the deep investing fascia by numerous heavy bands and septae that divide the fat into smaller compartments. At the sides of the back the skin and fat gradually thin and soften as they merge with the chest wall and abdominal layers.

As mentioned in Chapter 9, the deep fascia includes the nuchal fascia and vertebral fascia down to the lumbodorsal (thoracolumbar) fascia. All these fasciae merge anterolaterally into the pectoral and costal fascia and inferolaterally into the aponeurosis of the external oblique muscle and the fascia lata of the hip and thighs. Fascial septae form intermuscular clefts that enclose muscles into compartments.

The numerous cutaneous nerves in the back are derived from the anterior and posterior rami of the cervical, thoracic, and lumbosacral spinal nerves (Figure 10-3). These nerves radiate from the spine in a segmental pattern.

Strategic Considerations

Expanders are positioned in the subcutaneous fatty plane about 1 cm under the skin. When expanders are located just above the deep fascia in an obese patient, the unyielding tissue of fat and skin may be difficult to expand.

Expanded tissue may be more efficiently advanced in a transverse direction than with vertical movement. Two or more expansion processes may be re-

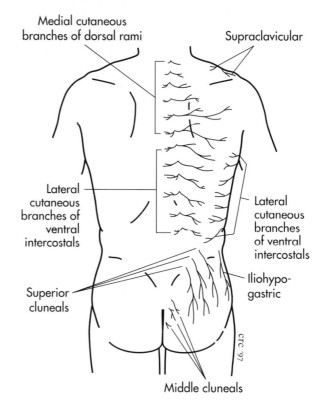

Figure 10-3 Cutaneous nerves of the back.

quired to cover a defect in a series of cephalad or caudad flap advancements. Reexpanded skin may appear thin and atrophic with a minimal subcutaneous fat cushion but an increased reactive hypervascularity.

Incisions 2 to 4 cm long may be hidden under the posterior axillary folds or between the intergluteal cleft. Long scissors, cutting suction devices, and elevators can facilitate dissection of the pockets for the expanders. If the defects are wide enough, an intralesional incision can be effectively used to dissect the pockets for balloon and valve placement.

Expander Selection

Round, rectangular, and crescent shapes may be effectively used to resurface defects on the back. These expanders are smooth-wall units with remote or incorporated valve systems.

Surgical Technique

After the lesion's configuration and the designated donor sites are determined, the expander units are outlined on the skin in relation to the defect. Locations of incisions are also marked to determine reasonable paths for dissection of the subcutaneous pockets. The skin is prepared with an antibiotic solution, and the tissues are infiltrated with large volumes of Xylocaine (0.5%) and epinephrine (1:400,000) to aid in dissection and improve hemostasis. The incision is made 1 cm into the subcutaneous layer, where soft tissue dissection forms a tunnel to the edge of the proposed implant pocket.

The tissues are elevated by blunt and cutting dissection according to the dimensions of the outlined implant. The partially filled, smooth-wall expander is inserted from the incision to the pocket with the help of a blunt-tipped, slightly curved, large, plastic Yankow suction device. The implant is filled further with methylene blue–colored bacitracin solution by inserting a 23-gauge scalp vein needle into the remote valve. The implant is manuevered into its final position by manual pressure. The remote valve is placed into its own pocket. The implant is then filled to tissue tolerance to decrease hematoma formation, reduce implant folds, maintain pocket size, and finally to test the system for imperfections and leaks.

Serial expansion is begun 1 to 2 weeks after insertion on a weekly or every-other-week basis. When sufficient tissue has been stretched (three times width of defect), the second stage of reconstruction is scheduled. At the final phase, capsulectomy and capsulotomies open the expanded flap to maximize tissue coverage. Subcutaneous fat under the defect is preserved and used as autogenous filler material to reduce the anticipated concave deformities from expansion. Any residual capsules, if present, should be at least scored with a cautery to permit closure of the new pocket and reduce the risk of pseudobursa formation. A surgical drain may be required to remove fluid after extensive tissue dissection and mobilization and to collapse the potential spaces.

Case Results

Since 1979 the author completed 31 expansions in the upper back and 29 in the lower back. The defects included scars, nevi, and unsightly skin grafts (Table 10-3). Thirty-seven percent of patients underwent two or more expansions because of the defect's size and the direction of flap advancement.

Complications of back reconstruction included minor difficulties (8%) and major problems (5%) that terminated the procedure (Table 10-4). The incidence of complications increased with expansion in children and in conditions that warranted multiple expansion procedures. Delayed changes in sensation and concave deformities were minimal and did not require corrective procedures. Scars were revised for hypertrophy and widening in about 10% of patients.

■ **Table 10-3** Types of Defects in 60 Back Reconstructions

Area/type	Number
Upper back	
Scar	15
Skin graft	5
Nevus	11
Lower back	
Scar	13
Skin graft	7
Nevus	9

■ **Table 10-4** Complications in 60 Back Reconstructions

Type	Number
Minor (8%)	
Implant failure	2
Balloon exposure	1
Dehiscence	2
Major (5%)	
Infection	2
Ischemia	1

CASE REPORT AND ANALYSIS: Back Reconstruction

Hypertrophic Burn Scar to Back, Shoulders, and Upper Extremities

History (Figure 10-4, *A*)

This 7-year-old patient sustained a flame burn injury to the upper half of his back, posterodorsal aspects of both brachia, left side of face, and left scalp at age 3. At age 6 the patient had the 3 × 5 cm skin graft on his midface replaced with normal skin and a 7 × 15 cm area of frontal temporoparietal alopecia replaced with hair-bearing tissue by the author using expansion techniques. After these procedures the patient wanted further reconstruction of burn scars on his body. The goals of surgery were to (1) excise the remaining scarred skin on his upper back and the posterodorsal areas of both upper extremities and (2) minimize the new scar lines.

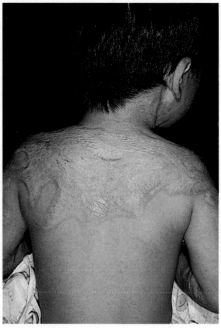

10-4A

Surgical Procedure (Figure 10-4, *B* to *G*)

A 1000 cc rectangular expander was inserted under uninvolved back skin below the 10 × 30 cm scarred scapular tissue. A 640 cc rectangular expander was placed under normal skin on the posterior aspect of each brachium from the elbow to the axilla adjacent to the 7 × 15 cm patch of scarred posterodorsal skin. All expanders were located in the subcutaneous fatty plane and were positioned through a 3.5 cm transverse incision at the top of the back scar. Each valve was placed under the scarred tissue on the back. Intraoperative filling of each expander lessened the chance for hematoma formation.

Serial expansion of each expander began 3 weeks after their insertion on a weekly basis for 4 months. A 20 cm hemispheric back flap was created to permit 10 cm of cephalad advancement to cover the 10 cm–wide scarred back skin. A 15 cm hemispheric brachial flap was generated on each extremity for 7.5 cm of advancement to replace the 7 cm–wide scarred patch. At surgery, intraoperative expansion of each expander gained 2 to 3 cm of tissue. Capsulectomies and base capsulotomies opened the flaps for maximal coverage. The scarred skin was de-epithelialized and used for soft tissue filling to minimize concavities.

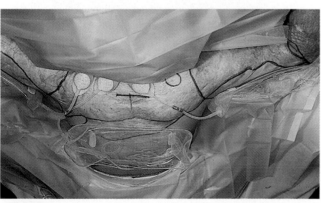

10-4B

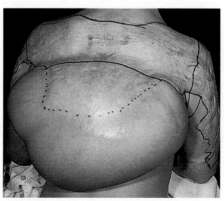

10-4C

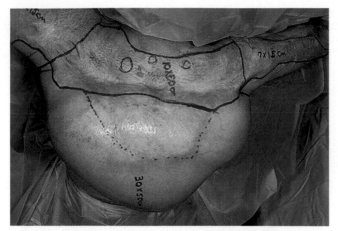

10-4D

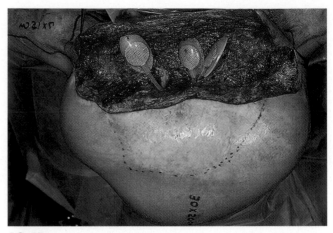

10-4E

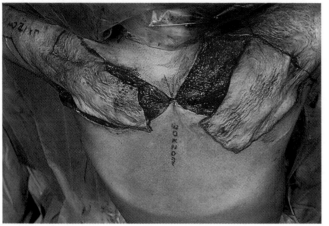

10-4F

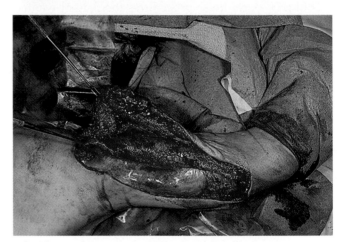

10-4G

Results (Figure 10-4, *H* and *I*)

The patient is shown 1 year after surgery with all the scarred tissue excised and replaced with supple normal skin. The scar lines of skin closure have matured and softened with the help of steroid-laden tapes. Skin sensation has slowly returned.

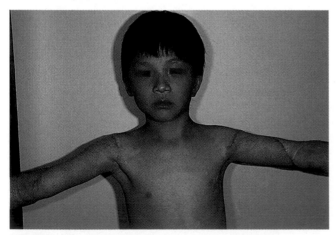

10-4H

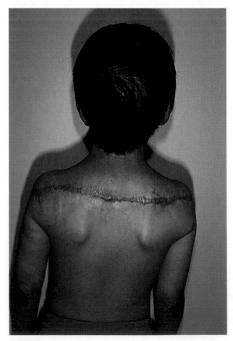

10-4I

CASE REPORT AND ANALYSIS: Combined Abdominal and Back Procedures

Congenital Giant Nevus on Abdomen, Back, and Buttock

History (Figure 10-5, *A* and *B*)
A 5-year-old patient had a congenital giant nevus that involved the left half of her abdomen with extension across her back and down to the left buttock. Because of the potential for malignant degeneration, a series of fractional expansion reductions were planned. The goals of surgery were to (1) excise the entire pigmented lesion; (2) preserve the anatomic relationships of the umbilicus, pubis and inguinal line, and buttock; and (3) minimize the surgical scars.

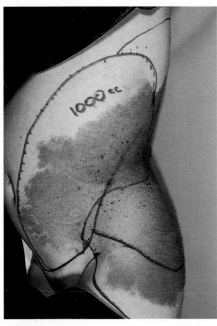

10-5A

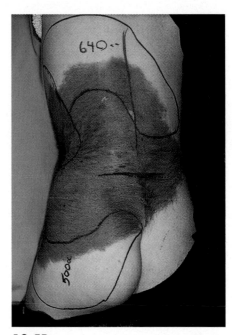

10-5B

First Surgical Procedure (Figure 10-5, *C* to *F*)
A 1000 cc rectangular expander was placed under the normal and involved skin of the left abdomen from the pubis, lateral to the umbilicus, and up to the side of the trunk. A 640 cc rectangular expander was positioned under the skin of the high back, across the midline, and down along the lateral extension of the nevus over the right back. A 500 cc crescent expander was positioned lateral to the groin line, under the skin of the upper lateral thigh, and across the upper half of the left buttock. All expanders were located in the subcutaneous fatty plane through a 3.5 cm incision within the nevus at the level of the superior iliac crest. The remote valves of the upper two expanders were under upper back skin, and the lower expander's valve was positioned under the midanterior thigh skin. Intraoperative filling with saline prevented hematoma formation.

Serial expansion was begun 3 weeks later on an every-other-week basis for 4 months until sufficient tissue was generated for the first reduction. Intraoperative expansion at surgery gained 2 to 3 cm of tissue. Capsulectomies of the hemispheric flaps along with base capsulotomies unfurled the tissue for maximal advancement. Strategic salvaging of the underlying subcutaneous fat aided in filling the depressed reconstructed areas.

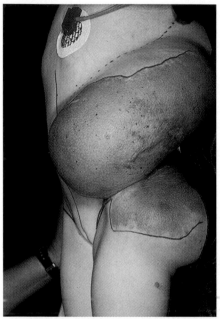

10-5C

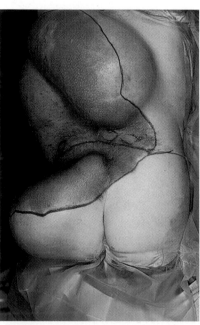

10-5D

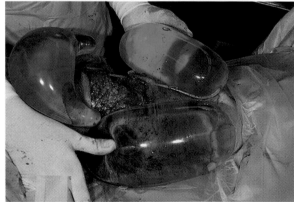

10-5E

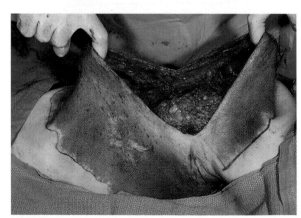

10-5F

Results (Figure 10-5, *G* and *H*)

About 70% of the nevus was removed with the first expansion process. Hypertrophic scars developed along the lines of closure. The umbilicus was temporarily displaced toward the left side of the abdomen.

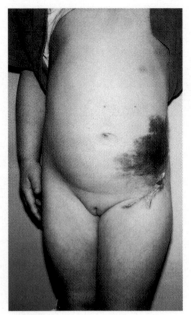

10-5G

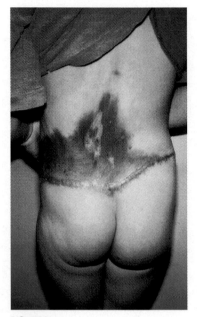

10-5H

Second Surgical Procedure (Figure 10-5, *I*)

About 6 months later, three tissue expanders of the same size and shape were reinserted through the same scar incision. Intraoperative filling of the expanders with saline prevented any hematoma formation.

Serial expansion continued for 3 months until sufficient tissue was obtained for completion of the reconstruction. Intraoperative expansion at surgery provided an additional 2 to 3 cm of flap for advancement. Capsulectomies, capsulotomies, and salvage of adipose tissue were done to maximize procedural effects.

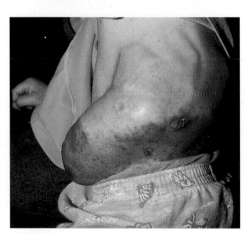

10-5I

Results (Figure 10-5, *J* and *K*)

The patient is shown about 1 year later with all the nevus removed. The umbilicus was relocated to its normal midline position. Slight scar hypertrophy has occurred, but maturation and softening of the scar are evident. The pubis, groin crease, and buttocks have been repositioned to their normal sites. Scar revisions may be attempted in the future after the patient completes her adolescent growth phase.

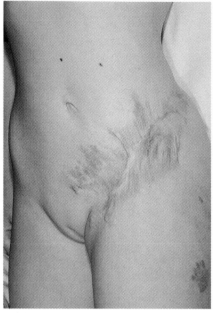

10-5J

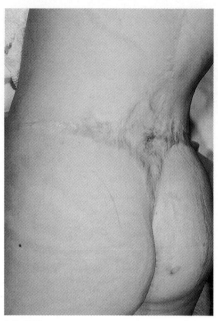

10-5K

11 Scrotal Reconstruction

The use of tissue expansion in male genital reconstruction is limited by the elastic and loose characteristics of the genital skin. Expansion of such donor skin is also difficult because of the special anatomic relationships of the penis and scrotum. Expansion of genital tissue may also be painful because of the sensitivity of the organs (Figure 11-1). The author has performed a single reconstruction of the scrotum after extensive loss of skin from Fournier's gangrene (see Case Report and Analysis).

Extensive necrotizing fasciitis from mixed aerobic and anaerobic organisms can lead to significant loss of skin and soft tissue in the scrotum, penis, and perineum. Debilitation, poor hygiene, diabetes mellitus, and local infections are predisposing factors that result in Fournier's gangrene. A repetitive series of débridements and translocation of the testes may be required to control the infection.

The author completed a successful scrotal reconstruction in two stages by elevating expanded skin flaps from the medial aspects of the thighs. The expanded skin maintained the form of a scrotal sac and contained the translocated testes. Although the expansion process was performed without infections to the expanders, the patient required pain medication during each filling period because of local pain.

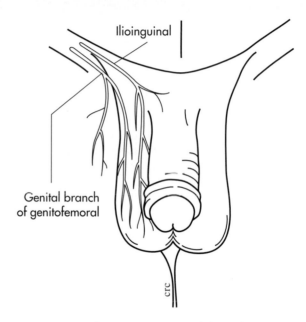

Figure 11-1 Cutaneous nerves of the male genitalia.

CASE REPORT AND ANALYSIS: Scrotal Reconstruction

CASE 1: Fournier's Gangrene

History (Figure 11-2, *A*)

This 27-year-old patient developed a mixed infection of his perineum and scrotum that resulted in loss of his scrotal, perineal, and groin tissue. The testes were translocated under tissue of the medial thighs. After multiple débridements, healing by secondary intention occurred. The patient requested scrotal reconstruction.

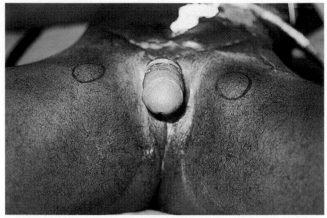

11-2A

First Surgical Procedure (Figure 11-2, *B*)

A 300 cc round expander was inserted under the skin of each medial thigh through a 2 cm incision. Serial expansions were performed over 6 weeks with saline injections of 20 to 25 ml weekly. The patient required sedation and pain medication at each filling period because of pressure pain. When 16 cm hemispheric flaps were obtained, the patient was returned to surgery for the final reconstruction.

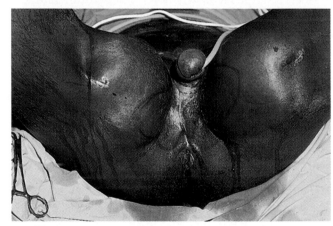

11-2B

Second Surgical Procedure (Figure 11-2, *C* and *D*)

The designed flaps were elevated after removal of the expanders. The testes were relocated from their thigh positions to the groin under the thinned-out flaps that were designed to form the scrotal sac. The donor thigh sites were approximated by primary closures.

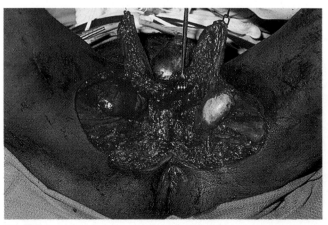

11-2C

11-2D

Result (Figure 11-2, *E* and *F*)
The patient is shown 4 weeks after completion of his reconstruction. The flaps resisted significant contrac-

tion with the testes in place. Sperm motility studies and counts were normal.

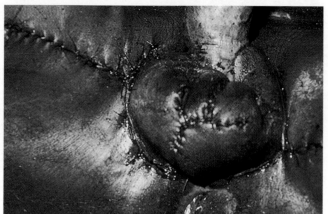

11-2E

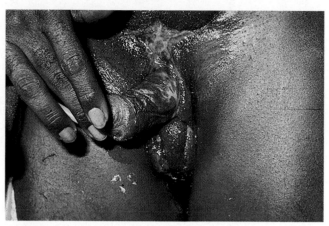

11-2F

12 Breast, Nipple, and Areolar Reconstruction

Current reconstruction of the postmastectomy deformity by tissue expansion technique culminates a series of evolutionary steps that has concentrated on expanding residual tissue to form a ptotic mound matching the opposite breast.[1-14] The temporary expander has been applied in a variety of postmastectomy, burn, and congenital defects[15] by stretching remaining chest wall tissue to a larger-than-desired size and then substituting it with a smaller implant.

During the formative years in tissue expansion technique, Radovan[1] and Lapin, Daniel, and Hutchins[2] performed delayed reconstructions of breast mounds with temporary expanders solely in the subcutaneous plane. The reconstructions initially were symmetric to the opposite breasts for at least the following three reasons:

1. The expansion site was controlled by locating the expander precisely at or above the preserved inframammary fold, which later provided a fulcrum for the creation of a pendulous mound.
2. Delayed reconstructions provided advantages over immediate reconstructions because (a) blood flow to the overlying skin flap was stable and (b) the axillary pocket had healed, thereby removing the possibility of lateral migration of the expander unit.
3. Expansion of chest wall skin was more effective than expansion of skin and muscle because of less tissue resistance to the stretching forces.

Unfortunately, a significant incidence of capsular contracture developed after insertion of the permanent implant in the subcutaneous plane.

The technique of tissue expansion was altered thereafter by inserting expanders under the submuscular plane.[3,5,6] The rationale for this location change was to permit the safe insertion of an expander at mastectomy. The muscle layer provided an additional protective barrier between the implant and the dissected skin flaps. Expander placement under both the pectoralis major muscle and the pectoralis minor–serratus anterior unit prevented lateral migration during the expansion phase. These maneuvers increased the safety and

efficacy of the expansion process. A major drawback of a submuscular expansion, however, remained its inability to yield consistently a natural-appearing breast reconstruction, despite variations in techniques to overcome this phenomenon, as discussed next.

EXPANSION TO MATCH OPPOSITE BREAST MOUND

Initial efforts at submuscular expansion of the new breast mound were performed until inspection determined close symmetry to the remaining breast. The expanded mound was then intentionally maintained in that state for up to 3 months with the hope that minimal tissue contraction would occur after the exchange procedure. Such efforts universally resulted in the development of a hemispheric mound without significant ptosis.

Overexpansion Technique

Overexpansion of tissue beyond the opposite breast's volume was attempted next to counter the stretchback phenomenon[16] observed after expansion. Again the results were disappointing, because hyperexpansion of tissue did not translate into lax tissue to provide ptosis.

Releasing Procedures of Pectoralis Major Muscle

The unyielding nature of the muscular plane limited the expansion process and also contributed to the stretchback phenomenon. Thus attempts to detach the muscle's lower costal origins and extend the plane beneath the rectus abdominis fascia usually resulted in a larger, softer, and more normally positioned mound.[8] These improvements were largely nullified, however, by the eventual appearance of a hemispheric mound without the benefit of a defined inframammary fold.

Creation of Inframammary Fold

Finally, an inframammary fold was created to produce a stable fulcrum from which the reconstructed mound could descend. The new inframammary fold was constructed through an external incision that permitted cephalad advancement and fixation of a crescent of de-epithelialized upper abdominal skin to the rib periosteum along the new fold.[17,18] A new fold could also be formed by an internal approach that mobilized the epigastric skin down to the umbilical level and then advanced and fixed the dermis by sutures to the rib periosteum along the new fold.[12] These additional techniques occasionally produced the appearance of a ptotic mound, but the results were unpredictable.

CONSERVATION MASTECTOMIES

The current concept of conservation mastectomies recommends complete tumor extirpation while preserving as much skin and breast tissue as possible to avoid mutilation. This surgery has been referred to as a *segmental mastectomy, partial mastectomy, lumpectomy,* or *tylectomy.* When the volume of breast tissue removed is insignificant, insertion of an expander or permanent alloplastic implant would be unnecessary to enhance the reconstruction.

Since conservation mastectomies are followed by radiation therapy to assist in sterilizing the field of residual local and multicentric cancer, the healing of the reconstructive site remains a concern. Radiation produces sufficient fibrosis that jeopardizes the softness and contour of the breast mound. Radiation injury also compromises the skin's ability to resist bouts of cellulitis or breakdown.

If an alloplastic permanent breast implant or a tissue expander is required to correct tissue shortage after a conservation mastectomy, the addition of radiation therapy will complicate the reconstructive efforts. Radiated tissue resists the forces of expansion. Premature loss of the expander may occur either from skin breakdown with expander exposure or from a periprosthetic infection. After insertion of the permanent implant, progressive scar contracture, malformation, mound displacement, implant exposure, and infection may be observed in the immediate or late follow-up period. The use of autogenous nonradiated tissue with the transverse rectus abdominis myocutaneous flap or microsurgical transfer of composite tissue transplantation may provide more acceptable aesthetic results than those obtained by expansion surgery.

This chapter outlines a predictable method for reconstruction of a ptotic breast mound by expansion technique. The approach integrates the advantageous aspects of the procedures just discussed. After a natural mound is achieved, alternative methods for nipple and areolar reconstruction are offered to the patient to complete the goals of breast reconstruction.

PREOPERATIVE ASSESSMENT

After needle or open biopsy indicates a diagnosis of breast cancer, the patient may request a consultation with the reconstructive surgeon, who discusses the different types of surgical procedures available. The surgeon then specifies those most suitable to the patient's desires, technical considerations, and donor sites, based on the patient's history, mammographic and sonographic findings, tumor pathology, and physical examination.

Management of the uninvolved breast focuses on premalignant changes, de novo development of breast cancer, and asymmetry to the reconstructed breast mound. A subcutaneous mastectomy may be suggested for premalignant findings, while a simple mastectomy would be recommended for in situ cancer. Asymmetric findings may be corrected by performing an augmentation mammoplasty, mastopexy, or reduction procedure on the uninvolved breast.

History

A strong family history of breast cancer (mother, sister) or "premalignant" changes of severe breast dysplasia in the patient increase the risk of cancer in the contralateral breast. The patient may consider a prophylactic subcutaneous mastectomy or conservative parenchymal mastectomy. Reconstruction of that breast can be performed by the insertion of an alloplastic implant under the pectoralis muscle with or without a skin-tightening procedure (Figure 12-1). Since the remaining breast skin brassiere (tissue covering) is not deficient, staged tissue expansion would not play a significant role in these cases.

Mammographic and Sonographic Findings

Abnormal mammographic and sonographic findings of a solid mass or clustered microcalcifications in either breast are indications for tissue biopsy. A diagnosis of breast cancer may be managed by lumpectomy and radiation therapy, simple mastectomy, or a modified radical mastectomy, depending on the stage of disease found in the specimen. A subcutaneous mastectomy is indicated whenever severe dysplastic changes are observed on biopsy. A prophylactic mastectomy may be more urgent when these findings are associated with a breast that is difficult to assess by physical examination (large, multinodular, fibrous breast) or mammography (radiodense tissue).

Tissue expansion plays an insignificant role in patients whose retained skin brassiere, including areola,

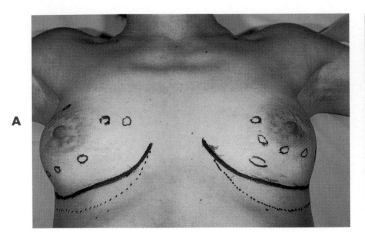

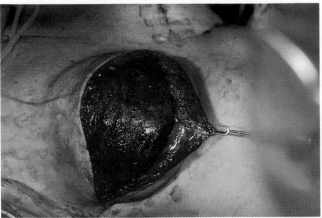

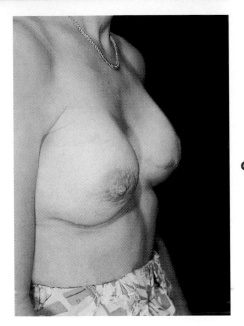

Figure 12-1 A, This 35-year-old patient had multinodular fibrocystic disease in both breasts. The number, size, and density of the nodules complicated ultrasonographic and mammographic interpretation. Since the patient's mother developed an invasive ductular carcinoma at age 53, prophylactic subcutaneous mastectomies were recommended. **B,** Through an inframammary approach, a total glandular mastectomy was performed with preservation of the nipple-areolar complex. A primary reconstruction was performed with insertion of a textured gel implant under the pectoralis major muscle. **C,** An acceptable ptotic breast resulted because no change occurred in the skin brassiere (breast covering).

has not been removed. If removal of the nipple along with the glandular tissue is required, the dimensions of the skin brassiere essentially remain intact. A permanent implant is positioned under the pectoralis major muscle (see Figure 12-1).

Tumor Pathology

The information from the previous biopsy provides the patient with the type of cancer (ductal vs. lobular), stage of invasion (in situ, invasive), stage of involvement (intralymphatic, intravascular, perineural, or intramuscular invasion), and degree of local dysplasia. These findings significantly influence the management protocol for this patient, which may include partial mastectomy, complete mastectomy (simple, modified, or radical), radiation therapy or chemotherapy/immunotherapy, and surgical treatment to the uninvolved breast (mirror-image or mammographically directed biopsy, prophylactic mastectomy). The surgeon's role is to delineate the types of reconstructions

recommended for the involved breast and the opposite side.

Physical Examination

Physical examination of a breast that has undergone a needle or open biopsy still assesses the essentials of an untouched mound, which is mostly symmetric to the contralateral side. The components include soft and ample skin coverage, symmetrically positioned nipple-areolar complex, projecting parenchymal mound, and functioning pectoralis major and minor muscles, which, along with fat, contribute to the formation of the infraclavicular fill, anterior axillary fold, and inframammary fold.

By virtue of a subcutaneous mastectomy, partial mastectomy (lumpectomy), or total mastectomy (modified, radical), the patient will sustain a variable loss of tissue on one side. The reconstructive surgeon's experience can closely predict the amount and distribution of tissue loss anticipated from each of these surgical

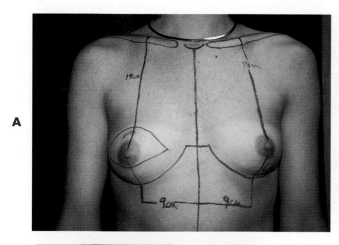

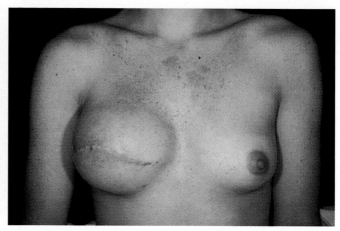

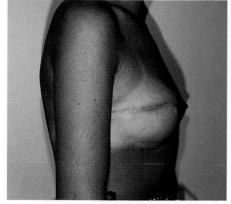

Figure 12-2 A, This 33-year-old patient underwent a right breast biopsy that revealed invasive ductular carcinoma. The 3 cm incision site was located at the 11- to 12-o'clock position. A modified radical mastectomy was planned through a 7 × 12 cm elliptic skin excision that included the nipple-areolar complex and the biopsy skin site and represented about 50% of the skin brassiere. **B,** Tissue expansion was required for 3 months to replace the amount of skin removed from an A-cup breast mound. **C,** At the second stage the expander was exchanged for a permanent, textured gel implant.

procedures. When this information is subtracted from the anatomic measurements of the biopsied breast (see later section on anatomic assessment), the surgeon should be able to give the patient an approximation of the final tissue losses and identify the reconstructive procedures to correct them.

In a patient scheduled for a subcutaneous mastectomy, for example, the replacement fill could be either a submuscular implant or an autogenous fill from a de-epithelialized transverse rectus abdominis flap. If a patient is to have a lumpectomy and radiation therapy, the anticipated loss of parenchyma and skin may be minimal, thus avoiding any need to replace them. The amount of tissue loss from these procedures contrasts sharply to that from a modified radical or radical mastectomy.

In a small-breasted patient scheduled for a modified radical mastectomy, the area of remaining skin may be tight when the biopsied skin incision site is removed in continuity with the nipple-areolar complex (Figure 12-2). This contrasts with a large-breasted patient scheduled for a similar surgical procedure, who is left with an ample skin brassiere (Figure 12-3). The former patient may be a suitable candidate for tissue expansion or flap replacement, whereas the latter may require only implant insertion. Usually the infraclavicular fill, anterior axillary

fold, and inframammary fold are intact after a modified radical mastectomy. The axillary hollowness from node dissection may be corrected with autogenous fill from a flap. The nipple-areolar complex may be reconstructed later.

After a radical mastectomy the reconstructive surgeon may need to create the axillary and infraclavicular fill (removal of fat, lymph glands, and pectoralis major muscle), axillary and inframammary folds, and skin and parenchymal tissue. The nipple-areolar complex may be replaced by a secondary procedure. These patients are usually candidates for a flap procedure (transverse rectus abdominis or latissimus dorsi myocutaneous flap) with or without an implant.

Indications for Tissue Expansion

The primary indication for breast reconstruction by tissue expansion is a chest wall with quantitatively insufficient but qualitatively adequate tissue. Usually these patients have intact pectoralis major, pectoralis minor, and serratus anterior muscles with sufficient infraclavicular fill. Tissue expansion is best indicated for construction of a small to medium-sized breast mound that lacks significant ptosis.

Secondary indications for expansion surgery may involve (1) patient preference in using only the chest

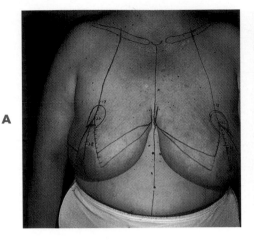

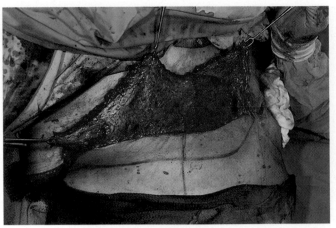

Figure 12-3 **A,** This 44-year-old patient was scheduled for bilateral modified mastectomies for invasive ductular carcinomas. The mastectomies were performed through a Wise pattern to remove the nipple-areolar complexes and to tighten the skin brassieres. **B,** Large dermal flaps were created from the inferior skin flaps. These flaps were sutured to the inferior edges of the pectoralis major muscles to provide a dermal sling. This extra tissue created a ptotic breast mound to support the textured adjustable saline-gel implants. **C,** The ptotic breast mounds underwent nipple-areolar reconstructions with the insertion of silicone implants (see section on nipple-areolar reconstruction). Intradermal tattooing was performed 3 months later.

wall tissue for the reconstruction and (2) inadequate or compromised distant donor sites. The transfer of distant tissues, such as the latissimus dorsi or transverse rectus abdominis myocutaneous flaps, is indicated in patients whose chest wall tissues are of poor quality and insufficient quantity, such as those covered by skin grafts or extensively damaged by radiotherapy. Distant flaps may also provide tissue for filling the skeletonized axilla, reconstructing the anterior axillary fold, correcting the infraclavicular hollow, and replacing insufficient pectoralis muscle coverage.

Advantages

The advantages of tissue expansion surgery include the following:

1. The surgical procedure is confined to the anterior chest wall and obviates the creation of additional distant donor site scars and morbidity (e.g., changes in adduction strength to the shoulder and flexion strength to the abdomen, potential formation of abdominal hernias).
2. The reconstructed tissue closely matches the rest of the chest wall in regard to color, texture, hair distribution, and sensation.
3. As a two-stage procedure, expansion surgery provides greater latitude in the size and shape of the re-

constructed breast, because the expansion volume can be adjusted to the proposed permanent implant volume that will achieve symmetry to the opposite breast.
4. In general, expansion surgery represents less surgical time, anesthesia, hospital stay, and potential flap complications compared with distant flap surgery.

Disadvantages

The disadvantages of expansion surgery involve foreign body complications during the insertion and reconstruction phases. These occur with a permanent implant during latissimus dorsi myocutaneous flap reconstruction but not with reconstructions using autogenous tissues during a transverse rectus abdominis myocutaneous flap. Disadvantages include the following:

1. Exposure of a silicone expander may result in infection if skin flap necrosis occurs immediately after a primary reconstruction. Skin ischemia from dissected flaps is more likely to occur after a mastectomy than during expander insertion under established tissue at a delayed reconstruction.
2. Exposure and infection of the expander or permanent implant may occur from dehiscence at the suture line. These complications may also develop

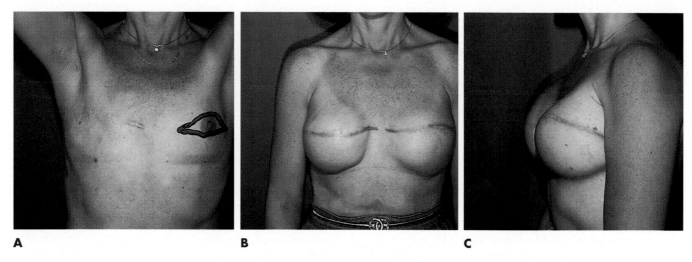

A   **B**   **C**

Figure 12-4 **A,** This 46-year old patient is scheduled for a left modified radical mastectomy for invasive ductular carcinoma. The nodule is located at the 3-o'clock position about 2 cm from the areolar border. A conservative skin excision is outlined and includes the nipple-areolar complex (2.5 cm diameter) and the skin biopsy site. The patient had undergone 2 years of chemotherapy before a standard radical mastectomy on her right breast. **B** and **C,** In the first stage the right mound was reconstructed after 4 months of expansion (600 cc expander) under the pectoralis muscle. In the second stage the Shoji skin-muscle technique along with recreation of the inframammary fold produced a ptotic breast mound. In contrast, the left breast underwent a primary reconstruction with the insertion of a 450 cc smooth-wall gel implant under the pectoralis major and minor and anterior serratus muscle flap. Since a minimal amount of the skin brassiere was excised, expansion of the remaining tissue was not necessary.

with a permanent implant using a latissimus dorsi myocutaneous flap reconstruction.

3. Expander and permanent implant failures and malpositions are always a concern when a reconstructive procedure involves a silicone prosthesis.

4. Multiple sessions to fill an expander or adjust filling of a permanent implant (if a removable reservoir and tubing are an integral part of the prosthesis) are required in the two-stage expansion procedure. Percutaneous needle sticks increase the potential for periprosthetic infections because of a break in sterile or aseptic technique.

5. Capsular contracture may mar the benefits of a fill with a permanent silicone implant.

6. Tissue expansion surgery may not succeed in providing either a ptotic mound or a large breast to match the contralateral side. As previously mentioned, expansion surgery does not provide tissue for reconstruction of a deficient infraclavicular fill, absent axillary fold, or malformed lateral axilla.

SURGICAL TECHNIQUE

The key element in the reconstruction of a deformed or absent breast mound is the *maximal preservation or restoration of the original skin envelope,* which once fell gracefully from the clavicle to the nipple and continued downward with a generous undercupping to the stable inframammary line. When adequate skin is present, the skilled surgeon can shape the skin into a ptotic mound that can drape over an anatomically shaped implant. The addition of a projected nipple

and areolar component completes the aesthetic conization of the reconstructed ptotic mound. Secondary restored features may include a straight anterior slope and a symmetric axillary fold and hollow.

Use of a tissue expander to gain extra tissue implies not only that a skin shortage exists, but also that a need exists for functioning pectoralis major, pectoralis minor, and serratus anterior muscles. The introduction of a "foreign body" silicone expander emphasizes the requirement for muscle coverage to protect the prosthesis from exposure and control its position during and after expansion. The provision of these two key elements (adequate skin and muscle) forms the basis of expansion reconstruction. If a significant amount of the original skin envelope can be preserved by the oncologic surgeon (conservation skin-removal mastectomies), the shape of the final breast mound should be almost identical to the opposite side (Figure 12-4). The challenge of expansion surgery therefore is creating a symmetric mound in tissue deficient cases. A systematic approach provides greater control of surgical and tissue variables, which in turn should result in a more predictable result.

STAGE I

Anatomic Assessment
(Figure 12-5, *A*)

In most clinical situations the surgeon has the diseased breast (primary reconstruction) or the opposite normal breast (delayed reconstruction) available to serve as a template model. The dimensions of the newly reconstructed breast are derived from measurements taken from the uninvolved breast (Figure 12-5, *B*). The author has used these anatomic measurements since 1979 to assess the preoperative dimensions of the breast, to assist in determining the end points of the expansion process, and to aid in the final stage of surgically defining the symmetric dimensions of the newly reconstructed breast mound.

The necessary equipment to standardize and identify the anatomic landmarks include various measuring devices (Figure 12-6). To duplicate the shape and length of the inframammary fold, a malleable draftsman's ruler is bent to conform to the uninvolved fold. The outline of the curved ruler is traced on unexposed radiographic film, which is then reflected as a replicate for the mastectomy site (Figure 12-7).

The relevant breast measurements that guide the reconstructive surgeon include the following:

> **AC** Breast position
> **DCE** Inframammary line
> **ABC** Vertical meridian line
> **DBE** Transverse breast line
> **CG** Nipple-midsternal line
> **HBC** Vertical breast line
> **DHE** Superior parenchymal line

Breast Position

The breast position (AC) on the chest wall can be determined relative to the midclavicular point (A) and the inframammary fold line (C). This distance is best measured with an obstetric caliper.

Inframammary Line

The inframammary fold line represents the neck or fulcrum of the ptotic breast mound. This fixed line or fold is a critical structure in breast reconstruction. It should be either preserved during the mastectomy procedure or restored at the reconstruction phase to produce a ptotic or drooping breast mound. The inferior edge of the tissue expander is located at or slightly below the inframammary line to mimic the length and curvature of the breast neck during the expansion phase. The inframammary line (DCE) begins at a medial point (E), usually 1 to 2 cm from the midsternal line. The closer and higher (cephalad) point E is to the parasternum, the greater the degree of cleavage created. Laterally the inframammary line divides at its *splay point* (D) into the upwardly directed lateral breast curve and the posteriorly directed brassiere line.

Vertical Meridian Line

The vertical meridian line (ABC) represents the length of drooping or ptosis of the breast, as measured downward from the midclavicular point (A), across the nipple (B), and to the inframammary line (C). The dimensions of this line become one of the most significant parameters to follow during the expansion process. Expansion is usually terminated when the meridian line on the reconstructed side is 2 to 3 cm longer than that on the normal side. This extra length compensates for skin contraction once the expander is removed.

The meridian line is further divided into an upper segment (AB) from the midclavicle to the nipple and a

Figure 12-5 **A,** Cutaneous nerves of the breast. **B,** Dimensional profile of the normal breast delineates measurements that should be achieved on the mastectomy side during the expansion and reconstructive phases.

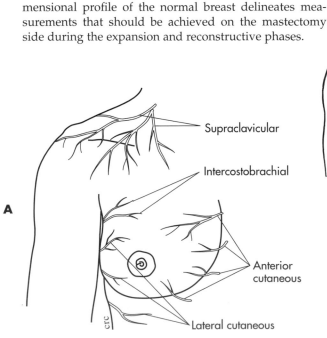

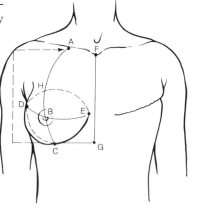

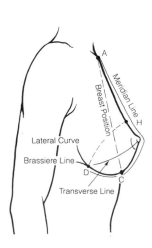

BREAST POSITION (AC) = Level of breast
INFRAMAMMARY LINE (DCE) = Fulcrum neck
   Medial Point (E)
   Lateral Splay Point (D) - Divided into Lateral Breast Curve and Brassiere Line
MERIDIAN LINE (ABC) = Degree of ptosis
   Mid-clavicle to nipple (AB)
   Nipple to inframammary point (BC)
TRANSVERSE BREAST LINE (DBE) = Degree of projection
NIPPLE-MIDSTERNAL LINE (CG) = Nipple position
BREAST SKIN HEIGHT (HBC) = Breast height
SUPERIOR PARENCHYMAL LINE (DHE) = Upper limits of breast

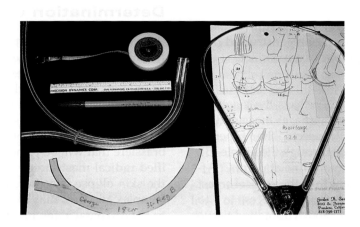

Figure 12-6 Devices such as the tape measure, straight ruler, and obstetric caliper *(right)* are useful to record the normal and mastectomized anatomic landmarks (see Figure 12-5, *B*). A malleable draftsman's ruler, shown below the marking pen, can duplicate the normal inframammary fold outlined on radiographic film.

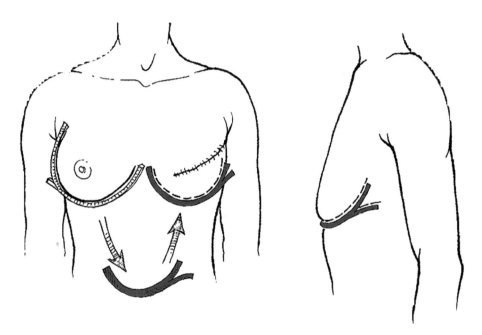

Figure 12-7 Film template is reversed on the reconstructed site and traced to recreate the outline of the new inframammary fold. Internal suture fixations to the undersurface of the dermis along the designated fold will recreate the fulcrum of the reconstructed ptotic breast mound (see section on inframammary line).

lower segment (BC) from the nipple to the inframammary line. This lower segment is accentuated during expansion to produce more undercupping for the reconstructed mound.

Transverse Breast Line

The length of the transverse breast line (DBE) represents the amount of breast projection. The longer its distance, the larger may be the volume of the inserted implant. The transverse breast line extends from the splay point D, through the nipple (B), and to the medial point E on the inframammary line.

Nipple-Midsternal Line

The nipple position is located not only on the meridian line but also from its lateral distance from the midsternal line (CG). An additional horizontal line (BE) from the medial point (E) on the inframammary line to the nipple (B) represents another reference landmark. In the last stages of reconstruction, these measurements ensure an approximate visualization of the reconstructed nipple-areolar complex on the new breast mound. In practical terms, however, nipple-areolar position is optimally located on the apex of the reconstructed mound and slightly higher (1 cm) than the contralateral complex. This location represents a

surgery or adjusted after surgery by filling or removing saline through a percutaneous needle stick into the buried remote valve system. The author prefers this type of implant to obtain optimal softness, smoothness, and projection of the implant.

Moderate or Significant Skin Loss

In patients with anticipated moderate (15% to 30%) or significant (more than 30%) skin loss after mastectomy, a tissue expander is necessary to restore lost skin. The technique for insertion of a tissue expander depends on whether a primary or delayed reconstruction is performed.

In a primary reconstruction the expander is inserted completely under the pectoralis major muscle and the mobilized pectoralis minor–serratus muscle flap (Figure 12-10). The surgical approach and dissection are identical to those used when a permanent implant is positioned under complete muscle coverage in patients with modest skin shortage. The expander must be localized under tissue that will directly contribute to the developing breast mound. The expander must be prevented from migrating toward the lateral gutter and upward into the axillary apex or infraclavicular region of the chest wall.

In a delayed reconstruction the lateral aspect of the mastectomy scar is opened 2.5 to 3 cm (Fig-

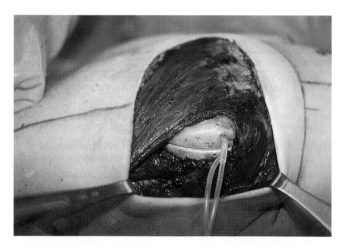

Figure 12-10 In this immediate reconstruction a double-lumen tissue expander with remote valves has been inserted under the elevated pectoralis major muscle. The pectoralis minor–serratus anterior muscle flap has been mobilized laterally to the desired extent of the expander pocket. The medial edge of this combined muscle flap is approximated to the lateral border of the pectoralis major muscle to contain the expander completely under a muscular plane. The expander is prevented from entering the exposed lateral gutter of the axillary dissection by its muscular containment. Since each compartment of this expander can be separately filled through its own valve system, an effective differential expansion of tissue is possible. However, the potential for implant complications is doubled with this type of expander unit.

ure 12-11). The lateral border of the pectoralis muscle is elevated under direct vision or endoscopic control. The subpectoral pocket is developed in the parasternal area with release of the pectoralis muscle from its origins on the fourth to sixth ribs. The pocket is dissected downward under the distal extensions of the pectoralis major fascia to a level 1 to 2 cm below the inframammary fold. It is not necessary to elevate the pectoralis minor–serratus anterior muscle flap because the lateral gutter is closed. The expander is inserted into this surgically defined space, whose lower half consists of pectoralis fascia, subcutaneous fat, and skin. Intraoperative expander filling with saline is performed to tissue tension to encourage hemostasis, maintain the pocket size, reduce implant folds, and begin the tissue stretching process (Figure 12-12).

Selection of Tissue Expander. The surgeon may select from various tissue expanders, all of which are capable of stretching sufficient amounts of tissue. For example, expanders may be constructed with a smooth or textured surface, an incorporated or remote valve system, and a round or anatomical shape. The author prefers an anatomically shaped, textured expander with an incorporated valve (Figure 12-12) for the following reasons:

1. A textured-surface expander may facilitate relative immobility of the implant in its pocket (deterring lateral migration) and creation of a thinner capsule (encouraging stretching).
2. An incorporated valve reduces the risk of potential problems that can occur with a remote system. Re-

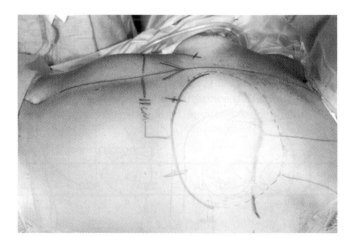

Figure 12-11 In this delayed reconstruction the anatomic breast markings are outlined on both sides. Expander dimensions and location are drawn on the skin. The access incision is located on the previous mastectomy scar beyond the lateral extent of the expander pocket to reduce the chance for implant exposure postoperatively. In most cases the incision length can be limited to 2.5 to 3 cm, which provides adequate access for pocket dissection.

mote valves may overturn, become inaccessible to needle penetration, separate from their tubing, or leak from vulnerable sites in their construction. However, inadvertent injury to the main expander unit may occur during needle puncture into the soft spot on the incorporated valve.

3. An anatomically shaped expander tends to stretch differentially the lower hemisphere of the developing breast mound more than the tissue in its upper pole. Although this maneuver may contribute extra tissue for a ptotic mound, the surgeon will be more successful in achieving this goal by defining the inframammary fold and surgically releasing restrictive tissue layers in the lower hemisphere of the reconstructed breast (see following discussion).

Filling of Expander.   In the immediate postoperative period the tissues are allowed to recover from surgical trauma. Expansion may begin about 3 weeks after insertion. Initially, larger saline volumes are injected weekly until tissue resistance is encountered. At that point the amount of saline injected is based on patient (pain) and tissue (pallor) tolerance. Preparation for saline injection uses aseptic technique, with Betadine, sterile gloves and saline, 23-gauge scalp vein needle, and 30 cc (ml) syringe.

Duration of Expansion.   The duration of expansion should be less for patients with moderate skin loss and longer for those with significant skin removal. The anatomically shaped expander is kept filled for

about 3 months to permit the overlying tissue to accommodate to the unit's contour and to resist contraction forces. The best criterion to determine the end point of expansion is not the final fill volume but the length of the vertical meridian line (Figure 12-13). This line should be at least 2 cm longer than the opposite uninvolved side. This extended length is necessary to compensate for the anticipated degree of tissue contraction after expander removal.

STAGE II

After expansion is completed in patients with moderate and significant skin loss, measurements of the reconstructed and uninvolved breast profiles are recorded, as described earlier. These dimensions help guide the surgeon to achieve a well-proportioned mound and symmetric match. At surgery, intraoperative balloon expansion further stretches the tissue before balloon removal. The expander is filled to maximal tissue tolerance (skin pallor) to gain a small amount of tissue to resist tissue contraction.

Shoji Technique: Creation of a Ptotic Mound

The entire length of the previous mastectomy scar is incised down to the pectoralis major muscle (the muscle fascia probably was removed during the mastectomy). The oncologic surgeon should have retained as

A
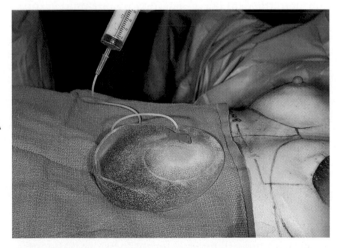

B
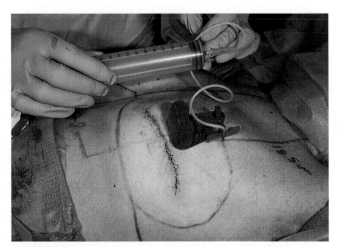

Figure 12-12   **A,** Anatomically shaped textured tissue expander with an incorporated valve for a patient undergoing a delayed breast reconstruction. The expander is being filled with saline through a 23-gauge scalp vein needle inserted into the metallic valve. The saline is colored with methylene blue dye to detect any holes within the implant. The expander's textured surface immobilizes the expander within its muscular pocket and also promotes formation of a thinner capsule. **B,** After the expander is inserted under its muscular coverage, the site of the implant's metallic valve is located and marked on the skin with the magnetic valve finder. The "sweet spot" on the valve is percutaneously entered with a scalp vein. The expander is filled with saline to tissue tolerance to reduce hematoma formation, maintain pocket size, assist in immediate tissue stretching, and elevate the access valve closer to the skin. The initial 2.5 cm lateral incision was lengthened along the previous mastectomy scar line because significant fibrous tissue was encountered. In most delayed reconstruction cases a limited lateral incision (2.5 to 3 cm) provides adequate access for the subpectoral dissection.

A
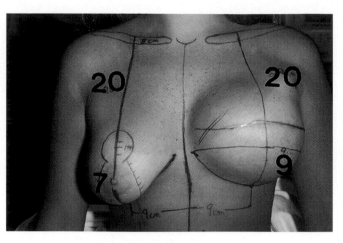
B

Figure 12-13 **A,** This 34-year-old patient underwent a left radical mastectomy for invasive colloidal carcinoma. A delayed reconstruction will use a 600 cc incorporated-valve expander positioned under the subpectoral plane through a 2.5 cm lateral incision (see Figure 12-11). **B,** After 3 months of expansion the vertical meridian line measured 29 cm from the midclavicle to the inframammary fold. At the second stage of reconstruction a mastopexy design was drawn on the right breast. The vertical meridian line measured 20 cm from the midclavicle to the proposed new position of the nipple. The distance along the vertical meridian line measured 7 cm from the nipple to the inframammary fold. The reconstructed breast mound was expanded about 2 cm more (29 cm) than the combined vertical meridian distance (27 cm) on the corrected ptotic right breast. This overexpansion was performed to account for an unknown degree of tissue contraction after expander removal.

much fat (not strands of breast tissue) as possible under the skin during the mastectomy. Preservation of maximal adipose tissue, consistent with the criteria for a complete mastectomy, should be discussed with the oncologic surgeon before expansion surgery to enhance the reconstructive results. Since tissue expansion always reduces adipose tissue from compression hypoxia, a compromise exists regarding final mound softness and contour and a skate-flap type of nipple reconstruction (see later discussion).

The cephalic skin-fat flap is elevated by cautery from the incision's level to the expander's superior margin (Figure 12-14, *A*). Further suprapectoral dissection may be done below the infraclavicular level to free tissue for skin-draping enhancement of the lower reconstructed mound. The caudal skin-fat flap is similarly elevated from the mastectomy incision down to the level of the inframammary fold (Figure 12-14, *B*).

In primary reconstructions, dissection is performed above both the extended fascia of the pectoralis major muscle and the pectoralis minor–serratus muscle flap, temporarily leaving the capsule intact over the expander's inferior half. In delayed reconstructions, when no attempt was made to cover the inferior half with this muscle flap, the caudal flap is raised off the inferior border of the pectoralis major muscle and the expander's capsule down to the level of the inframammary fold.

Next an incision is made along the entire inferior border of the pectoralis major muscle through the capsule of the expander, freeing its connection to the inferior layer consisting of capsule and extended fascial sheets (Figure 12-14, *C* and *D*). This inferior layer may

be considered a physical restraint that prevents the creation of adequate undercupping and ptosis to the breast profile. The author prefers excision, rather than multiple capsulotomies, of this unfurled "scar" capsule to ensure skin contouring to the shape of the permanent implant.

A subpectoral base and/or dome capsulotomy is usually performed to encourage downward muscle draping over the permanent implant. At times a subpectoral capsulectomy may be necessary to unfurl the restricting contour of the capsule that surrounded the expander. These surgical maneuvers permit maximal draping of tissue over the implant. In so doing, three flaps are created: cephalic skin-fat flap, pectoralis major muscle flap, and caudal skin-fat flap (Figure 12-14, *E* and *F*).

Re-creation of Inframammary Line

Since 1979 an internal suture technique has evolved to define the inframammary fulcrum, over which the ptotic mound droops. The author prefers this internal approach rather than an external incision at the inframammary line to which the upper abdominal tissue is advanced. Disadvantages of the external method include an additional scar, distortion, and another possible source for a suture line or implant infection.

To create a natural fold, 10 to 12 O-proline sutures are individually placed into the dermis outlining the inframammary line, starting from its medial point to its lateral splay point (Figure 12-14, *G* and *H*). Each suture is secured to the capsular floor, forming skin dimples about 1 cm apart that will disappear within 3 months.

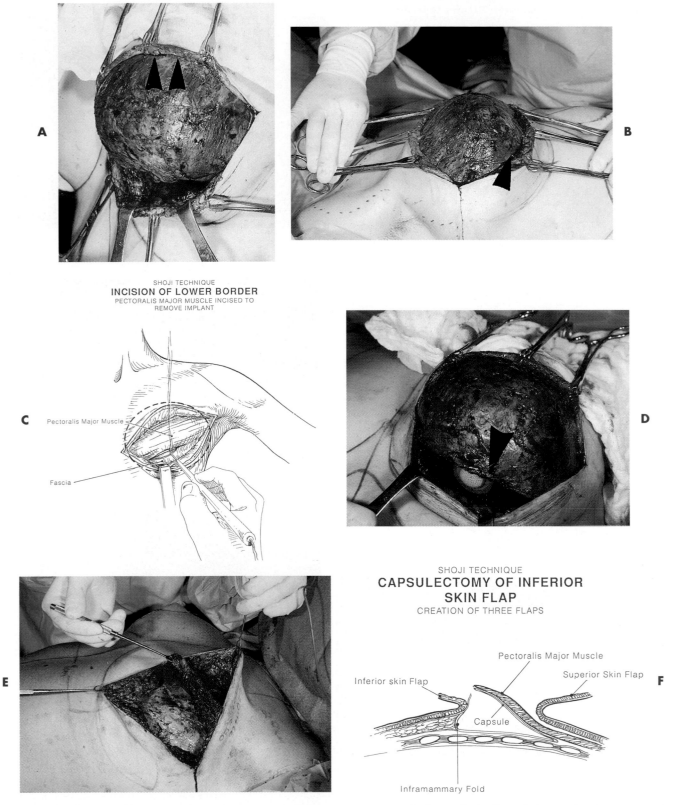

SHOJI TECHNIQUE
INCISION OF LOWER BORDER
PECTORALIS MAJOR MUSCLE INCISED TO
REMOVE IMPLANT

Pectoralis Major Muscle

Fascia

SHOJI TECHNIQUE
**CAPSULECTOMY OF INFERIOR
SKIN FLAP**
CREATION OF THREE FLAPS

Pectoralis Major Muscle

Inferior skin Flap

Superior Skin Flap

Capsule

Inframammary Fold

Figure 12-14 **A,** After the entire transverse mastectomy scar is reopened, the cephalic flap of skin and subcutaneous fat *(arrows)* is elevated off the pectoralis major muscle. The dissection is performed at least to the expander's superior border but often continues upward to a level below the inferior clavicular border. **B,** When a primary reconstruction was performed, the caudal flap *(arrow)* is raised off the inferior aspect of the pectoralis major muscle and the continuation of the capsule down to the level of the inframammary fold. Laterally the flap is elevated from the pectoralis minor–anterior serratus muscle coverage, following the expander's curvature. **C** and **D,** Expander capsule and extended pectoralis major fascia (if present) are transected with a cutting cautery, allowing the expander to be removed from its pocket. After this inferior capsule is excised, minimal restrictive tissue is present in the lower hemispheric skin flap. A dome capsulectomy and base capsulotomy unfurl the muscle flap so it can drape over the permanent implant. **E** and **F,** These surgical maneuvers have created three flaps: a cephalic skin-fat flap, muscle flap, and caudal skin-fat flap that has been freed of its restraining capsule.
Continued

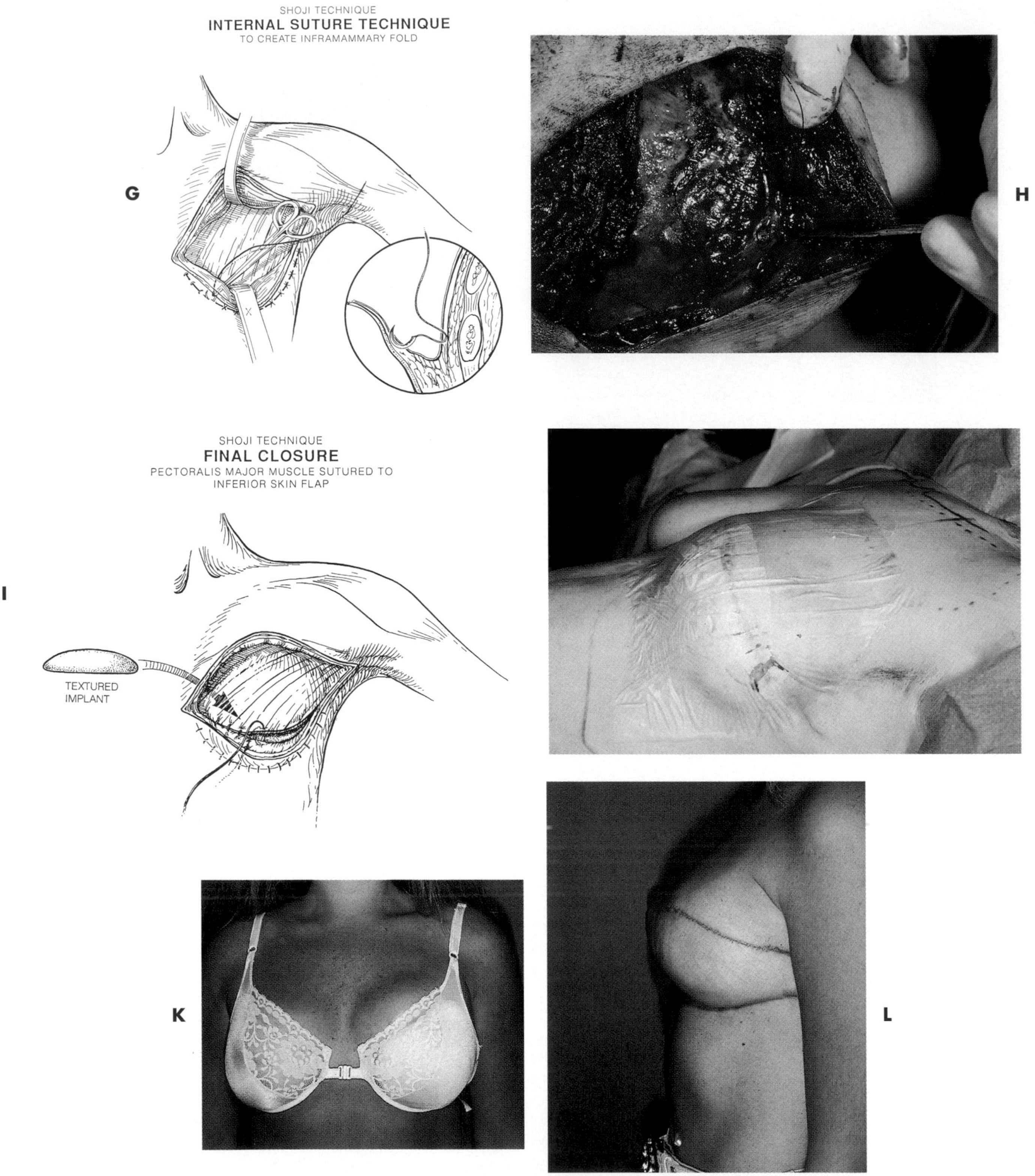

SHOJI TECHNIQUE
INTERNAL SUTURE TECHNIQUE
TO CREATE INFRAMAMMARY FOLD

G

H

SHOJI TECHNIQUE
FINAL CLOSURE
PECTORALIS MAJOR MUSCLE SUTURED TO
INFERIOR SKIN FLAP

I

TEXTURED
IMPLANT

J

K

L

Figure 12-14, cont'd   G and H, New inframammary fold is created with permanent sutures (O-proline) that extend from its medial point to its lateral splay point. Each suture is meticulously passed from the floor of the remaining capsule into the dermis of the flap, tracing the outline of the inframammary fold. Each suture must demonstrate a slight skin dimple, indicating secure skin tacking to the outline of the inframammary line and to the capsular floor. I, Released pectoralis muscle is allowed to drape over the inserted permanent implant. Its inferior edge is tacked with a few absorbable sutures to the undersurface of the inferior skin flap. The repositioned muscle should cross the skin line of closure to protect the implant from suture line exposure. Ideally the muscle should be at a level lower than the anticipated level of nipple reconstruction. The muscle layer can add protection between the reconstructed nipple and the permanent implant. J, An adhesive transparent drape temporarily fixes the approximated skin flaps in a downward position for a week. This manuever may contribute to a more ptotic appearance of the reconstructed breast mound. K and L, Three months after the first stage of reconstruction, a ptotic left breast mound has been created symmetric to the right breast, which has undergone a mastopexy. Once the optimal breast mound has been achieved by the Shoji technique and implant adjustment, the nipple may be reconstructed to complete the breast's appearance.

Suction-assisted lipectomy of a thickened fold will further create a ledge for the breast mound and implant.

Type of Implant

The reconstructive surgeon has a variety of permanent implants available to insert into the tailored pocket. This newly created skin-fat-muscle brassiere, however, possesses two critical characteristics that must be considered in implant selection: (1) the stretched tissue is thinner after expansion with less subcutaneous fat, which contributes to implant folds or discrepancies; and (2) the final pocket is larger than that before expansion. Smaller-based implants do not adequately fill the medial and lateral aspects of the pocket. To compensate for these anatomic changes, an implant with a larger base dimension and a softer "feel" is recommended over an implant with a more limited width that is firmer to palpation.

The surgeon may recommend a silicone gel implant, saline implant, or a double-lumen implant. The author recommends adjustable saline or saline-gel implants with a remote valve system that enables the surgeon to match the opposite breast by changing volume, tension, and to some degree, projection of the implant. This feature also permits the surgeon to reduce palpable and visible implant folds that may become sites for implant rupture. If early development of capsular contracture is recognized, the surgeon may be able to inject a steroid (triamcinolone [Kenalog], 20 to 30 mg/10 ml) into the implant to reduce capsular activity.

Implant surfaces may also be smooth or textured. Textured surfaces may provide a firmer "feel" and reflect implant irregularities from textured folds on the skin surface. Whether textured surfaces significantly reduce capsular contracture is still under clinical investigation.

When the patient is satisfied with the appearance and "feel" of the reconstructed mound, nipple-areolar reconstruction may be considered. The remote valve and tubing are removed with the patient under local anesthesia when reconstruction is completed.

Implant Insertion and Closure

After the selected implant is positioned in its pocket, it should be seated as far down as possible onto the reconstructed inframammary line. The patient sits upright for inspection of implant base regularity and symmetry to the opposite side. Further adjustment of sutures or pocket dimensions may be necessary.

At final closure the pectoralis major muscle is allowed to drape downward over the seated implant and is fixed at that level to the inner surface of the inferior skin flap with a few absorbable sutures (Figure 12-14, *I*). The muscle should be under the skin closure and even 2 to 3 cm below it. This muscle position

ensures that the implant will be protected when a nipple reconstruction is performed using the skate technique (see later).

The skin flaps are approximated in a layered closure and temporarily stabilized in a downward position for a week with an adhesive drape (Figure 12-14, *J*). A surgical drain exits from under the axilla.

After skin sutures are removed within 3 weeks, the permanent implant may be adjusted with saline through its remote valve to produce optimal projection, softness, and reduction of implant folds and irregularities (Figure 12-14, *K* and *L*).

NIPPLE-AREOLAR RECONSTRUCTION

The patient views nipple-areolar reconstruction as the completion of her reconstructed ptotic breast mound. It complements the shape of the breast mound and provides symmetry to the opposite side. A well-constructed nipple-areolar complex reassures the patient that the physical and psychologic stigmata of a mastectomy are behind her. The patient will exhibit more confidence both clothed and undressed.

Nipple Reconstruction

Nipple-sharing techniques remain an attractive alternative because of the near-identical characteristics that the donor tissue confers regarding texture, color, and topography. This technique is considered if the patient has minimal concerns about the anticipated changes in sensation and possesses a projected nipple on the donor site. Most patients even find that normal sensation eventually returns to the donor site. Some women may also appreciate similar projection of both nipples from the sharing procedure.

Nipple sharing may not be appropriate for patients who consider it violation of the remaining normal breast. In addition, the remote possibility exists that a pagetoid-like cancer may be transferred from the donor site to the reconstructed mound. Once the composite graft has survived and matured in its new environment, the transplanted nipple will undergo minimal reduced projection and size.

Local flap techniques are indicated when the patient is psychologically unwilling to share her opposite nipple or possesses an insufficient donor nipple. Numerous flap techniques have been described, including the quadrapod flap, double-opposing flaps, dermal fat flaps, and a nipple pull-out with wraparound graft. The *skate flap* or any of its modifications has advantages in terms of reliability, simplicity, and predictable projection. It is the author's method of choice for nipple reconstructions on mounds produced by tissue expansion or transverse rectus abdominis muscle flap techniques.

Surgical Techniques

Nipple reconstruction is performed with local anesthesia as an outpatient surgical procedure 3 months at the earliest after completion of the breast mound. The patient sits upright on the operating room table for measurements. The most appropriate site for nipple placement may be challenging because location is based on mound symmetry and balance with the opposite side. Thus midclavicular-to-nipple and midsternal-to-nipple measurements are obtained on the normal side and replicated on the reconstructed side.

A nipple-areolar pasty may be positioned on a selected site, then adjusted to a more optimal location based on the normal excursion of the uninvolved breast in or out of a brassiere (Figure 12-15, *A*). The final spot represents a compromise location based on the artistic perception of the surgeon and patient. A 1 cm circle is drawn around the selected nipple site, with an outer concentric circle approximating the proportions of the opposite areola.

If a nipple-sharing procedure is elected, the inner concentric nipple area is de-epithelialized. The transected composite nipple graft is transferred from the normal side and sutured into the prepared recipient site (Figure 12-15, *B*). The nipple graft is covered with protective dressing. Intradermal tattooing may be performed at least 3 months later to provide areolar and nipple pigmentation (Figure 12-15, *C*).

If a skate flap is selected for nipple reconstruction, the optimal nipple location is determined by the same methods outlined earlier (Figure 12-15, *D*). Three triangular flaps are drawn at the 3-, 6-, and 9-o'clock positions such that the apex of each triangle touches the outer limit of the areolar concentric ring and the base of each flap is in continuity with the nipple site (Figure 12-15, *E*). The tangent and orientation of these three flaps may be rotated (1) to align them with the areas of greatest laxity on the mound to permit closure of the defects and (2) to avoid crossing scar lines of the mastectomy incision.

Once the design pattern is determined, full-thickness incisions are made through the skin of the 3- and 9-o'clock flaps, which are elevated to their bases (Figure 12-15, *F*). The 6-o'clock flap is incised and elevated with attached subcutaneous fat to the nipple's midpoint. This limb is purposely raised beyond its base so that the three-pronged flap is elevated as a skin-fat flap with its base located at the 12-o'clock position. The surgeon must ensure that sufficient subcutaneous tissue remains attached to the flap at its base to provide bulk and blood supply. Thus the skate flap's blood supply is from central subcutaneous fat and adjacent subdermal sources.

The apex of the 6-o'clock flap is sutured to subcutaneous tissue under the center of the nipple, creating an elevated nipple body. Each full-thickness skin defect created by elevation of the three limbs is closed primarily by subdermal approximation. The 3- and 9-o'clock flaps are trimmed, wrapped, and sutured around the centrally constructed nipple to cover bare areas (Figure 12-15, *G*). A protective dressing is applied over the reconstructed nipple.

Areolar Tattooing

Three months after the nipple reconstruction, intradermal tattooing with pigments may be done to camouflage the donor scars and nipple and adjust areolar size and shape to ensure symmetry (Figure 12-16, *A* and *B*). The

Figure 12-15   A, This 37-year-old patient underwent immediate tissue expansion reconstruction of her left breast for invasive ductular carcinoma. At the second stage a ptotic breast mound was created by the Shoji technique, which removed the restricting tissue from the lower flap and developed the inframammary fold line. Nipple reconstruction began by determining its optimal position on the left mound through measurements and adjustments. **B,** After the outer concentric circle is outlined in the shape of the opposite areola, the 1 cm nipple site is de-epithelialized. The large donor nipple is transected in a horizontal direction and transferred as a composite graft to the prepared recipient site. A few interrupted skin sutures secure the graft in place. **C,** Intradermal tattooing of the areolar-nipple complex may be performed about 3 months later to match it to the opposite side. **D,** After bilateral mastectomies, nipples may be constructed on the breast mounds by the skate technique. The optimal nipple site is determined by visual symmetry and balance on each of the reconstructed mounds. The premastectomy distance of the nipple along the vertical meridian line from the midclavicular point may assist in estimating its position on the new mound. The application of pasties on the chosen sites corrects the final adjustments. In this 5-foot, 7-inch-tall patient the location of the nipples before mastectomies was 22 cm (9 inches) from the midclavicular point and 10 cm (4 inches) lateral from the midsternal line. This nipple location was closely duplicated on the reconstructed mounds. **E,** The skate design consists of three triangular flaps outlined at the 3-, 6-, and 9-o'clock positions. The base of each triangle is continuous with the 1 cm nipple circle. The apex of each flap touches the edge of the concentric areolar ring. This design may be changed, however, to accommodate the findings on the breast mound. For example, the orientation of the flaps may be rotated to align them in the direction of greatest skin laxity. The 3- and 9-o'clock flaps can be shorter than the 6-o'clock flap. **F,** The skate flap is elevated by incising the 3- and 9-o'clock limbs as either split-thickness or full-thickness flaps. The 6-o'clock limb is raised as a skin-fat flap with its base at the 12-o'clock position. Injury to the breast implant should be prevented by coverage from its capsule and overlying pectoralis muscle. **G,** Flap closure begins by attaching the apex of the thick 6-o'clock flap to the deep fatty tissue under its base. The 3- and 9-o'clock limbs are trimmed and wrapped around the bare sides of the 6-o'clock flap. Each of the triangular defects are undermined and approximated to create three radiating incision lines. A protective dressing covers the nipple reconstruction for 5 days.

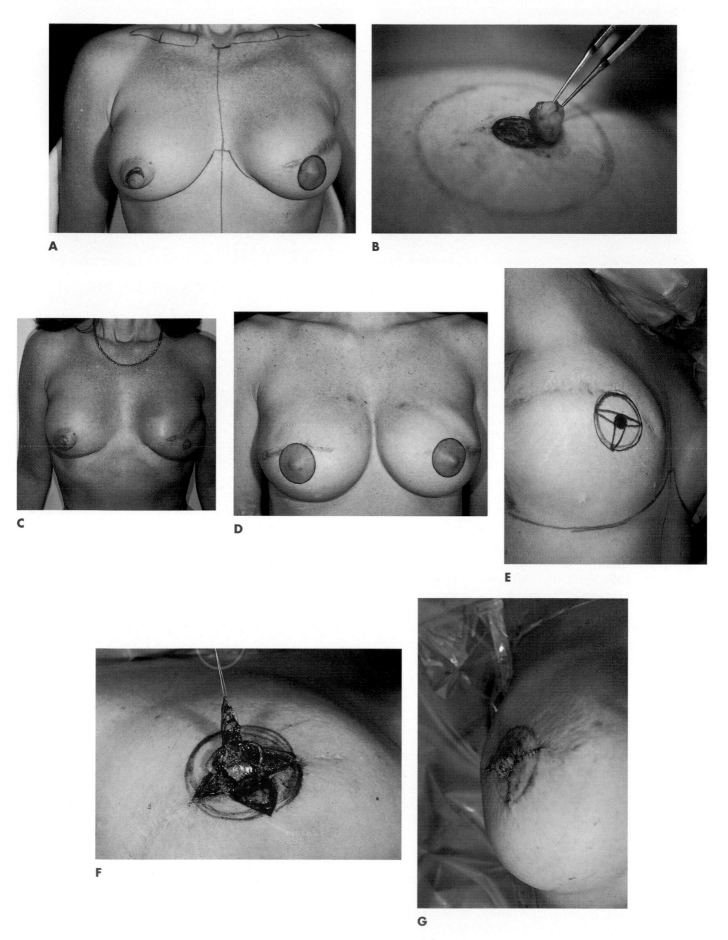

Figure 12-15, cont'd For legend see opposite page.

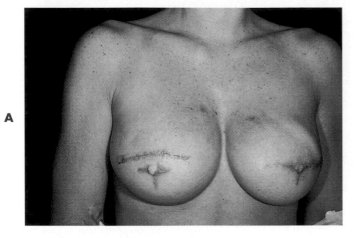

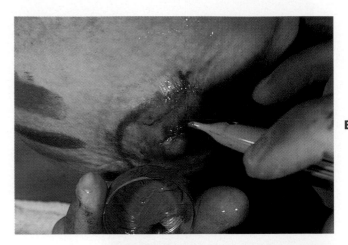

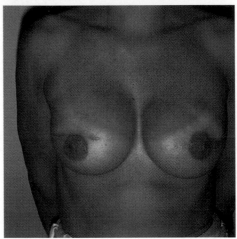

Figure 12-16   A, Three months after nipple reconstructions the patient is prepared for intradermal tattooing to recreate the original nipple-areolar complexes, camouflage the donor scars, and adjust areolar shape and size. **B,** Seven-pronged needle device drives the pigments into the dermis for permanent coloring. The treated areas are covered daily with an antibiotic cream until the scab disappears. **C,** The patient has completed her breast procedure with a nipple-areolar reconstruction. Secondary tattooing was performed 6 months later to achieve optimal pigmentation.

author uses a seven-pronged needle tattooing device that drives into the dermis the selected colored pigments that were blended to match the opposite or both sides. Darker pigment spots may be introduced randomly into the areola to simulate Montgomery's glands. The treated areas are covered daily with an antibiotic ointment until healing occurs. The tattoo pigments may appear lighter and less defined over time. Secondary treatments may be required 3 to 6 months later to achieve the optimal color match (Figure 12-16, C).

Secondary Procedures

Nipple projection is initially overcorrected to allow for tissue contraction at a later stage. If the final amount of nipple projection and bulk is insufficient to match the opposite side, secondary procedures to add tissue (crushed cartilage) under the nipple will restore symmetry.

Areolar Filling
Reconstruction of an areolar mound to provide apical fullness to the reconstructed ptotic breast with a nipple has not been emphasized after mastectomy. The benefits of an areolar fill include conversion from a globular

to a more conical-shaped breast. Areolar projection is possible with an alloplastic implant or autogenous fill.

Alloplastic Areolar Implant.   After nipple reconstruction is completed, areolar projection may be considered 3 months later at the earliest. The primary indication is to obtain improved symmetry with the opposite breast by creating a more conical shape. Many patients, however, who either possess a modestly projected nipple on the normal breast or do not want any nipple reconstruction, may prefer only the insertion of an areolar-nipple implant. A permanent implant suggests a modest nipple or enhances the projection of a previously reconstructed nipple complex (Figure 12-17).

A solid but pliable silicone elastomer implant can be easily carved into an areolar disk with scissors and smoothly buffed with a wire brush (Figure 12-18). The implant is designed to be about 1 cm thick at its apex, which may represent a 1 cm–wide and 1 cm–high nipple, and sloped at its periphery. If an autogenous nipple reconstruction is already present on the breast mound, the alloplastic areolar disk may be designed not to include the nipple projection on its apex. An additional foreign body under the skin may be associated with a higher complication rate from implant exposure and infection. The areolar implant is safe to insert only

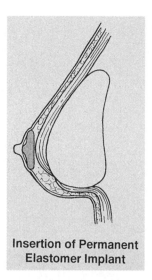

Insertion of Permanent
Elastomer Implant

Figure 12-17 Alloplastic silicone areolar implant may be inserted under the reconstructed nipple to give the reconstructed breast mound a more conical shape. The solid but pliable elastomer implant may be shaped with an apical projection that either suggests a nipple or further emphasizes the constructed nipple (shared nipple or skate flap). The implant may be a permanent areolar fill or a temporary framework for creation of a capsule into which autogenous tissue is transplanted.

when the overlying skin is stable and the subcutaneous fat is substantial to protect the implant. The implant may be inserted as either a permanent fill or a temporary template for creation of a capsule into which autogenous tissue is transplanted (see next section).

A 3 cm incision is made in the lateral extent of the mastectomy scar at least 2.5 cm from the concentric outline of the areolar marking (Figure 12-19, *A*). The incision is purposely located away from the implant's edge to reduce the risk of exposure and infection. The incision is carried down to the pectoralis major muscle. Blunt dissection of the circular areolar pocket under the nipple is developed above the muscle, leaving maximal subcutaneous fat adherent to the dermis. If a 4 cm, round intraoperative expander is available, the expander may be filled within this dissected pocket to assist in creating an adequate and symmetric pocket for the implant (Figure 12-19, *B*). An areolar expander usually is not required to produce a space for the elastomer implant.

The areolar implant is inserted in a flat position and inspected for symmetry (Figure 12-19, *C*). The incision is closed in layers. If skin tattooing has not been done, intradermal pigments may be introduced into the dermis 3 months later at the earliest (Figure 12-19, *D*). It is preferable to complete the nipple-areolar tattooing first, before insertion of the elastomer implant, to avoid possible bacterial contamination of this foreign body.

The permanent elastomer implant produces an areolar-nipple projection to complement the breast mound (Figure 12-19, *E* and *F*). The removal of an

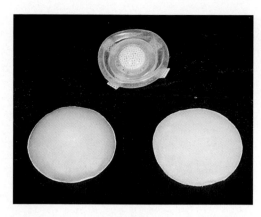

Figure 12-18 Lower-left implant is a soft silicone wafer in the form of a tapered areola with an apical nipple projection. The lower-right implant has a similar shape except without a nipple prominence. The top implant is an intraoperative round expander (4 cm diameter) with an incorporated valve that may be useful to develop the areolar pocket.

infected areolar implant does not jeopardize the breast implant because of its coverage with the muscle flaps.

Autogenous Fill
After nipple reconstruction has been successfully completed by either nipple-sharing or skate-flap techniques, the areolar mound can also be built up with autogenous tissues. In most patients the use of autogenous tissue is preferable to insertion of a permanent alloplastic implant. The autogenous material is usually accepted by the surrounding tissue and less subject to early or delayed bacterial contamination. Autogenous tissue eventually becomes softer with time and thus more natural to palpation.

However, a major drawback remains the unpredictable rate of absorption of lipoinjected fat or adipofascial tissue. The use of lipoinjected fat for breast augmentation is contraindicated because of legitimate concerns of liquefaction, reactive inflammation, and organization that may lead to calcification. The presence of macro- or microcalcifications from fat in breast tissue may be interpreted as being associated with breast cancer. The use of lipoinjected fat to augment the contour of a breast mound reconstructed after a mastectomy may provide, at best, filling in the form of scar replacement tissue. At worse, calcifications in a lipoinjected area may trigger concerns of persistent breast cancer in unnoticed parenchymal tissue after a mastectomy. This is an unlikely scenario because radiologists, pathologists, and surgeons are confident that a mastectomy removes all or 95% of the breast tissue. Postmastectomy discovery of a calcification by mammography or ultrasonography is unusual because the need to follow a mastectomy site with these modalities is rarely indicated.

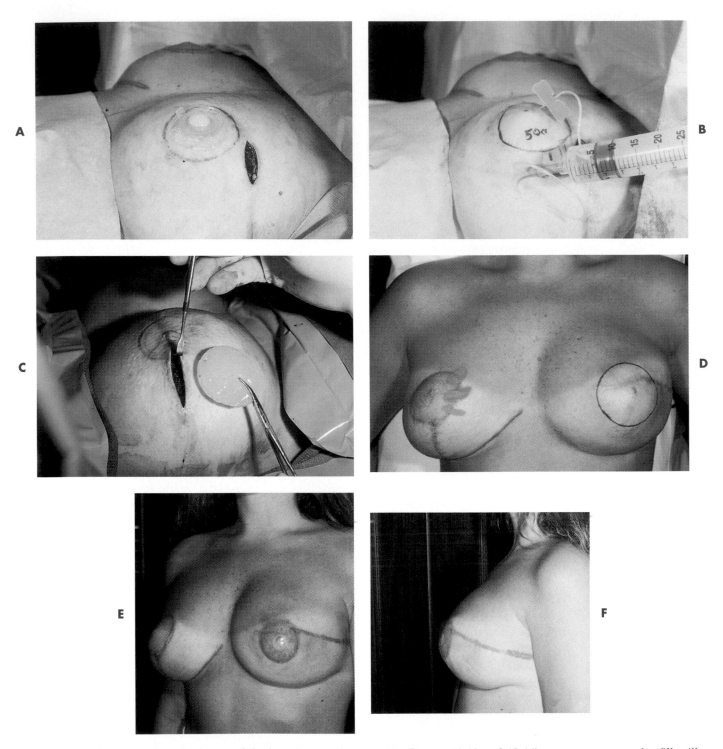

Figure 12-19   **A,** After completion of the breast mound (patient in Figures 12-13 and 12-14), a permanent areolar fill will convert the globular mound into a more conical breast. First, a 3.0 cm incision along the lateral extent of the mastectomy scar permits dissection of an areolar pocket above the pectoralis major muscle. An intraoperative areolar-shaped expander is about to be inserted into its pocket. **B,** Intraoperative expansion with the areolar expander assists in stretching the overlying tissue and ensuring a symmetric pocket for the implant. **C,** The areolar implant is inserted into its created pocket for a permanent fill. The incision line is placed about 2.5 cm from the lateral edge of the permanent implant to reduce the opportunity for implant exposure. **D,** Intradermal tattooing of the right areola camouflages the mastopexy scar and adjusts areolar shape, size, and location. The reconstructed left areolar mound and nipple will also be tattooed to match the opposite side. **E** and **F,** Six months after her left breast reconstruction the patient's ptotic mound approximates the shape of the right breast because of its defined inframammary fold and apical fill.

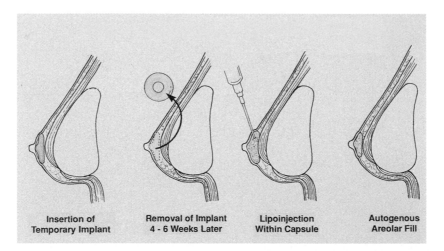

| Insertion of Temporary Implant | Removal of Implant 4 - 6 Weeks Later | Lipoinjection Within Capsule | Autogenous Areolar Fill |

Figure 12-20 Lipoinjected tissue may provide autogenous fill under the reconstructed areolar-nipple complex that converts the globular mound to a more conical shape. The sequential steps include (1) the insertion of a temporary nipple-areolar silicone implant to create a 4 to 6-week-old capsule and (2) injection of fat into the vacant contoured capsule after implant removal. The capsule is overfilled with fat because of the anticipated but unpredictable rate of its absorption. Fat may be injected into the subareolar space 3 to 6 months later for additional fill.

Nevertheless, the use of added fat in the subareolar space should be discouraged. Identical concerns may also be raised when calcifications are discovered in a breast mound reconstructed with a transverse rectus abdominis flap. Nonviable fat may liquefy and organize into calcifications that are rarely mistaken for persistent foci of cancer. Open or needle biopsies may be necessary to resolve this issue.

Lipoinjection (Figure 12-20)

At the first stage the silicone areolar implant is inserted in the manner previously described. The implant is to be removed after a fresh capsule has developed around it within 4 to 6 weeks. An immature capsule contains an increased blood supply, which is more likely to support the imported autogenous tissue fill.

At surgery the implant is removed through the same insertion incision. Adipose tissue is syringe-suctioned with a large-bore cannula from the abdomen or thigh. The aspirate is immediately decanted on a moist sponge. The fatty material is recovered and deposited into the barrel of a syringe, which is capped by reinsertion of the plunger. The fat-filled syringe is placed into a cool-water bath and used immediately to limit prolonged exposure to ambient temperature and air. The prepared fat is injected through a 14-gauge catheter, filling the contoured-shaped capsule with about 20 to 30 cc of adipose tissue. The incision is closed in layers. Since an unknown portion of the fat will not survive, additional fat may be lipoinjected into the subareolar space 3 to 6 months later.

Adipofascial Flaps (Figure 12-21)

Adipofascial flaps offer an improved alternative for autogenous fill other than fat aspirates from liposuction.

The flap provides a variable and random blood supply, which increases the chances for tissue survival. When this tissue is transferred within the vascularized molded capsule of the areolar implant, tissue viability may be enhanced.

Adipofascial flaps may be elevated from redundant tissue along the inframammary fold line at the 3- or 9-o'clock position. Either flap is based at the intersection of the vertical meridian line and the inframammary fold. These flaps may include a portion of the extended pectoralis major fascia or rectus abdominis fascia. A more conventional adipofascial flap is based cranially at the juncture of the vertical meridian line and inframammary fold and is drawn downward as a tongue of tissue 3 cm wide and 7 to 10 cm long. A skin incision is made along the central portion of the inframammary fold. A second 3 cm horizontal incision is made at the distal limits of the sketched flap. The flap is developed first by undermining subcutaneous fat to a depth of 3 or 4 mm from the inframammary incision to the flap's end. The distal incision permits the fat and anterior sheath of the rectus abdominis muscle to be cut in an elliptic shape. The surgeon grasps the tip of the tonguelike flap with a forceps and cuts along both edges of the flap, which includes the anterior rectus fascia. The distal flap is pulled upward through the upper incision as far as the inframammary line and includes a few perforators from the pectoralis major muscle.

The elevated adipofascial flap is reflected in a cephalad direction through a subcutaneous tunnel under the skin and enters the capsule of the areolar implant. The flap's distal end may be folded on itself by sutures into the shape of the areolar mound. Two absorbable sutures are incorporated into the flap's distal portion and passed through the tunnel to exit percutaneously from the areolar pocket. The flap is secured in the

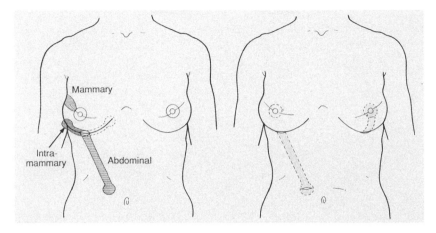

Figure 12-21 An adipofascial flap may offer an alternative autogenous fill under the reconstructed areolar-nipple complex. The distal flap may be configured into a rounded end that resembles the shape of the areolar bud. This fabricated tip may be either (1) transposed into the contoured, 4 to 6-week-old capsule created from a temporary areolar implant or (2) simply positioned under a constructed nipple. In the first method the capsule serves to isolate the flap's end. In the second the flap must be held in position under the nipple by a series of sutures. The adipofascial flap may be elevated from any site with tissue redundancy that is based on the inframammary fold in line with the vertical meridian line. Flaps may be based along each side of the inframammary fold. A common donor site extends into the upper abdomen as a tongue of tissue 3 cm wide and 7 to 10 cm long based on the rectus abdominis fascia. The flaps are tunneled under the subcutaneous plane of the breast mound to the areolar site.

areolar pocket by securing or tying down the sutures. The incisions are closed in layers.

CASE RESULTS

From 1979 to 1997 the author performed 1113 breast reconstructions in 909 patients. A single breast reconstruction was completed in 705 patients, and 408 patients underwent bilateral procedures (Table 12-3).

The major problems were the congenital deformities found in the nine patients with Poland's syndrome (absence of breast parenchyma or pectoralis muscle) and the ablations resulting from 68 subcutaneous, 251 simple, 646 modified radical, and 139 radical mastectomies. The age range extended from 18 to 79 years. Delayed reconstructions were performed in 258 patients and primary reconstructions in 846 patients.

Subcutaneous mastectomies were reconstructed with only alloplastic implants: 12 silicone gel, 13 saline, 20 saline adjustable, and 23 gel-saline adjustable types. The adjustable implant consisted of a remote valve and tubing system that was removed after sufficient volume, symmetry, and softness were obtained without implant folds. Skin ptosis was present in 12 of the 68 patients with subcutaneous mastectomies. These patients had their skin brassiere reduced, nipple-areolar complex elevated, and a subpectoral implant inserted to correct the ptosis.

Of the 253 breasts that underwent a simple mastectomy, 72 were reconstructed with a saline adjustable or saline-gel adjustable implant. In these patients the residual skin brassiere was adequate to receive an implant only. However, 181 breasts underwent tissue expansion after a simple mastectomy because of skin loss. The removal of the nipple-areolar complex and skin biopsy site resulted in such a degree of skin inadequacy that implant insertion would not create a ptotic or symmetric mound.

Of the 646 breasts that underwent modified radical mastectomies, 373 were reconstructed by tissue expansion technique, 250 by the transverse rectus abdominis myocutaneous (TRAM) flap, and 23 by latissimus dorsi muscle flap. After tissue expansion was completed, replacement implants comprised 79 gel, 53 saline, 61 saline-adjustable, and 180 saline-gel adjustable types of prosthesis. In TRAM flap-reconstructed breasts, 211 had sufficient autogenous dermal-fat fill. Patients with insufficient fat received implants to create the desired appearance: 8 gel, 7 saline, 11 saline adjustable, and 13 saline-gel adjustable types. Latissimus dorsi flap reconstructions were employed in only 23 breasts, which were augmented by 12 gel, 2 saline, 4 saline adjustable, and 5 saline-gel adjustable prostheses.

Of the 139 breasts managed by a radical mastectomy technique, their reconstructions were either by TRAM flaps, latissimus dorsi flaps, or buttock free-flap method. Most TRAM flaps contained sufficient tissue to avoid the use of an implant, but 25 were augmented with 7 gel, 2 saline, 5 saline adjustable, and 11 saline-gel adjustable implants. In 53 latissimus dorsi flap reconstructions, added implants comprised 31 gel, 4 saline, 5 saline adjustable, and 13 saline-gel adjustable prostheses. Only two breasts were reconstructed by a buttock flap. Each possessed enough tissue to match the opposite breast.

■ **Table 12-3** Type of Implants for Poland's Syndrome and Mastectomy Reconstructions*

		Mastectomy			
Implant	Poland's syndrome	Subcutaneous	Simple	Modified radical	Radical
Alloplastic					
Gel		12			
Saline		13			
Saline adjustable		20	28		
Saline-gel adjustable		23	44		
Tissue expansion					
Gel	2		36	79	
Saline			29	53	
Saline adjustable			51	61	
Saline-gel adjustable	7		65	180	2
TRAM† flap					
No implant				211	57
Gel				8	7
Saline				7	2
Saline adjustable				11	5
Saline-gel adjustable				13	11
Latissimus dorsi flap					
Gel				12	31
Saline				2	4
Saline adjustable				4	5
Saline-gel adjustable				5	13
Buttock free flap					2
TOTAL	9	68	251	646	139

*Cases from private practice and two university practices.
†Transverse rectus abdominis myocutaneous.

The author preferred implants that could be adjusted postoperatively over implants whose volumes were determined at surgery. The adjustable type eliminated concerns of volume, projection, symmetry, softness, and folds.

Tissue Expansion

The author employed tissue expansion technique for reconstruction of 554 breasts that were determined to have insufficient skin after mastectomy (see Table 12-3). Patients underwent 181 simple or 373 modified radical mastectomies. In 115 cases, gel implants were used as the permanent prostheses, and 82 breasts received saline implants. In most cases, saline adjustable (112 breasts) or saline-gel adjustable (245 breasts) implants were selected as the final permanent prosthesis.

From 1979 to 1986, 265 breasts underwent tissue expansion technique, 213 of which had nipple reconstruction procedures (Table 12-4). From 1987 to 1997 an additional 289 breasts completed similar expansion procedures, 252 of which advanced to secondary nipple reconstructions. Almost all patients requested intradermal tattooing, but 89 of 554 breasts (16%) were not reconstructed by a nipple procedure. Thus 465 of

■ **Table 12-4** Types of Breast and Nipple Reconstructions in 554 Breasts

	Number of breasts	
Type	1979-1986	1987-1997
Mound only	52	37
Nipple sharing	39	79
Core skin graft	63	0
Quadripod flap	75	0
Double-opposing tab	25	0
Dermal-fat flap	11	0
Skate flap	0	173
TOTAL	265	289

554 cases (84%) included some type of nipple procedure and areolar tattooing.

In 12 of the 554 cases, however, the tissue to be expanded was less than optimal in quality because of radiation injury either during or after expansion. Results were compromised by radiation changes that resisted expansion forces, promoted skin contraction, and enhanced capsular contracture. Secondary procedures, such as nipple-areolar reconstructions and intradermal tattooing, were not performed within radiated tissue to

Surgical Procedure (Figure 12-22, *C* to *F*)
Six months after the mound reconstructions, areolar filling was provided by a silicone cushion implant (Figure 12-22, *C*). A 3 cm incision was made within a previous transverse biopsy scar above her right areola (Figure 12-22, *D*). A pocket was deeply dissected under the areola to accommodate a 4 cm intraoperative expander. Intraoperative filling of the temporary expander was repeated three times to a volume of 30 cc. The permanent implant (4.5 cm diameter) was positioned under the areola. A similar intraoperative expansion procedure was performed under the left areola using a 3.0 cm incision through a previous axillary scar (Figure 12-22, *E* and *F*). Another permanent cushion areolar implant replaced the expander.

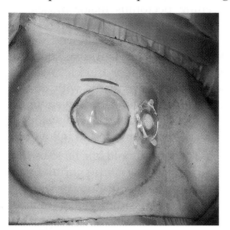

12-22C

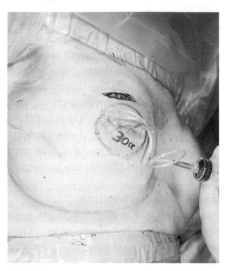

12-22D

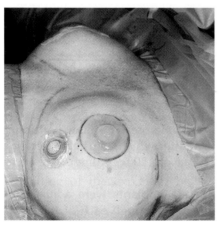

12-22E

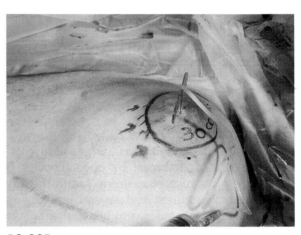

12-22F

Results (Figure 12-22, *G* and *H*)

The patient is shown 1 year after her breast expansions and insertion of areolar cushion implants. The patient achieved a C-cup size with apical fullness of the areo-lae. The remote fill valves and their tubing were removed after the patient was satisfied with her reconstructed breast mounds and areolar fills.

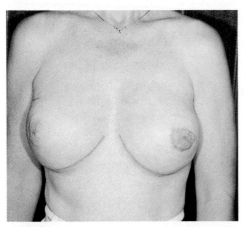

12-22G

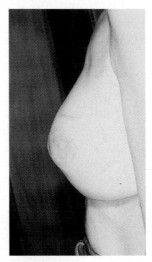

12-22H

CASE 2: Right Simple and Left Modified Radical Mastectomies

History (Figure 12-23, *A* and *B*)

This 45-year-old patient underwent a left modified radical mastectomy for invasive ductular cancer and a prophylactic right simple mastectomy. A 350 cc gel implant was inserted under the pectoralis major muscle to create the right breast mound. A 600 cc expander was inserted in a submuscular plane under the left breast tissue. Radiation therapy was required for the left breast mound because of cancer's invasive nature. Tissue expansion of the radiated tissue was performed slowly as appropriate over 4 months until sufficient tissue was obtained. A left implant exchange for the expander resulted in completion of the bilateral mound reconstructions. Skate flaps constructed the nipples 6 months later, followed by intradermal tattooing of the areolae.

A capsular contracture developed in the radiated left breast within a year. The patient requested a larger and softer breast mound. A capsulectomy and exchange for a larger implant (550 cc) were performed. A prosthetic infection occurred in the immediate postoperative period and resulted in implant removal. The patient was referred about 1 year later for further reconstructions.

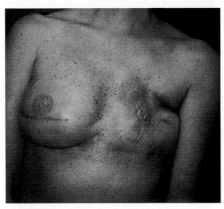

12-23A

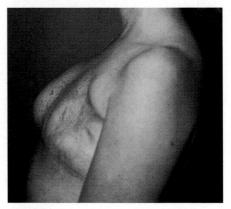

12-23B

Surgical Procedure (Figure 12-23, *C* to *J*)

A bipedicle transverse rectus abdominis myocuta-neous (TRAM) flap reconstructed the patient's breast mound (Figure 12-23, *C* and *D*). The nipple-areolar complex was replaced by the transposed skin flap. The right breast implant was also replaced with a tissue expander to increase breast size and manage the progressive Baker III capsular contracture (Figure 12-23, *E*).

Serial expansion of the right breast expander was performed over 3 months (Figure 12-23, *F*). When sufficient tissue was obtained, a Becker saline-gel implant (200 cc gel : 200 cc saline) was inserted with redefinition of the inframammary fold (Shoji technique).

The patient requested a nipple-areolar reconstruction by areolar filling with lipoinjected fat. She did not want to undergo another skate flap reconstruction for the nipple projection. The original right nipple-areolar reconstruction had to be disregarded because of its high position on the new breast mound. The placement of areolar pasties on each of the breast mounds determined their optimal locations (Figure 12-23, *G*).

Insertion of temporary silicone implants under the selected areolar sites was aided by the intraoperative expanders (Figure 12-23, *H*). The areolar wafer implants were removed after 6 weeks, when vascularized capsules had conformed to the implants' shape. Thirty to 45 cc of suctioned fat from the hips was injected into each of the vacant capsules as autogenous filler material (Figure 12-23, *I* and *J*). Intradermal tattooing 6 months later provided pigmentations to simulate the areolar-nipple complexes.

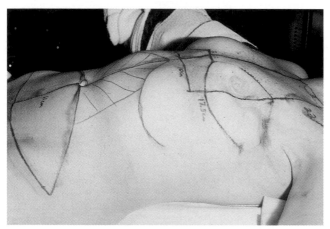

12-23C

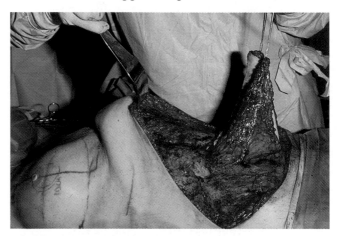

12-23D

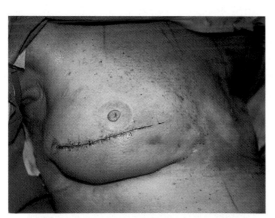

12-23E

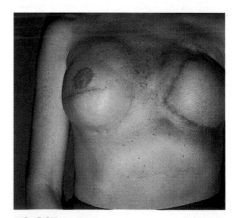

12-23F

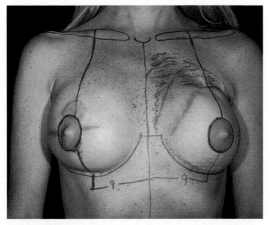

12-23G

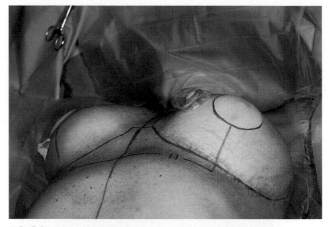

12-23H

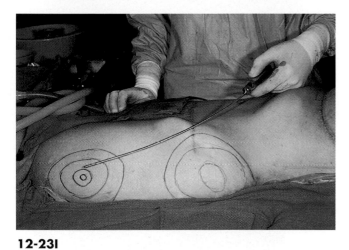

12-23I

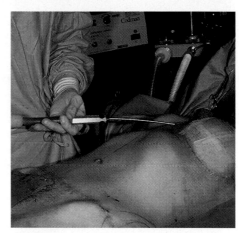

12-23J

Results (Figure 12-23, *K* to *N*)
Two years after her reconstructions the patient demonstrates symmetric breasts with apical fullness under

the areolar tattooing. An Nd:YAG 1064 nm laser lightened the pigmentations within the original right nipple-areolar complex.

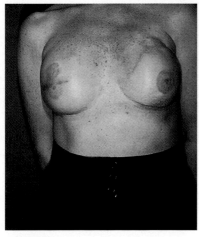

12-23K

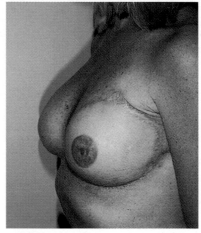

12-23L

Continued

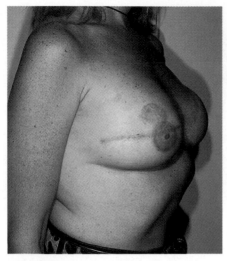

12-23M

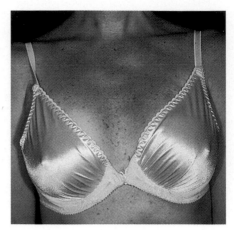

12-23N

CASE 3: Left Modified Radical Mastectomy in Small Breast

History (Figure 12-24, *A* and *B*)

This 34-year-old patient was diagnosed with invasive ductular carcinoma in the tail of her left breast by open biopsy. The biopsy site was at the 2-o'clock position about 13 cm from the nipple. A modified radical mastectomy was planned through a 4 cm–wide skin ellipse that included the nipple-areolar complex and the skin biopsy site. The amount of skin removal was estimated at 40% of the skin brassiere of the breast mound.

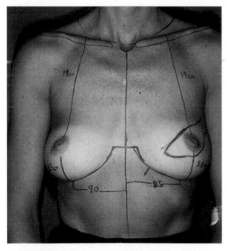

12-24A

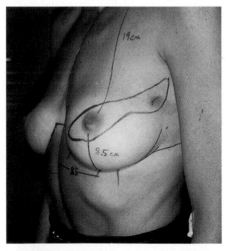

12-24B

Stage I: Mastectomy and Expander Insertion
(Figure 12-24, *C*)
After mastectomy a double-balloon expander system was positioned under complete coverage by the pectoralis major, pectoralis minor, and serratus anterior muscles. Each of the two remote valves was buried under the lateral axillary skin.

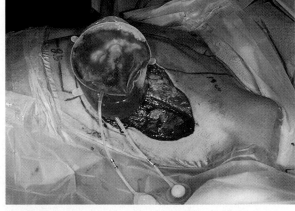

12-24C

Expansion Course (Figure 12-24, *D*)
The patient's balloons were filled with saline weekly over 3 months. The anterior balloon contained 300 cc, and the posterior balloon was filled to 400 cc by the end of expansion. The vertical meridian line on the expanded breast mound measured 30 cm from the midclavicle to the inframammary fold. A similar plumb line on the uninvolved right breast measured 28 cm. Expansion may be terminated when the reconstructed breast mound is at least 2 cm longer along the vertical meridian line than on the normal side.

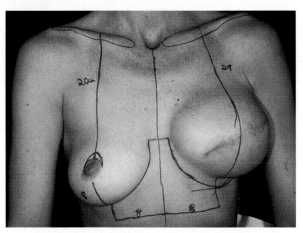

12-24D

Stage II: Implant Exchange with Shoji Technique
(Figure 12-24, *E*)
The Shoji technique was used to reconstruct a ptotic breast mound that was close in appearance to the opposite side. The final pocket was lowered by 3 cm, with redefinition of the inframammary fold by the internal suturing technique. An adjustable saline textured implant was filled through its buried valve postoperatively until optimal prosthetic volume, projection, softness, and smoothness were obtained.

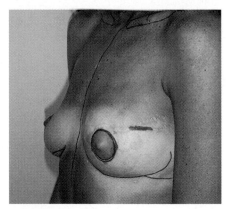

12-24E

Nipple-Areolar Reconstruction
(Figure 12-24, *F* and *G*)

The patient requested a more natural-appearing breast mound that would include a nipple-areolar complex. This was accomplished by the insertion of an areolar silicone wafer with a modest central prominence for a nipple (Figure 12-24, *F*). A 3.0 cm incision along the transverse mastectomy scar permitted dissection of a 4.5 cm circular pocket at the proposed areolar site. A 4 cm intraoperative expander stretched the overlying skin and created a uniform pocket for the permanent implant. Intradermal tattooing was performed about 4 months later after wound healing (Figure 12-24, *G*).

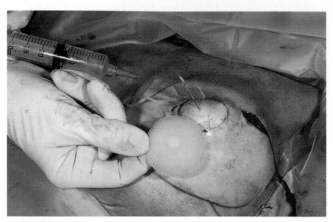

12-24F

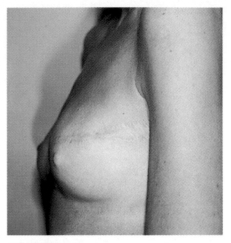

12-24G

Results (Figure 12-24, *H*)

About 3 months later the patient has a soft ptotic breast mound, classified as a Baker II encapsulation. Minimal implant irregularities are present along its medial lower border. The remote valve and tubing were removed 6 months after the nipple-areolar tattooing. The reconstructed breast remains in close symmetry to its opposite side.

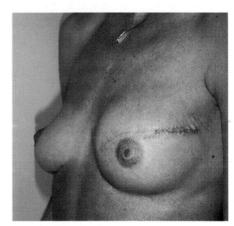

12-24H

CASE 4:   Left Modified Radical Mastectomy in Moderate-Size Breast

History (Figure 12-25, *A*)

This 38-year-old patient was diagnosed with an infiltrating ductal carcinoma in her left breast. A 4.5 cm–wide skin ellipse, which included the nipple-areolar complex, was planned for excision during her modified radical mastectomy. This amount of skin removal was estimated at 35% of her tissue brassiere.

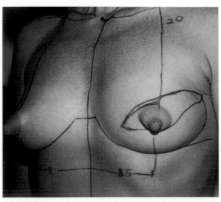

12-25A

Stage I: Mastectomy and Expander Insertion
(Figure 12-25, *B*)

After the modified radical mastectomy a 600 cc textured breast expander was placed under coverage of the pectoralis major, pectoralis minor, and serratus anterior muscles. Intraoperative filling with 350 ml of saline initiated the expansion process. The surgical drain was removed 5 days after surgery.

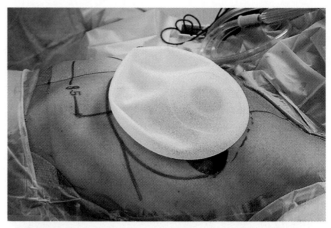

12-25B

Expansion Course (Figure 12-25, *C*)

Serial expansion with 25 to 30 ml of saline was performed weekly by a percutaneous needle stick into the incorporated valve. The length of the vertical meridian line was measured after each week of expansion. When its distance on the left mound exceeded that of the right breast by at least 2 cm, the hyperexpanded state (800 cc) was maintained for an additional 4 to 6 weeks.

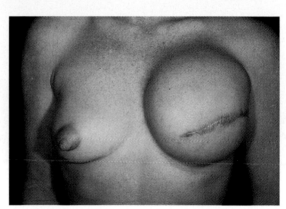

12-25C

Stage II: Implant Exchange with Shoji Technique
(Figure 12-25, *D* and *E*)

The Shoji technique redefined the inframammary fold and created a ptotic breast mound with a 350 cc saline adjustable implant. The remote valve was located below the lateral aspect of the inframammary line. Saline injections postoperatively adjusted the implant's volume, projection, smoothness, and softness to match the opposite breast.

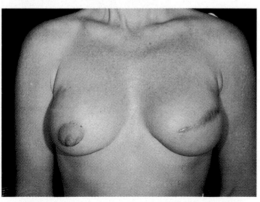

12-25D

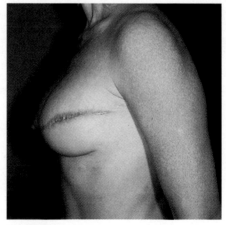

12-25E

Nipple-Areolar Reconstruction (Figure 12-25, *F* to *I*) Six months after completion of the breast mound, nipple-areolar reconstruction was requested to produce an appearance similar to the right breast. The nipple position was sighted with the aid of a pasty. The right nipple was transected and transferred to the left breast mound (Figure 12-25, *F*). After 4 months, apical filling was scheduled to create a cone shape to match the opposite breast.

At surgery an intraoperative expander was inserted into the 4 cm areolar pocket, which was dissected from a 2.5 cm incision along the mastectomy scar (Figure 12-25, *G*). Intraoperative stretching created a symmetric round cavity that received the temporary silicone areolar implant (Figure 12-25, *H*). When the implant was removed about 6 weeks later, the vacant capsule was filled with 30 cc of fat obtained by syringe liposuction from the abdomen (Figure 12-25, *I*). Intradermal tattooing was performed 3 months later to approximate the color of the opposite areolar complex.

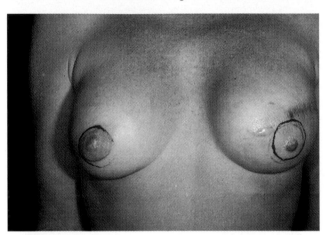

12-25F

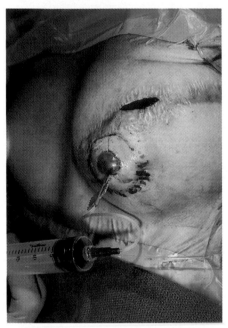

12-25G

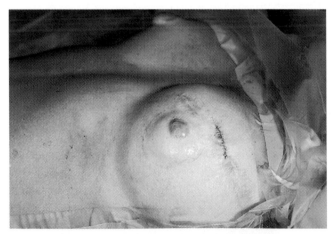

12-25H

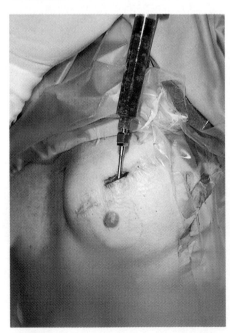

12-25I

Results (Figure 12-25, *J* and *K*)

Three years after her breast reconstruction the patient's implant has remained mobile and soft with a Baker II/III encapsulation. A setback procedure re-

duced the prominence of the right areola through a circumareolar incision that permitted removal of subareolar tissue.

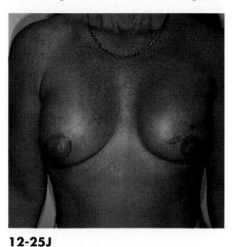

12-25J

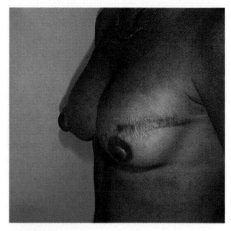

12-25K

CASE 5: Bilateral Modified Radical Mastectomies in Small and Moderate-Size Breasts

History (Figure 12-26, *A*)

This 47-year-old patient was diagnosed with bilateral invasive ductal carcinomas. The skin ellipses, which included the biopsied sites and nipple-areolar complexes, removed about 50% of the skin brassieres.

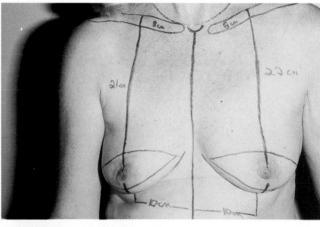

12-26A

Stage I: Mastectomies and Expander Insertion
(Figure 12-26, *B*)

After the modified radical mastectomies, 600 cc textured round expanders were inserted under complete coverage by the pectoralis major and minor and serratus anterior muscles. The expanders were filled intraoperatively with 300 ml of saline through their incorporated valves.

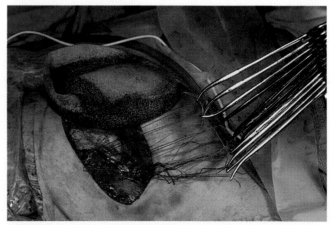

12-26B

Expansion Course (Figure 12-26, *C*)

After 3 months of weekly expansions with 20 to 25 ml of saline, the vertical meridian lines (midclavicle to inframammary fold) measured 32 cm on each side. This amount of tissue expansion would result in a C-cup breast mound.

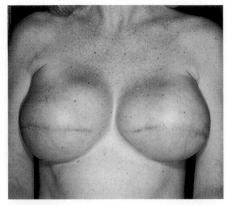

12-26C

Stage II: Implant Exchange with Shoji Technique (Figure 12-26, *D* and *E*)

At surgery the mastectomy scar was reopened to allow the cephalic and caudal skin flaps to be dissected off the muscle coverage (Figure 12-26, *D*). After the pectoralis major fascia was incised parallel to the muscle's lower border, the expander was removed. Three flaps (two skin flaps and a muscle layer) were avail-able to create a ptotic breast mound (Figure 12-26, *E*). The inframammary fold was defined by internal sutures from the dermis to the deep capsule on the chest wall. A 450 cc saline adjustable implant was inserted under the muscle layer, which was tacked 3 to 4 cm below the edge of the lower skin flap. The remote valve was buried in the subcutaneous fat lateral to the inframammary fold.

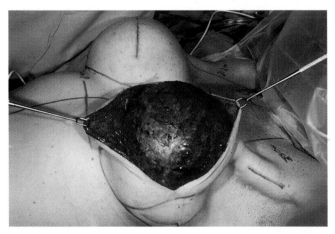

12-26D

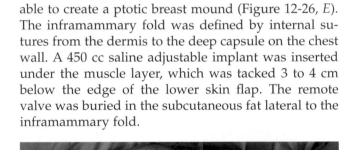

12-26E

Nipple-Areolar Reconstruction
(Figure 12-26, *F* to *O*)

The breast mounds were adjusted by saline filling to the desired volume, projection, and softness (Figure 12-26, *F* and *G*). Implant folds were visible because of the thinness of overlying tissue and the final fill volume, which resulted in fold production. The patient accepted the appearance of implant irregularities.

Bilateral skate flaps constructed nipple projections at measured sites on the breast mounds 1 year after the mastectomies (Figure 12-26, *H*).

The patient wanted to convert the mounds' globular appearance into a more conical shape through apical filling. Areolar pockets were dissected from 2.5 cm incisions in the medial mastectomy scars. After intraoperative expansion with areolar expanders created symmetric round pockets, temporary silicone areolar wafers were inserted (Figure 12-26, *I* and *J*).

After 6 weeks, reactive capsules had developed around the implants (Figure 12-26, *K*). The areolar pockets and the donor adipofascial flaps were outlined (Figure 12-26, *L*). The tissue sources for the areolar fill were redundant skin on the lateral aspects of each breast mound (Figure 12-26, *M*). Each flap, based medial to the areolar site, was de-epithelialized and inserted into the emptied subareolar capsule (Figure 12-26, *N* and *O*). The donor sites were approximated in a layered closure over the muscle.

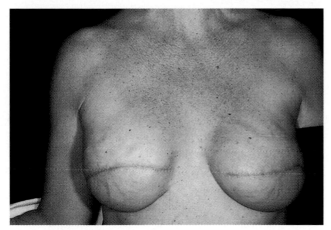

12-26F

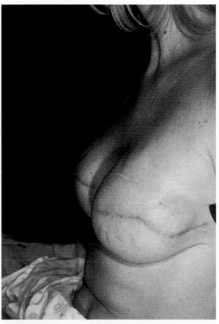

12-26G

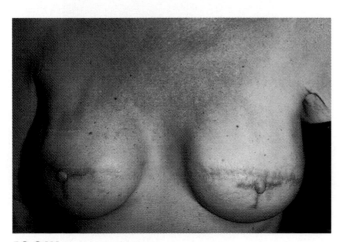

12-26H

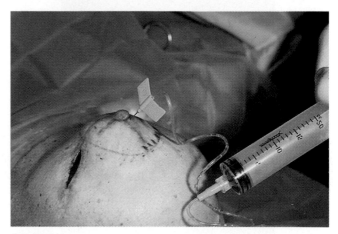

12-26I

Continued

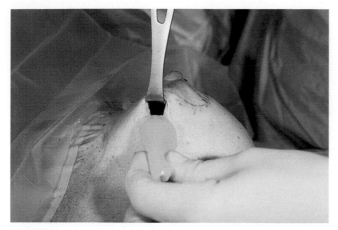

12-26J

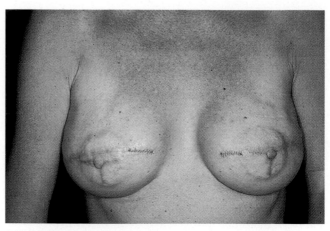

12-26K

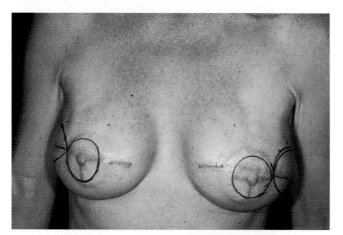

12-26L

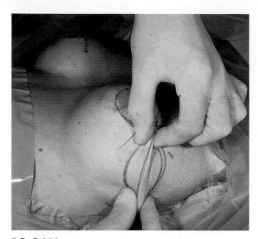

12-26M

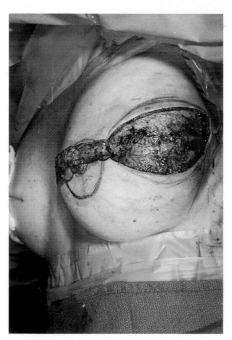

12-26N

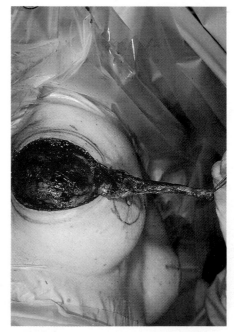

12-26O

Results (Figure 12-26, *P* and *Q*)

The patient is shown 3 months after completion of her breast reconstructions. Intradermal tattooing of the nipple-areolar complexes was performed 3 months after the adipodermal flaps were transferred for apical projection. The remote valves for the permanent mam-

mary implants were removed with the patient under local anesthesia 4 months after tattooing. The breast implants remained soft with a Baker II encapsulation. Implant folds persisted to the same degree without further deepening.

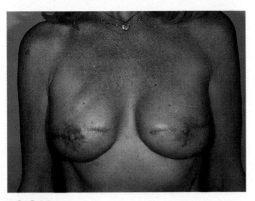

12-26P

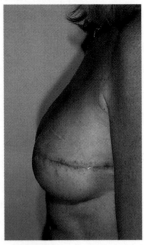

12-26Q

CASE 6: Bilateral Modified Radical Mastectomies in Moderate-Size and Large Breasts

History (Figure 12-27, *A*)

This 48-year-old patient was diagnosed with invasive multifocal ductal carcinomas in both breasts. She had a strong family history for breast cancer and had undergone a number of biopsies for suspicious mammographic lesions in past years. The amount of skin removal, which included the nipple-areolar complex and skin biopsy site, was estimated at 40% to 45% of the breast skin brassiere (38-full C-cup).

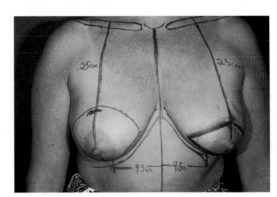

12-27A

Stage I: Mastectomies and Expander Insertion
(Figure 12-27, *B*)

After the modified radical mastectomies were completed, 600 cc smooth round expanders were positioned under muscle coverage from the pectoralis major and minor and serratus anterior. The remote valves were located in the subcutaneous fat under the lateral axillary skin. Each expander was filled with 300 ml of saline at surgery to maintain the pocket dimensions.

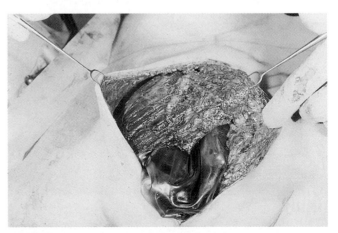

12-27B

Expansion Course (Figure 12-27, *C*)

Serial expansions with 20 to 30 ml of saline were completed weekly for 3 to 4 months, resulting in a total volume of 700 cc within each expander. The most significant measure of expansion, however, was indicated by the length of the vertical meridian line over time. When the distance from the midclavicle to inframammary fold reached 34 cm, the patient was scheduled for her exchange procedure.

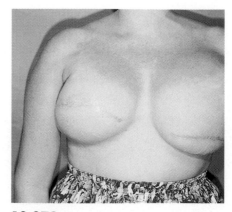

12-27C

Stage II: Implant Exchange with Shoji Technique
(Figure 12-27, *D*)

At surgery the entire lengths of the horizontal mastectomy scars were incised to elevate the thick skin flaps from the muscular layer. The fascial extension of the pectoralis major muscle was transected to remove the expander and to create the third flap (muscle) in the Shoji technique. The inframammary fold was constructed by multiple internal sutures. A 550 cc textured gel implant was positioned in its pocket, over which the pectoralis major muscle draped. The muscle's inferior edge was sutured to the subcutaneous fat 4 cm inside the lower skin flap's border. The muscle was purposefully sutured below the skin closure line so that the implant would remain isolated after wound separation and areolar reconstruction would occur above the muscle layer.

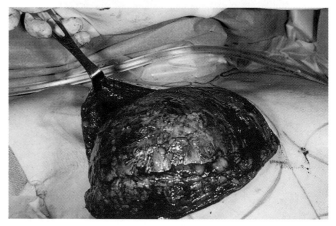

12-27D

Nipple-Areolar Reconstruction
(Figure 12-27, *E* to *J*)

Four months after construction of ptotic breast mounds, optimal locations of the nipple-areolar complexes were sighted by measurements and pasty adjustments (Figure 12-27, *E* and *F*). Bilateral skate flaps constructed the projected nipples (Figure 12-27, *G*).

Bilateral adipofascial flaps (2 × 12 cm) from the rectus abdominis fascia were elevated and based on the inframammary folds (Figure 12-27, *H* to *J*). The distal end of each flap was sutured into a mound that resembled an areolar cushion. A subcutaneous tunnel was created from the inframammary fold to the designated site for apical filling under the reconstructed nipple. The club end of the adipofascial flap was passed through the tunnel and fixed by sutures in the subareolar pocket. A prefabricated capsule may not be required to contain the club end of the transferred flap.

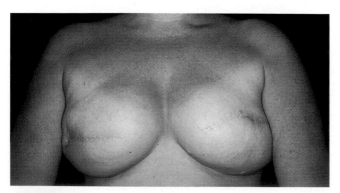

12-27E

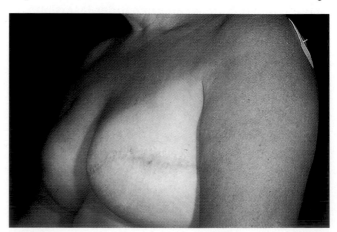

12-27F

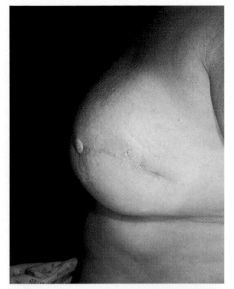

12-27G

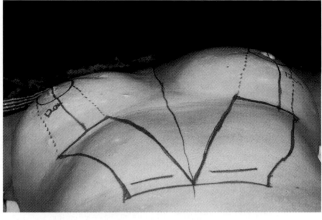

12-27H

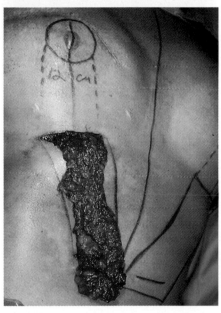

12-27I

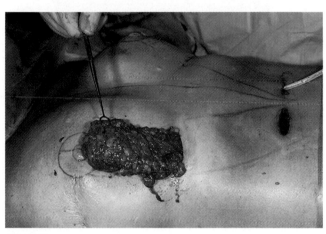

12-27J

Results (Figure 12-27, *K* and *L*)

Three years after her breast reconstructions the patient has a 38 C-cup size. The breast implants are soft and classified as a Baker II/III encapsulation. The mounds have remained ptotic and symmetric. Nipple-areolar tattooing was completed 3 months after the adipofascial flaps were transferred.

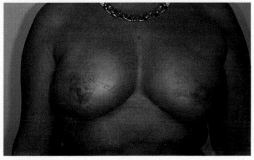

12-27K

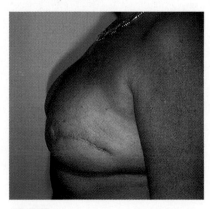

12-27L

CASE 7: Delayed Reconstruction after Left Modified Radical Mastectomy and Right Augmentation Mammoplasty

History (Figure 12-28, *A* and *B*)

This 39-year-old patient requested a delayed reconstruction of her left breast and an augmentation mammoplasty to her right breast. A modified radical mastectomy for invasive ductal carcinoma was performed 2 years earlier, removing a portion of the pectoralis muscle from its origins on the fourth to sixth ribs. The pathology report listed the dimensions of the skin el-

lipse as 6 × 15 cm, about 40% of the left breast brassiere. The patient had received a year of multidrug chemotherapy and was taking an antiestrogenic agent. Surveillance studies did not demonstrate abnormalities within the right breast. The patient was a candidate for expansion surgery for the left breast mound and an augmentation of her right breast (34-A cup).

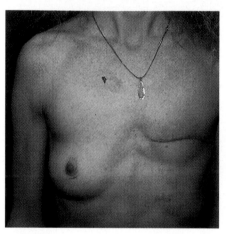

12-28A

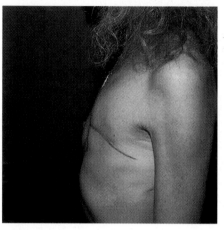

12-28B

Stage I: Expander Insertion and Mammoplasty
(Figure 12-28, *C* and *D*)

A 3.5 cm transverse incision in the midaxilla permitted dissection under the pectoralis major muscle with a lighted retractor and electrocautery (Figure 12-28, *C*). The generous pocket extended 1 cm from the midsternal line, 2 cm below the previous inframammary line, and up to the level of the third rib. A custom-made stacked expander, consisting of an elliptic base unit (250 cc) and a smaller anterior unit (200 cc), was inserted into its prepared pocket (Figure 12-28, *D*). The separated ex-

panders were smooth walled with an incorporated valve (upper unit) and a remote valve (lower unit). Intraoperative filling of the lower unit with 100 ml of saline maintained the pocket size, and 50 ml of saline in the upper unit provided anterior expansion.

A subpectoral augmentation mammoplasty through an axillary approach permitted the insertion of a 250 cc smooth-wall gel implant. Dissection was achieved 1 cm below the inframammary fold with a lighted retractor and an extended suction cautery.

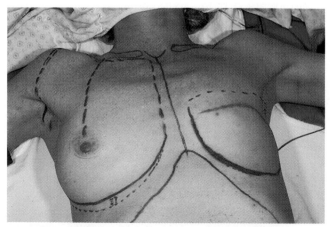

12-28C

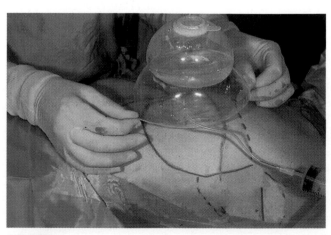

12-28D

Expansion Course (Figure 12-28, *E*)
Serial weekly fillings of saline to both stacked expanders produced an anatomically shaped breast mound with a degree of ptosis. The final fill volumes at the end of 3 months were 340 cc for the top round expander and 225 cc for the bottom elliptic expander.

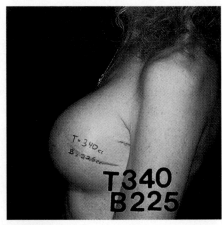

12-28E

Stage II: Implant Exchange with Shoji Technique (Figure 12-28, *F* to *H*)
At surgery the transverse mastectomy scar was reopened on the left breast mound (Figure 12-28, *F*). Three flaps were created with the Shoji technique after removal of the stacked expander. The inframammary fold was defined by internal sutures. A smooth-walled Becker implant (250 cc gel:250 cc saline) was inserted under the muscle flap. A minimal amount of saline (75 ml) was introduced into the saline compartment at surgery.

Saline was added to the Becker implant within a year after surgery to match the shape, projection, and softness of the augmented breast with a 34-full B-cup size (Figure 12-28, *G* and *H*).

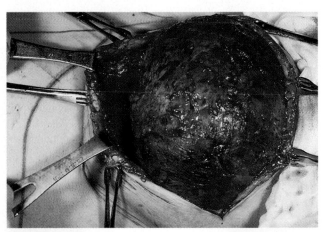

12-28F

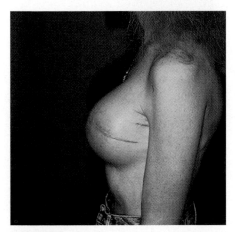

12-28G

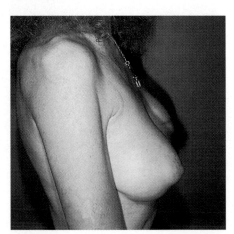

12-28H

Nipple-Areolar Reconstruction
(Figure 12-28, *I* and *J*)
The optimal location of the nipple-areolar complex on the left breast mound was determined by sighting with a pasty and from measurements reflecting the reference positions of the right complex (Figure 12-28, *I*). A 2.5 cm incision within the mastectomy scar above

the proposed site allowed a deep dissection above the pectoralis muscle in the shape of the outlined areola (4.5 cm diameter). Intraoperative expansion with an areolar expander up to 20 cc created a symmetric pocket (Figure 12-28, *J*). The contoured silicone elastomer implant (4.5 cm) with nipple projection was inserted to produce apical fullness.

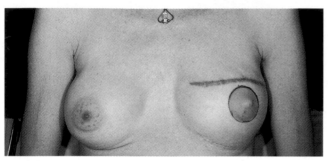

12-28I

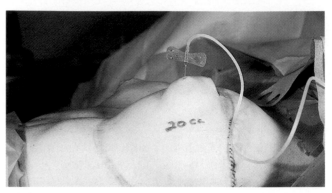

12-28J

Results (Figure 12-28, *K* and *L*)
The patient is shown 3 years after completion of her left breast reconstruction and right augmentation mammoplasty. Intradermal tattooing of the nipple-areolar outline was performed 4 months after the are-

olar silicone implant was positioned. The remote valve for the Becker prosthesis was removed with the patient under local anesthesia after optimal breast symmetry was achieved.

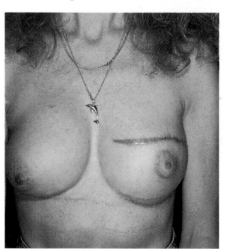

12-28K

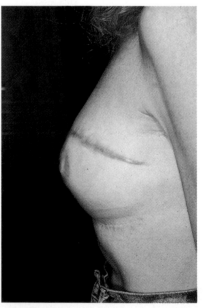

12-28L

CASE 8: Left Modified Radical Mastectomy and Right Subcutaneous Mastectomy

History (Figure 12-29, *A* and *B*)

This 36-year-old patient was diagnosed with an invasive lobular carcinoma in her left breast. A contralateral mirror-image biopsy, performed on her right breast

through a periareolar incision, revealed dysplastic changes. A left modified radical mastectomy and simultaneous right subcutaneous mastectomy with preservation of the areola were recommended.

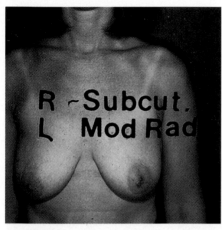

12-29A

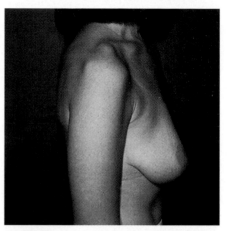

12-29B

Stage I: Mastectomies and Expander Insertion
(Figure 12-29, *C* and *D*)

The right subcutaneous mastectomy was done through an inframammary approach that removed the nipple in continuity with the parenchymal tissue (Figure 12-29, *C*). A smooth-walled Becker prosthesis (250 cc gel : 250 cc saline) was inserted under the elevated pectoralis major muscle. A small amount of saline (50 ml) was added through the buried remote valve at surgery.

The left modified radical mastectomy removed a skin ellipse that included the biopsy site and the

nipple-areolar complex (Figure 12-29, *D*). This amount of skin represented about 45% of the breast brassiere. A custom-made stacked expander, consisting of an anterior balloon (300 cc) and a posterior elliptic balloon (450 cc), was inserted under total muscle coverage. This involved suturing the elevated pectoralis minor–serratus anterior muscle flap to the inferior border of the pectoralis major muscle. The stacked expander was filled during surgery with saline through a remote valve system for each expander (150 cc anterior balloon, 200 cc posterior balloon).

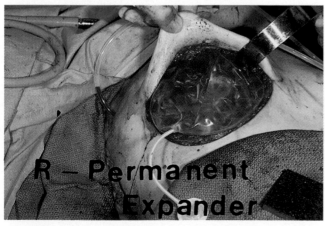

12-29C

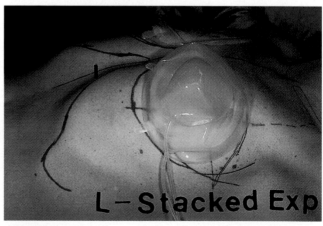

12-29D

Expansion Course (Figure 12-29, *E* and *F*)

Weekly serial fillings with 20 to 25 ml of saline to each of the stacked expanders for 3 months achieved sufficient tissue for left breast reconstruction (Figure 12-29, *E*). The final volume of both the anterior and the posterior expander was 450 cc. The vertical meridian line from the midclavicle to the inframammary fold measured 2 cm longer than the identical reference line on the right breast after the expansion process.

In the right breast the final saline volume in the Becker permanent implant was 250 cc, giving a total implant volume of 500 cc (Figure 12-29, *F*). The additional saline was injected in increments of 30 ml over 3 months after surgery. The patient helped to determine the projection, softness, and smoothness of the breast mound during the filling periods.

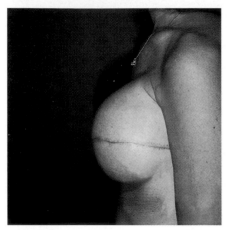

12-29E

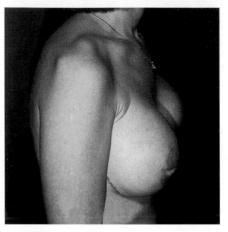

12-29F

Stage II: Implant Exchange with Shoji Technique (Figure 12-29, *G* to *I*)

At surgery, three flaps were created when the stacked expander was removed from the left breast (Figure 12-29, *G*). The inframammary fold was developed by internal sutures following the outline of the reflected opposite fold. A Becker implant, identical to the right prosthesis, was inserted under the pectoralis major muscle. About 150 ml of saline was added to the implant at surgery. Final filling up to 250 ml of saline adjusted the projection, softness, and smoothness of the implant in the postoperative period (Figures 12-29, *H* and *I*).

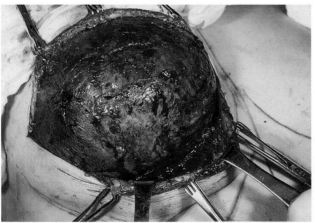

12-29G

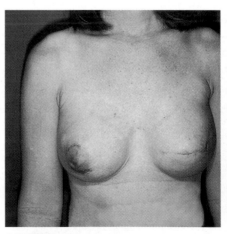

12-29H

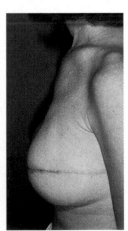

12-29I

Nipple-Areolar Reconstruction
(Figure 12-29, *J* to *L*)

Six months later a subareolar pocket above the pectoralis muscle was dissected through a 2.5 cm incision in the lateral aspect of the mastectomy scar (Figure 12-29, *J*). Intraoperative expansion with a 4.5 cm areolar expander created a symmetric pocket. A permanent silicone areolar implant was inserted to promote apical filling and provide suggestion of a nipple. A similar areolar cushion implant was inserted under the right areola for apical projection.

Four months after insertion of the left areolar implant (Figure 12-29, *K*), intradermal tattooing completed the breast reconstruction (Figure 12-29, *L*). Tattooing was also performed on the right areola to match the reconstructed side.

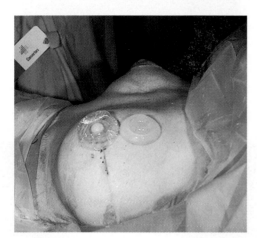

12-29J

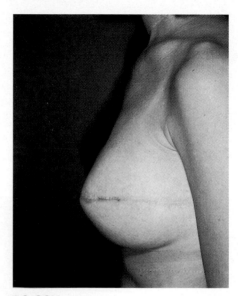

12-29K

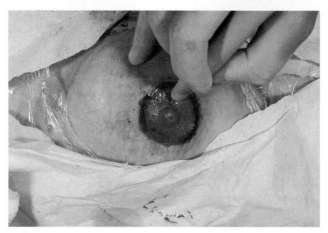

12-29L

Results (Figure 12-29, *M* to *P*)

Two years after surgery the patient has a ptotic left breast that closely approximates the opposite side. The breast remains soft with a Baker II/III encapsulation. Apical conization produces a more youthful mound under clothing.

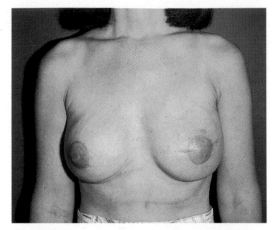

12-29M

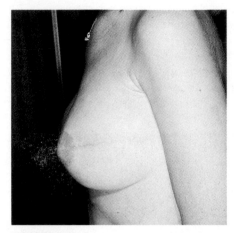

12-29N

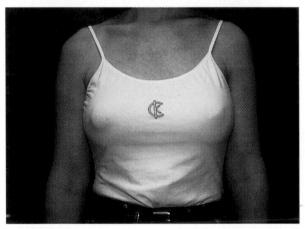

12-29O

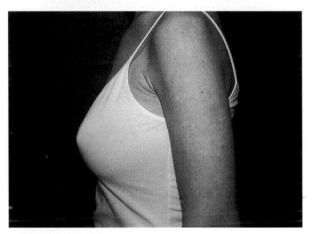

12-29P

CASE 9: Delayed Reconstruction After Left Modified Radical Mastectomy and Right Simple Mastectomy in Large Breast

History (Figure 12-30, *A*)

This 55-year-old patient underwent a left modified radical mastectomy for invasive ductal carcinoma with a year of chemotherapy. An in situ intraductal cancer was discovered in her large ptotic right breast (44-DD cup). A simple mastectomy was recommended for her comedocarcinoma. The patient requested bilateral breast reconstructions by expansion technique and did not consider a TRAM flap procedure.

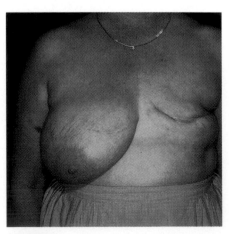

12-30A

Stage I: Delayed Reconstruction and Mastectomy (Figure 12-30, *B* to *F*)

A custom-made stacked expander was inserted through a 4 cm incision in the lateral aspect of the left mastectomy scar (Figure 12-30, *B*). The stacked expander consisted of a smaller 300 cc anterior round balloon ectopically positioned on the larger 500 cc posterior round balloon (Figure 12-30, *C*). Each balloon was filled with its own remote valve system. The retropectoral dissection was facilitated by a lighted retractor and suction cautery. The expander unit was positioned in its lower pocket by suture fixation tabs. Intraoperative filling with 100 ml of saline in the anterior balloon and 250 ml of saline in the posterior balloon maintained the dissected pocket.

The skin design for the right simple mastectomy resembled a Wise pattern, with the vertical limbs (12 cm) drawn outside the large nipple-areolar complex (Figure 12-30, *D*). The inferior skin flap would be de-

epithelialized to provide additional support under the skin closure (Figure 12-30, *E*). At surgery the central portion of the retained dermal flap was sutured in the shape of an areolar cushion to provide apical fullness under the inverted T-shaped skin closure (Figure 12-30, *F*). A Becker permanent prosthesis (300 cc gel : 300 cc saline) was inserted under the elevated pectoralis major muscle and the attached dermal flap, which was sutured to the muscle's inferior border. The implant was filled with 100 ml of saline at surgery.

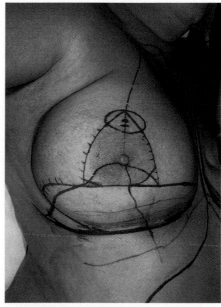

12-30D

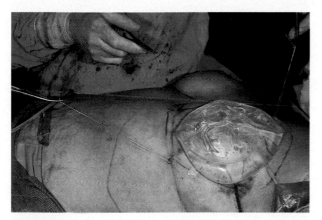

12-30B

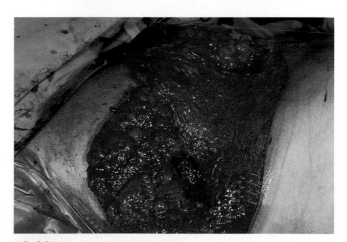

12-30E

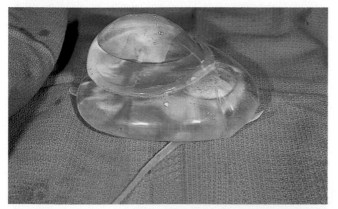

12-30C

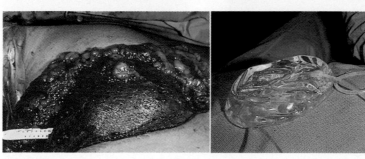

12-30F

Expansion Course (Figure 12-30, *G*)

Weekly serial expansions with 20 to 25 ml of saline in each balloon continued until sufficient tissue was produced in the left breast mound to match the right breast. When each of the stacked balloons contained 500 cc of saline, the vertical meridian line from the midclavicle to the inframammary fold was 3 cm longer than the right breast meridian line. The final amount of saline added to the right Becker implant was 300 ml, for a total implant volume of 600 cc.

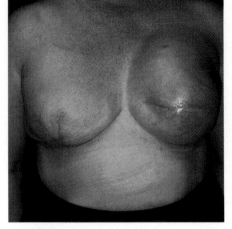

12-30G

Stage II: Implant Exchange with Shoji Technique (Figure 12-30, *H*)

At surgery, three flaps were created after removal of the stacked expander. The inframammary fold was recreated by a series of internal sutures placed along the marked line. A Becker permanent prosthesis (300 cc gel:300 cc saline) was inserted into the prepared pocket under the released pectoralis major muscle. About 250 ml of saline was added to the implant at surgery to fill out the skin brassiere.

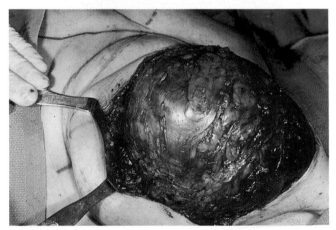

12-30H

Nipple-Areolar Reconstruction
(Figure 12-30, *I* and *J*)

Six months later the areolar sites were determined on each mound by the appearance of pasties and from measurements (Figure 12-30, *I*). Silicone areolar elas-

tomer implants with a central nipple projection were inserted into the subareolar pockets, which were dissected from 2.5 cm incisions along the mastectomy scars (Figure 12-30, *J*).

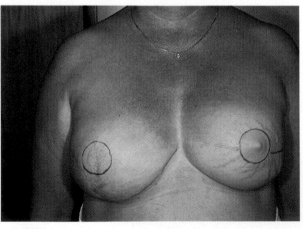

12-30I

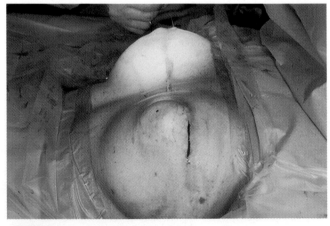

12-30J

Results (Figure 12-30, *K*)
Three years later the patient has D-cup-sized breast mounds that have a degree of ptosis and apical filling. Intradermal tattooing was performed 4 months after insertion of the areolar implants.

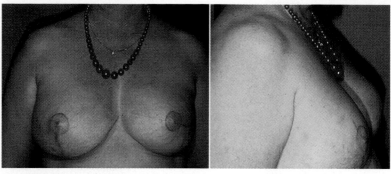

12-30K

CASE 10: Bilateral Modified Radical Mastectomies

History (Figure 12-31, *A left*)
This 56-year-old patient underwent bilateral modified radical mastectomies for invasive ductal carcinomas. A significant amount of the lower third of the pectoralis muscles was resected. The patient requested breast reconstruction by expansion technique.

Stage I: Expander Insertion (Figure 12-31, *A right*)
Two custom-made stacked expanders, each consisting of an anterior balloon (200 cc) and a posterior balloon (350 cc), were inserted through 3 cm incisions in the lateral aspects of the mastectomy scars under the subcutaneous tissue of the anticipated mounds' lower hemispheres. Each anterior balloon was filled with 75 ml of saline and each posterior balloon about 150 ml of saline.

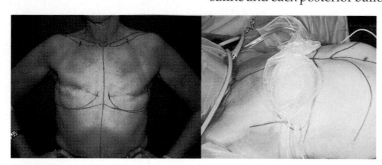

12-31A

Expansion Course (Figure 12-31, *B* and *C*)

Serial filling of the expander compartments averaged 20 to 30 ml of saline weekly. Expansion progressed rapidly over 2 months because stretching occurred under the thin skin flaps. At the end of expansion the anterior balloons contained 500 ml and the posterior balloons 435 (right) and 425 (left) ml of saline.

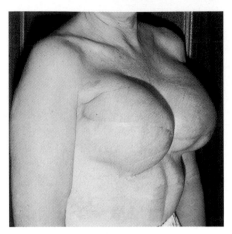

12-31B

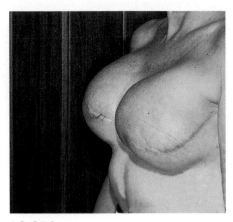

12-31C

Stage II: Implant Exchange with Shoji Technique
(Figure 12-31, *D*)

At surgery the mastectomy scar was opened across its extent. After the stacked expander was removed, the inframammary fold was defined with a series of internal sutures. Removal of the thin capsule adherent to the skin flaps' undersurface was not required. A Becker prosthesis (250 cc gel:250 cc saline) was inserted into the expanded pocket and filled with 100 ml of saline.

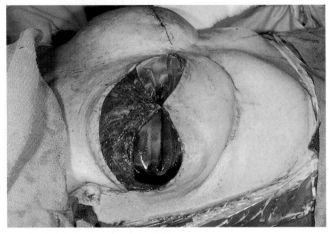

12-31D

Results (Figure 12-31, *E* and *F*)

Further adjustments in implant volume were performed postoperatively. A final implant volume of 550 cc was attained to produce a 36-full C-cup mound.

The patient did not request apical filling but had intradermal tattooing of the nipple-areolar complexes. The breast implants developed a Baker III encapsulation within 3 years after surgery.

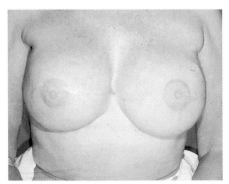

12-31E

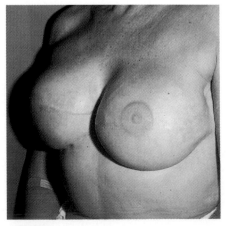

12-31F

CASE 11: Delayed Reconstruction After Left Modified Radical Mastectomy and Right Subcutaneous Mastectomy

History (Figure 12-32, *A*)

This 48-year-old patient underwent a left modified radical mastectomy for invasive ductal carcinoma. A right breast biopsy demonstrated dysplastic changes. The patient requested a delayed reconstruction for her left breast and proceeded with a prophylactic right subcutaneous mastectomy.

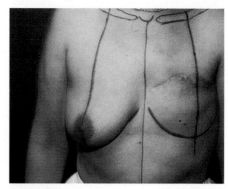

12-32A

Stage I: Delayed Reconstruction and Prophylactic Mastectomy (Figure 12-32, *B* to *E*)

The outline of the breast expander position was marked on the left chest wall (Figure 12-32, *B*). A 3 cm incision was drawn on the lateral aspect of the mastectomy scar. A stacked tissue expander, consisting of an anterior balloon (150 cc) and a posterior balloon (300 cc), was inserted under the pectoralis major muscle through the lateral incision (Figure 12-32, *C*).

A right prophylactic subcutaneous mastectomy was performed through an inframammary incision (Figure 12-32, *D*). A Becker permanent prosthesis (250 cc gel : 250 cc saline) was inserted under the pectoralis major muscle (Figure 12-32, *E*). The saline compartment was filled with 100 ml of saline.

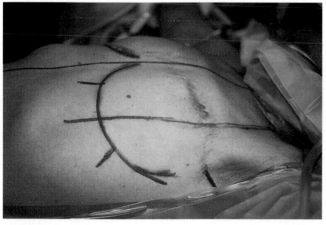

12-32B

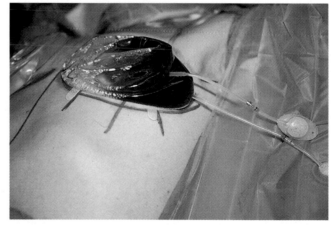

12-32C

Continued

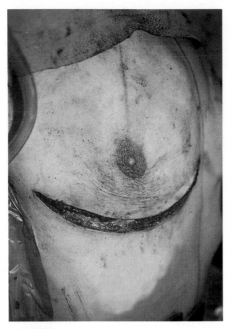

12-32D

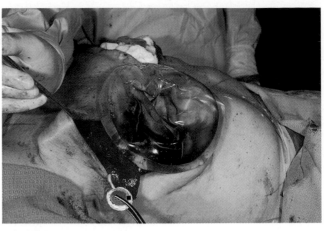

12-32E

Expansion Course (Figure 12-32, *F* and *G*)

In the immediate postoperative period, full-thickness skin loss occurred over the apex of the right breast (Figure 12-32, *F*). The saline was removed from the Becker implant to reduce skin tension. A full-thickness skin graft from the right groin resurfaced the exposed pectoralis major muscle. No periprosthetic infection developed.

Serial filling with 20 to 25 ml of saline to the left stacked expander progressed weekly over 3 months (Figure 12-32, *G*) to the final volume of 550 cc.

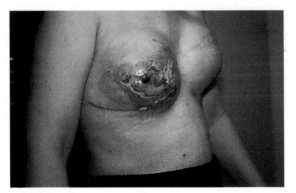

12-32F

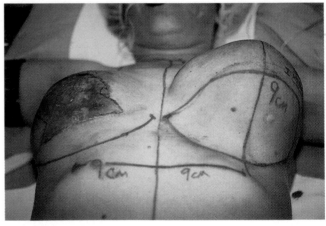

12-32G

Stage II: Implant Exchange with Shoji Technique (Figure 12-32, *H* to *J*)

At surgery, three flaps were developed after removal of the stacked expander (Figure 12-32, *H*). The inframammary fold was defined with internal sutures. A Becker prosthesis (250 cc gel:250 cc saline) was inserted into the prepared pocket and filled with 125 ml of saline.

During the interval surgery to the left breast, the right permanent expander was slowly filled to stretch the overlying skin graft over 5 months (Figure 12-32, *I* and *J*). The grafted right breast mound finally achieved close symmetry to the left reconstructed mound.

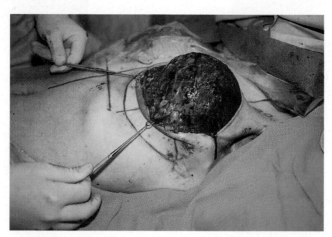

12-32H

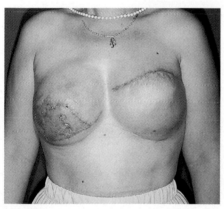

12-32I

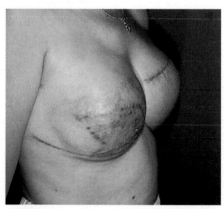

12-32J

Nipple-Areolar Reconstruction (Figure 12-32, *K*)

Six months later the optimal sites for the nipple-areolar complexes were located with pasties. Subareolar pockets were dissected deep under the skin graft on the right mound and under the skin flap on the left mound. Intraoperative filling of the areolar expanders created symmetric pockets. A 4.5 cm silicone areolar implant was inserted into each pocket for apical projection.

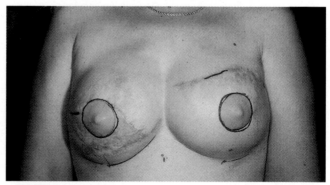

12-32K

Results (Figure 12-32, *L* and *M*)

Five years later the patient has ptotic breast mounds classified as a Baker III encapsulation. The areolar im-

plants have continued to provide apical fill. Intradermal tattooing was done about 1 year after the areolar implants were inserted.

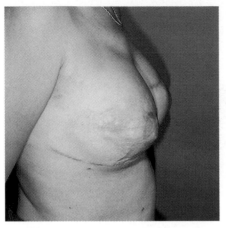

12-32L

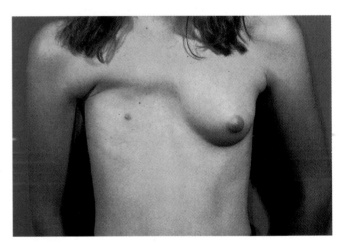

12-32M

CASE 12: Poland's Syndrome to Right Breast

History (Figure 12-33, *A*)

This 18-year-old patient had Poland's syndrome to the right chest wall that involved absence of the pectoralis major muscle, slight concavity to the right rib cage, and presence of a rudimentary nipple without an areola. The patient sought reconstruction because of the developing left breast mound with puberty.

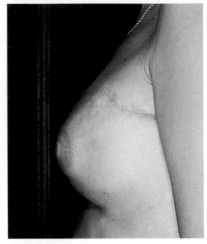

12-33A

Surgical Procedure (Figure 12-33, *B* and *C*)

A 4.5 cm inframammary incision permitted the dissection of a pocket for insertion of a Becker (150 cc gel : 150 cc saline) prosthesis (Figure 12-33, *B*). The volume was increased slowly with saline to adjust the implant to the enlarging left breast mound. One year after no further changes were observed in the left breast, the remote valve was removed (Figure 12-33, *C*).

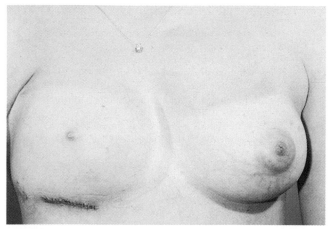

12-33B

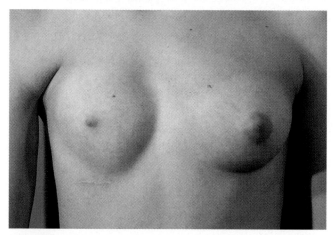

12-33C

Results (Figure 12-33, *D*)

Four years after the Becker implant was inserted, the patient's prosthesis remains soft with a Baker II/III encapsulation.

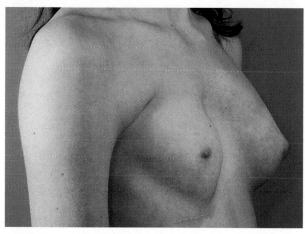

12-33D

SUMMARY

The long-term results of tissue expansion for breast reconstruction have been successful with acceptable rates of complications. Indications for expansion technique include patients with mild-to-moderate skin loss after mastectomy with remaining skin of good quality. The technique is safe and reliable for reconstruction of a mildly ptotic breast. Secondary procedures such as nipple reconstruction and areolar-filling techniques contribute to the completion of the breast mound to match the opposite side. In patients who require autogenous tissue for reconstruction, in declining preference, the TRAM, latissimus dorsi muscle, and buttock free flaps are recommended.

Avoidance of complications with improved techniques and indications should lower the incidence rates for perioperative problems of infection, ischemia, deflation, and malposition. A decreased capsular contracture rate can be achieved by minimizing postoperative complications such as large seromas, hematomas, and periprosthetic infections. The benefits of textured-wall implants in reducing capsular contractures require further study.

REFERENCES

1. Radovan C: Reconstruction of the breast after radical mastectomy using a temporary expander, *Plast Surg Forum* 1:41, 1978.
2. Lapin R, Daniel D, Hutchins H: Primary breast reconstruction following mastectomy using a skin expander prosthesis, *Breast* 6:20, 1980.
3. Gruber RP: Breast reconstruction following mastectomy: a comparison of submuscular and subcutaneous techniques, *Plast Reconstr Surg* 76:312, 1981.

4. Radovan C: Breast reconstruction after mastectomy using the temporary expander, *Plast Reconstr Surg* 69:195, 1982.

5. Argenta LC, Marks MW, Grabb WC: Selective use of serial expansion in breast reconstruction, *Ann Plast Surg* 11:188, 1983.

6. Bostwick J: *Aesthetic and reconstructive breast surgery*, St Louis, 1983, Mosby.

7. Gibney J: Tissue expansion. In Habal M, editor: *Advances in plastic and reconstructive surgery*, Chicago, 1984, Year Book.

8. Versaci AD, Balkovich ME: Tissue expansion. In Habal M, editor: *Advances in plastic and reconstructive surgery*, Chicago, 1984, Year Book.

9. Seckel BR, Hyland WT: Soft tissue expander for delayed and immediate breast reconstruction, *Surg Clin North Am* 65:383, 1985.

10. Becker H: Breast reconstruction following mastectomy using a permanent expander, *Plast Surg Forum* 9:20, 1986.

11. Gibney J: The long term results of tissue expansion for breast reconstruction, *Clin Plast Surg* 14:509, 1987.

12. Versaci AD: Reconstruction of a pendulous breast utilizing the tissue expander, *Plast Reconstr Surg* 80:387, 1987.

13. Versaci AD: Reconstruction of a pendulous breast utilizing a tissue expander, *Clin Plast Surg* 14:499, 1987.

14. Jurkiewicz MJ, Krizek TJ, Mathes SJ, Ariyan S: *Plastic surgery principles and practice*, vol 2, St Louis, 1990, CV Mosby Co.

15. Versaci AM, Balkovich ME, Goldstein SA: Breast reconstruction by tissue expansion for congenital and burn deformities, *Ann Plast Surg* 16:20, 1986.

16. Radovan C: Advantages and complications of breast reconstruction using temporary expander, *ASPRS Plast Surg Forum* 3:63, 1978.

17. Pennisi VR: Making a definite inframammary fold under a reconstructed breast, *Plast Reconstr Surg* 60:523, 1977.

18. Ryan JJ: A lower thoracic advancement flap in breast reconstruction after mastectomy, *Plast Reconstr Surg* 70:153, 1982.

PART
Three INTRAOPERATIVE EXPANSION

13 Intraoperative Expansion as Immediate Reconstructive Technique

A common goal of the plastic and reconstructive surgeon is to provide ideal tissue replacement with minimal scars. Since the concept of tissue expansion was introduced 30 years ago, the technique remains one of the few methods that satisfies both aesthetic and functional requirements. In the majority of cases, donor tissue is expanded over time from adjacent areas that provide near-perfect color match, texture, sensation, and retention of special adnexal structures (e.g., hair follicles, sweat and sebaceous glands).

The need for long-term judicious expansion over many weeks and months, however, has limited use of tissue expansion to elective reconstructive problems that require significant amounts of tissue replacement. Additional disadvantages of chronic expansion are the cosmetic and functional deformities that result from the long-term presence of an enlarging foreign body. Also, a silicone expander under thin and poorly vascularized tissue can lead to implant exposure and infection. Prolonged expansion involves two surgical procedures: one to insert the expander and the other to remove the expander, excise the defect, and advance the flap.

In contrast to long-term expansion, intraoperative expansion permits the surgeon to stretch skin within minutes. Rapid skin expansion is accomplished by cyclic loading (saline filling) of temporary silicone expanders or other external skin-stretching devices. The recruitment of extra tissue permits the surgeon to close small skin defects with minimal tension or distortion.

This chapter discusses the concept of rapid expansion, physiologic and histologic changes, surgical technique and results, and common complications associated with this innovative method. Intraoperative expansion may have a broader clinical application than long-term expansion in the daily practice of the plastic and reconstructive surgeon. The technique de-

livers added tissue that may be required for reconstructive purposes in a safe, reliable, uncomplicated manner. In aesthetic surgery, intraoperative expansion may be useful for removing additional tissue during rhytidoplasty (elimination of wrinkles) or producing more skin for draping after augmentation mammoplasty.

CONCEPT

Neumann[1] first reported on soft tissue stretching by means of buried balloons. Since then, surgeons have determined the duration, amount, and direction of expansion to generate large quantities of tissue for reconstruction. All these efforts have used the mechanism of gradual stretching of tissues by expander over many weeks and months.

In the past 16 years the author has employed rapid intraoperative ("booster") expansion at the end of long-term expansion cases (Figure 13-1). This maneuver often provided an additional 1 to 3 cm of tissue before flap advancement, depending on the site of expansion, age of patient, and local tissue factors. In more than 1000 cases, rapid expansion has not adversely affected the chronically expanded flap and its capsule (see Chapter 3). Such flaps have regained sensation, remained supple, and retained adnexal structures (e.g., hair follicles) to enhance the overall reconstruction. Minimal histologic differences were observed in all skin layers between chronically expanded tissues and those that underwent intraoperative expansion as the final step of long-term expansion before reconstruction.

The concept of incrementally elongating skin to its limits of inherent extensibility at surgery has been studied and applied to clinical problems.[2-5] *Mechanical tension* ("skin hooking"), however, minimally changes

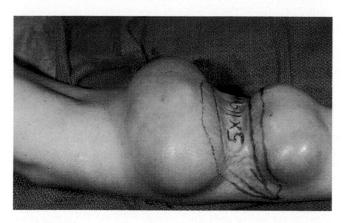

Figure 13-1 A 27-year-old patient sustained a dog-bite injury to her right forearm that resulted in a skin graft. After 1 year the patient wanted the graft removed and replaced with normal tissue. A 100 cc rectangular expander was inserted under the normal volar skin of the proximal forearm adjacent to the defect. A second, 50 cc rectangular expander was positioned in the distal volar forearm. After 3 months of longterm expansion, intraoperative filling of the expander beyond tissue tolerance was sustained for 3 to 5 minutes before opening the pocket to begin the reconstructive procedure. Intraoperative expansion temporarily produced skin ischemia and resulted in a closed capsulotomy. Both events increased the amount of available skin by 1 to 3 cm.

Net Surface Area Gain

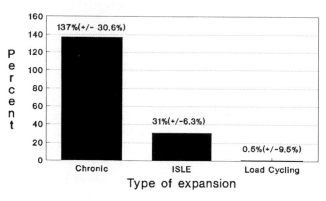

Figure 13-2 Summary of the percent gain in surface area of guinea pig skin that (1) was chronically stretched with a 40 cc expander over 6 weeks, (2) was subjected to intraoperative sustained limited expansion (*ISLE*) with a 40 cc expander over three cycles, and (3) was stretched by skin hooks (*load cycling*) over three cycles. Chronic expansion produced a 137% gain in surface area of the flap over its control measurement. Intraoperative expansion rapidly gained 31% in surface area over its control. Linear stretching with skin hooks over three cycles only provided a 0.5% gain in surface area over its control. (From Machida B, Liu-Shindo M, Sasaki GH, Rice DH: *Ann Plast Surg* 26:227-231, 1991.)

the viscoelasticity of skin because of the technical difficulties of applying a sufficient pull on the skin edge. Gibson and others[6] and Hirshowitz and colleagues[7] emphasized that cyclic loading of skin represents the most effective way to recruit extra tissue.

Intraoperative expansion by tissue expander balloons, as discussed in this chapter, thus is an outgrowth of the author's own experience and the significant contributions of other surgeons. Tissue expansion by inflating balloons produces more useful tissue than that obtained by using skin hooks (linear tension) because of expansion's more versatile means of tissue recruitment.

TISSUE CONSIDERATIONS

Experimental and clinical experiences with intraoperative balloon expansion raise at least four topics for discussion: (1) tissue gain, (2) origins and biomechanics of tissue gain, (3) pressure and blood flow changes, and (4) stretchback.

Tissue Gain

In loose skin animal models, intraoperative balloon expansion resulted in a 15% to 20% tissue gain. Machida and co-workers[8] inserted a 40 cc round ex-

pander (4 cm diameter) under the dorsal skin of a guinea pig. After repeating a 3-minute expansion and 3-minute rest cycle, the arc length and flap area were measured. Intraoperative expansion produced a 15% increase in flap length and a 31% gain in surface area (Figure 13-2).

Siegert and others[9] inserted a 200 cc round expander under the lateral flank in a dog. The expander was filled to a maximum volume of 300 cc until a tissue pressure of 100 mm Hg was maintained for at least 15 minutes. The expander was emptied for 20 minutes to ensure a return of circulatory perfusion. The serial expansion cycle was repeated up to 80 cycles. The maximal increase in flap length was 15% to 20% despite further increases in expander volume up to an average end volume of 1139 cc during the 3-hour course of the experiment.

In the author's clinical experience,[10,11] cyclic intraoperative balloon expansion for 1 to 3 minutes resulted in a 10% to 30% tissue gain. Up to a 2.5 cm tissue gain could be anticipated from each expander, depending on the patient's age and site of expansion.

Siegert and colleagues[9] also observed a 10% volume increase per hour in patients undergoing expansion for correction of severe microtia. Each of 30 patients had a 35 cc otoplasty expander filled at 5-minute intervals under a constant tissue pressure of 100 mm Hg for 4 to 16 cycles. The infusion volumes ranged from 16 to 95 cc on the first expansion cycle and increased slightly thereafter on subsequent fillings.

Although a preoperative assessment of the anticipated skin defect can be made, the degree of adjacent skin elasticity and glide to cover a defect is more difficult to predict in each patient. The ease of skin approximation depends on the defect's size, body site, patient's age, and local factors related to the donor skin. In general, defects larger than 4 cm in width are difficult to close by simple undermining and scoring the adjacent flaps without resorting to importation of tissue (e.g., skin grafts) or creation of larger local flaps (e.g., transposition flaps). Primary closure of smaller defects can still be problematic because of thicker and tethered donor skin, as found in the scalp, back, and plantar surfaces.

Sugihara,[12] Ohura,[13] and Stark[14] and their colleagues measured the extensibility of skin with a tensiometer from patients of different ages at various anatomic locations. Skin from patients less than 2 years of age possessed the greatest amount of intrinsic skin extensibility.

Chretien-Marquet[15] demonstrated that large skin defects involving at least 30% of an anatomic unit could be excised and closed with minimal undermining in one or several stages by taking advantage of an enforced position around flexible joints. The patients were children ranging in age from 4 months to 14 years.

Van Rappard and others[16] emphasized that tolerance to skin expansion varied according to the body site. Tissue expansion became less tolerant progressing from the scalp, breast, trunk, face, neck, back, upper leg, upper arm, forearm, and to the lower leg.

Origins and Biomechanics

The mechanisms that lead to an increase in skin length during intraoperative expansion are believed to involve the skin's intrinsic elasticity, "creep" behavior, interstitial fluid displacement, and biologic stimulation of cell division. The elastic properties of skin do not require preliminary stretching with an expander, and skin responds immediately after expansion forces are applied. An elastic deformation of the three-dimensional network of elastin and collagen fibers can readily account for an initial length increase of 15% to 20%.

Further elongation of skin length with additional expansion is believed to result from the phenomenon of *creep*, which is a time-dependent deformation of skin with each strain-volume curve obtained during serial expansion. Siegert and co-surgeons,[9] however, demonstrated that intact skin does not behave in vivo as a perfect viscoelastic material, and thus the strain-volume curves of the individual expansion cycles remain identical. Their data suggested that the phenomenon of creep did not contribute significantly to tissue gain.

Accordingly, an additional increase in expander volume results in a smaller incremental change in skin length by fluid displacement in tissues above and below the expander. This effect indirectly contributes to more skin advancement by reducing the thickness of skin, subcutaneous fat, and underlying muscles. Furthermore, as the expander volume progressively increases beyond its stated volume, the expander base diameter linearly increases and dissects with more undermining and mobilization, as described by Siegert and others.[9] These findings reinforce the results of Mackay and colleagues,[17] who believe that the major factor for wound closure depends more on extent of subcutaneous mobilization than on skin stretching.

Although Austad and associates[18,19] demonstrated an increased mitotic activity in the epidermis after chronic expansion, no study has reported on biologic growth after intraoperative expansion. If an increase in skin cell growth can be demonstrated above the anticipated level from a stimulus of trauma, such cellular activity may contribute to a critical gain weeks after immediate expansion has been completed.

Pressure and "Blood Flow" Changes

When tissue expanders are surgically inserted in their subcutaneous pockets, the adjacent skin flaps need to be undermined. Further damage caused by immediate mechanical expansion may narrow vessel diameters, occlude venous and lymphatic drainage, and produce endothelial disruption, leading to spasm and microthrombus formation. From this series of events, rapidly expanded flaps may not appear to be suitable for flap reconstruction. However, clinical experience with immediate expansion has shown the reliability of this technique to provide added tissue for coverage of most small and medium-sized defects.

Smaller volume expanders achieve a higher and steeper pressure-volume curve than larger volume expanders for a given volume. Since small expanders are filled rapidly, they reach a greater intraluminal pressure that affects the surrounding tissues. When the intraluminal pressure exceeds the perfusion pressure, blood flow decreases.

The author[11] studied "blood flow," as determined by laser Doppler scans, in skin before and during intraoperative serial expansion (Figure 13-3). Laser Doppler flow decreased rapidly to zero during the expansion phases. When the expander was deflated, the values recovered to near-normal levels within a minute. All flaps had satisfactory dermal bleeding at their leading edges before inset and survived in total length. In more than 840 intraoperative cases, flap ischemia was observed more frequently when flaps were located in the distal portions of the ex-

tremities (see section on complications). This complication can be prevented by cutting back to bleeding tissue at the dermis before the flap is sutured to the opposite side.

Stretchback

Skin stretchback results from forces exerted by elastic fibers and collagen that cause skin to return to its original state. The phenomenon of stretchback is observed after intraoperative and long-term expansion. *Immediate stretchback* refers to the amount of tissue shrinkage with expander removal. This area lost to immediate stretchback can be easily reestablished by advancing the flap.

Machida and others[8] calculated an immediate reduction of 15.4% surface area and 15.7% arc length after intraoperative expansion and a 24% surface area and 18.8% arch length decrease after chronic expansion in a guinea pig model (Figure 13-4). Nordstrom[20] also described delayed stretchback after scalp reduction in which one-third to one-half the effect of excision was lost during the 12-week postoperative period. This phenomenon may also be caused by wound contraction and contracture.

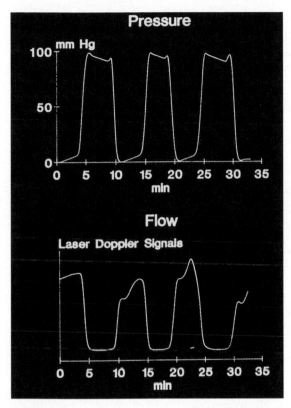

Figure 13-3 Graphs of "blood perfusion changes," as determined by laser Doppler measurements, in human forearm skin during removal of a tattoo by intraoperative expansion. Before insertion of the 100 cc round expander, the laser Doppler index of skin above the tattoo measured 45 units. A repeat measurement at the same site 10 minutes after expander insertion recorded a return of "blood flow" to the preinsertion level. Intraoperative expansion began by filling the expander with 100 ml of saline and sustaining the intraluminal pressure (by adding 10 ml saline) for 5 minutes to 100 mm Hg. During this initial fill the laser Doppler index dropped to 0 units of "blood perfusion." On balloon deflation the index gradually returned to prefill levels within 3 minutes. After a 5-minute break the balloon was again filled with 125 ml of saline for 5 minutes, during which a 100 mm Hg intraluminal pressure was maintained by adding 15 ml saline. The laser Doppler index again fell to 0. After a 5-minute deflation period the laser "perfusion index" slowly returned to prefill levels. The balloon was filled for a third time with 140 ml of saline for 5 minutes, during which an additional 10 ml of saline was required to maintain an intraluminal pressure of 100 mm Hg. The "perfusion index" returned more slowly to prefill levels within 5 minutes.

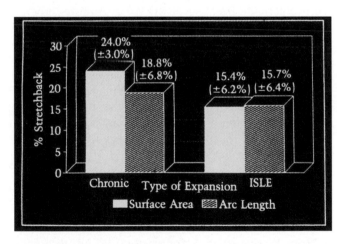

Figure 13-4 Calculated amount of immediate stretchback in guinea pig skin either intraoperatively expanded or chronically stretched with round expanders. After intraoperative expansion (three cycles of expansion and deflation) the tissue demonstrated an immediate stretchback of 15.4% in surface area and 15.7% in arc length. After chronic expansion the tissue contracted by 24% in surface area and 18.8% in arc length. No statistical significance was found between the two groups. These observations may have no relationship to the effects of delayed stretchback in expanded tissues. *ISLE,* Intraoperative sustained limited expansion. (From Machid BK, Liu-Shindo M, Sasaki GH, Rice DH: *Ann Plast Surg* 26:227-231, 1991.)

■ **Table 13-1** Intraoperative Expansion and Tissue Gain

Anatomic region	Average tissue gain (cm) per expander
Scalp	1.0-1.5
Forehead	1.0-2.5
Upper half of nose	1.0-1.5
Nasal tip	0.5-0.75
Midface	1.0-2.5
Neck	1.0-2.5
Chest/abdomen	1.5-2.5
Back/sacrum	1.0-1.5
Upper extremity	1.0-2.0
Lower extremity above knee	1.0-2.0
Lower extremity below knee	0.75-1.0

■ **Table 13-2** Sites of 844 Intraoperative Expansions

Site	Number
Head and neck	
Scalp	105
Forehead	94
Midface	117
Ear	5
Nose	147
Neck	24
Trunk	
Chest	43
Back	49
Breast	46
Upper extremity	
Upper arm	47
Forearm	67
Hand	13
Digit	7
Lower extremity	
Above knee	37
Knee	7
Below knee	26
Foot	10

CLINICAL INDICATIONS

In general, established or anticipated defects 2.5 to 3 cm in width can be simply closed by undermining the adjacent flaps without resorting to importation of tissue (e.g., skin grafts) or creation of local flaps (e.g., transposition flaps). Defects larger than 3.5 cm may be difficult to approximate because of overwhelming closing tension. If these larger defects are able to be closed, significant distortion of adjacent mobile structures may result. Primary closure of these larger defects may also be problematic because of thicker and more tethered donor skin, as found on the back, or a compromised blood supply from previous trauma, scarring, infection, or radiation. Even small defects (1 cm) located within thick sebaceous skin, such as found on the nasal tip, present challenges for simple linear closures. For this reason, nasal tip reconstruction frequently relies on local transposition or V-Y advancement flaps.

Indications for intraoperative expansion include the following:

- Primary closure for difficult defects that are overly wide or tight on trial closure
- Reduction or prevention of distortions and eventually widened hypertrophic scars
- Primary closure of a donor site from which a wide flap was transposed

The author's clinical experience with the intraoperative expansion technique in more than 840 cases indicated that up to 2.5 cm of tissue could be gained from each intraoperative expander (Table 13-1). Because of the thicker and nonelastic nature of skin from the scalp, nasal tip, and back, the average tissue gained by immediate expansion at these sites is less than that expected from other areas. Since two or more expanders can be positioned under opposite sides of a defect, more tissue can be generated with multiple expanders to approximate skin around larger defects. If the ad-

vantages of transposition flaps are preferred over the results of a linear or rotational advancement flap, intraoperative expansion of this donor flap may be useful (1) to expand a section of the transposition flap or (2) to facilitate closure of the donor site.

Intraoperative expansion has been used in almost all areas of reconstruction on the body surface (Table 13-2). In the author's experience the youngest patient was less than 1 year of age and the oldest patient in the ninth decade. Expansion has been well tolerated by all patients. Ecchymosis and rarely epithelial slough at the distal flap margins have not detracted from the overall results.

HISTOLOGIC FINDINGS

Light microscopy of skin tissues was performed using routine and special staining procedures in 10 patients who underwent intraoperative expansion. Reference samples were studied before and after expansion. No significant histologic changes in the epidermis, dermis, dermal appendages, adipose tissue, or muscle were observed in the tissues studied (Figure 13-5). Special collagen and elastin stains demonstrated slight malalignment but no evidence of microfragmentation. Shorter periods between expansions, larger volumes at each interval, and longer duration of expansion produced more inflammatory responses and ecchymotic changes.

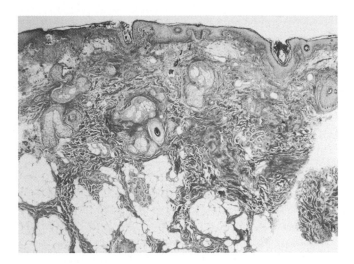

Figure 13-5 This trichrome-stained slide demonstrates the histologic findings in facial skin subjected to intraoperative expansion. This extra tissue was needed to resurface a defect produced after excision of a widened scar. No significant changes were seen in the epidermis, dermal appendages, collagen fibers, or adipocytes. Except for the infiltration of inflammatory cells from the trauma of the surgical procedure, the histology was similar to adjacent nonexpanded skin. Special elastin stains also did not show significant changes (e.g., microfragmentation, malalignment) in the elastin fibers in the reticular dermis.

EXPANDER UNITS

Intraoperative expanders consist of a silicone bag, tubing, and fast-fill remote valve. The volumes of standard expanders are 1, 2, 5, and 20 cc (Figure 13-6). Larger volume expanders may be selected for intraoperative use by changing the dome-shaped valve to the two-way fast-fill valve. These expanders may be round or rectangular. Custom-made expanders for unusual defects may be requested but generally are not required.

Most intraoperative expanders are used one time and should be discarded after the procedure is completed. However, a protective disposable sleeve around some expanders permits full standard autoclaving and thus multiple use of the implant in different patients.

PATIENT INFORMATION

The creation of a hemispheric mound adjacent to the site of reconstruction is inherent to tissue expansion. Most patients tolerate the temporary cosmetic and functional deformities associated with intraoperative expanders throughout the expansion period. Their acceptance of this temporary deformation increases when their concerns are anticipated and discussed in depth before the procedure. Because of rapid serial ex-

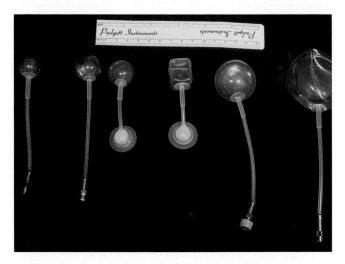

Figure 13-6 Small intraoperative expanders with either a fast-fill two-way valve or a standard remote valve. The expander volumes range from 1 to 20 cc. Larger conventional expanders used in long-term expansion are also available for intraoperative use with the substitution of a fast-fill valve. The addition of a disposable silicone sleeve around the expander allows repeated use.

pansions at surgery, the expanded skin may appear bruised with slight intradermal ecchymosis. Because intraoperative expansion results in an increased area of dissection, postoperative drainage of serosanguineous fluid may occur for a few days through the skin closure.

The experience of undergoing an intraoperative procedure should not be painful because the patient or the local field is anesthetized. Patients have not complained of increased pain or discomfort postoperatively. Variable degrees of paresthesias occur, but patients generally have normal return of sensation within 6 weeks after surgery.

Ischemia to the flap edge can occur after rapid expansion. Ischemia can lead to flap loss, wound separation, infection, and mixed pigmentation problems. The assessment of dermal bleeding at surgery is mandatory to preclude the complications of decreased flap perfusion. The surgeon should cut back on the expanded flap until satisfactory dermal bleeding is observed.

INTRAOPERATIVE PROCEDURE

After trial closure of a defect results in too tight an approximation or causes distortion of surrounding structures, intraoperative expansion should be considered. In most cases, however, preoperative planning, proper indications, and patient selection have already predetermined that the intraoperative procedure may be employed as part of the reconstructive process (Figure 13-7, *A*). The size and number of expanders needed to recruit adequate amounts of tissue to resurface the anticipated defect can be determined by (1) the size of the defect, (2) the size and location of available donor sites, and (3) the amount of advancement that can be expected from a hemispheric domed flap that has been serially expanded to its greatest limits.

General or local anesthesia may be employed, depending on the patient's age and preference and the lesion's location and size. Lidocaine (Xylocaine) with epinephrine (1:200,000 to 1:400,000) is used in patients to control bleeding. Epinephrine has not been known to contribute to flap ischemia.

When a benign lesion (scar, nevus, skin graft) is to be excised, a small incision (less than 1 cm) may be made parallel to the interface of the lesion and selected donor site(s) or radial within the lesion. A pocket(s) slightly larger than the base dimensions of the expander(s) is dissected under the donor tissue. When a suspected or known malignancy is to be removed, an excisional biopsy specimen is obtained first. After a tumor-free surgical margin is confirmed, a pocket(s) is developed adjacent to the defect larger than the size of the expander. A generous pocket helps contain the expander during serial expansions.

The intraoperative expanders may be placed under the skin at the subcutaneous level or under muscle (e.g., frontalis muscle of forehead) to replace similar tissue for an aesthetic and functional reconstruction.

Serial balloon expansion can then proceed, with the tubing positioned to exit through the defect site (Figure 13-7, *B*). A finger can be placed over the expander's entry site to prevent it from bulging out of its pocket during expansion. The use of sutures, skin clips, or towel clips to approximate temporarily the defect's edges may also be used to contain the expanders. Significant trauma during rapid expansion to the uninvolved skin edges may require them to be excised, leaving less tissue available for advancement.

The expander is filled with isotonic saline up to tissue tolerance, as determined by inspection (pallor) and palpation (firmness). Since the site has been anesthetized, patient intolerance to pain or pressure cannot be used as a reliable criterion to determine the end point of rapid expansion. The fill volume is maintained for 2 to 3 minutes during the first load cycle to initiate tissue stretch (Figure 13-7, *C*). The expander is deflated by withdrawing the saline to permit tissue perfusion for about 2 to 3 minutes. This procedure is repeated for two additional stress load cycles. The fill volume increases after each successive cycle, indicating effective tissue recruitment. A single expander filling for 10 to 15 minutes, especially in the extremi-

ties, may be too long and can produce sufficient tissue ischemia to lead to delayed necrosis.

After the expander(s) is removed from its pocket, a trial advancement is made for closure (Figure 13-7, *D*). Satisfactory bleeding from the dermis must be observed before flap approximation. In selected cases the expanded transposition flap (e.g., nasolabial or rhomboid flap) can be satisfactorily transferred to its recipient site with an easy donor site closure.

The sutures are removed at the appropriate time to prevent suture marks. An antibacterial ointment over the entire expanded flap for 3 to 5 days prevents dehydration and facilitates healing. Sunscreen lotions are recommended for at least 6 weeks postoperatively (Figure 13-7, *E*). Steroid-impregnated tapes may be useful to reduce hypertrophic scar formation.

COMPLICATIONS

The number of major complications associated with intraoperative expansion has decreased significantly with improvements in technique, patient indications, and clinical experience. In the author's series the complication rate was lowest in the head and neck (2%) and highest in the lower extremity (10%). A single case of marginal flap ischemia occurred in 492 reconstructions of the head and neck (0.2%), three cases in 138 expansions of the trunk (2%), and two cases in 134 upper extremity–resurfacing procedures (1%). Marginal flap necrosis developed in six of 80 cases (7.5%) of lower extremity reconstruction with intraoperative expansion. This complication was reduced after the technique of flap trimming for dermal bleeding was incorporated into the procedure.

After flap edge ischemia, small wound hematomas were the next most common problem. Intraoperative antibiotics are used to minimize the risk for infection; prolonged administration of antibiotics is not recommended. Topical ointment over rapidly expanded flaps is believed to reduce the rate of epithelial loss and subsequent flap loss.

CASE RESULTS: SCALP RECONSTRUCTION

The goal of scalp reconstruction is to provide (1) coverage similar to hair-bearing scalp tissue or (2) non-hairbearing scalp tissue to replace small scalp losses. Reconstructions using skin grafts or larger flaps create additional deficiences that may be unacceptable to the patient.

Intraoperative expansion of scalp tissue to resurface small defects less than 5 cm wide offers a practical

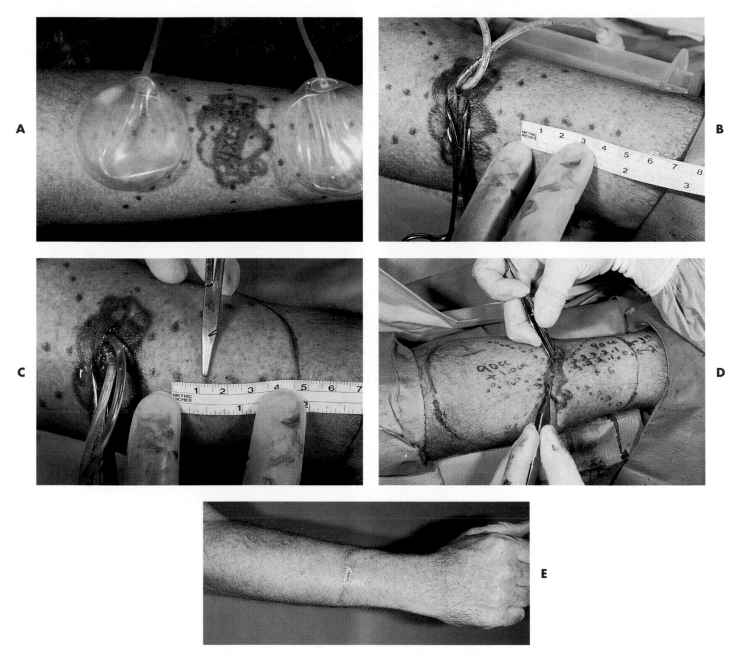

Figure 13-7 **A,** A 26-year-old patient had a 4 × 6 cm tattoo on the dorsum of his middle right forearm. Because of the tattoo's size and the axial direction of anticipated tissue closure, two 50 cc round expanders, one on each side of the tattoo, were required to gain sufficient tissue for closure. Rows of dots 1 cm apart were marked on the skin to demonstrate the amount of stretching during the expansion phases. A 2.5 cm intralesional incision is planned to permit pocket dissections in the subcutaneous fatty plane. **B,** Pockets have been generously dissected to contain the expanders during the serial expansion fills. The wound edges are approximated with a single towel clip. The distance between two dots over the apex of the distal expander is slightly more than 1 cm because the tissues have been injected with more than 50 ml of diluted local anesthetic (0.25% Xylocaine with 1:400,000 U epinephrine). **C,** In the third cycle of intraoperative expansion, each 50 cc round expander has been overfilled by 40 cc. Each serial expansion phase lasted about 3 minutes, with a 3-minute deflation period for reperfusion of tissues. The distance between the the same two dot markings has increased to 1.5 cm, indicating immediate tissue stretching. The amount of tissue stretch progressively diminishes from the apex to the periphery of the expanded tissue. The total amount of tissue gained at the end of intraoperative expansion was about 2 cm from each expanded area. **D,** Trial advancement of the rapidly stretched flaps was done after each expander was filled to 90 cc. The amount of gained tissue permitted a nontension closure after removal of the entire tattoo. Absorbing sutures from the dermis to the deep tissue advanced the flaps toward the incision closure and may help reduce the amount of delayed stretchback. **E,** Six weeks after reconstruction a hypertrophic scar has not developed, and sensation has returned gradually to presurgical levels. Some scar widening is anticipated and may require a scar revision in the future.

means to close them in a functional, aesthetic manner. The procedure has been successfully applied to reconstruct congenital defects, traumatic scars, premalignant lesions, malignancies, and hypertrophic widened scars. Long-term follow-up indicates not only reten- tion of hair density in the advancement flaps, but also creation of acceptable scars. With intraoperative expansion, however, a higher incidence of scar widening and alopecia occurs because of greater tension on skin closure.

CASE REPORT AND ANALYSIS: Scalp Reconstruction

Large Nevus on Scalp

History (Figure 13-8, *A*)

This 30-year-old patient had a 6 × 7 cm nevus on her left parieto-occipital scalp. A previous biopsy did not demonstrate malignancy. Because of the lesion's size and location, long-term expansion was discussed with the patient. However, she did not want a large scalp deformity during the expansion process. Intraoperative expansion was offered as an alternative method for reconstruction.

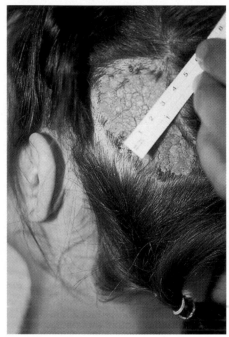

13-8A

Surgical Procedure (Figure 13-8, *B* and *C*)

At surgery a 2.5 cm incision was made within the nevus adjacent to the donor scalp skin. A subperiosteal pocket was dissected around the lesion to accommodate two 100 cc rectangular expanders. A series of three expansions of both expanders for 1 to 3 minutes gained enough tissue to advance the nor-mal scalp tissue across the defect. Each expansion filling was larger in volume than the previous one, indicating that additional tissue was being recruited (first fill, 100 cc/expander; second fill, 125 cc/expander; third fill, 150 cc/expander). The galea aponeurotica and periosteum were scored to release more tissue for the reconstruction.

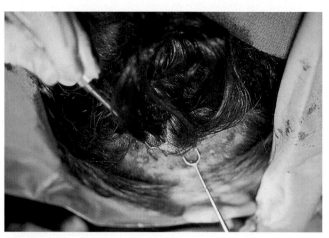

13-8C

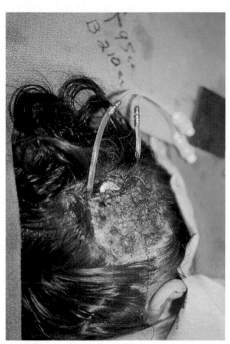

13-8B

Results (Figure 13-8, *D*)

The patient is shown immediately after scalp closure. The entire nevus was able to be removed. After a year, slight scar widening (7 mm) occurred along the seam line. No significant hair loss or thinning was observed in the rapidly expanded scalp.

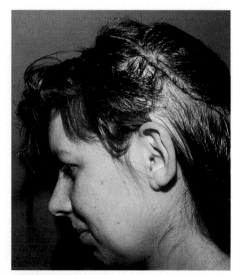

13-8D

CASE RESULTS: FOREHEAD RECONSTRUCTION

Forehead reconstructions usually involve the recruitment of either forehead skin or frontalis muscle and skin to resurface a defect. The goal of reconstruction in either case is to provide similar tissue with appropriate movement.

Intraoperative expansion of forehead skin or a frontalis myocutaneous flap with expanders can result in an aesthetic and functional reconstruction of defects 3.5 cm or more in width. At times, two expanders, one on each side of a median or paramedian defect, facilitate the recruitment of adequate amounts of tissue for an acceptable closure. Flap advancement can be made in either a vertical (midline defect) or a horizontal (lateral defect) direction to achieve the optimal aesthetic result. Long-term follow-up of forehead reconstructions demonstrated a functioning frontalis muscle unit and an acceptable nonhypertrophic scar.

CASE REPORTS AND ANALYSES: Forehead Reconstruction

CASE 1: Mohs' Surgical Forehead Defect for Basal Cell Cancer

History (Figure 13-9, *A left*)
This 56-year-old patient had a neglected sclerosing basal cell cancer on her forehead that was removed by Mohs' surgery. Although the anticipated 4 × 5 cm (actually 3.5 × 4 cm) defect could have been closed by a skin graft, local flaps, or chronic expansion, intraoperative expansion was suggested to provide like-tissue coverage with minimal scarring.

Surgical Procedure (Figure 13-9, *A right*)
The defect is shown immediately after excision and frozen section. Maximal undermining and releasing were performed with a trial closure. The defect was unable to be approximated in its lower half, and malposition of the brows occurred.

A 20 cc expander was positioned on each side of the forehead tissue in the subperiosteal plane. Both expanders were filled with 20 cc for 1 to 3 minutes and then deflated for the same period. The balloons were reinflated with 40 cc for 1 to 3 minutes, then deflated to permit vascular perfusion. The final fill volume of 50 cc into each balloon for 1 to 3 minutes gained 2 cm of tissue.

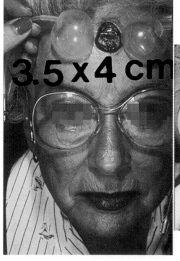
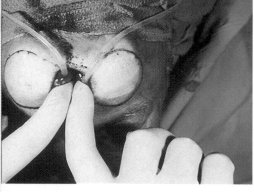

13-9A

Results (Figure 13-9, *B*)

One year later the patient has no persistence of cancer, an acceptable scar, and no changes to the brow complexes. The interbrow distance is slightly less than before surgery. The frontalis muscles demonstrate a normal 1 to 1.5 cm elevation of the brows.

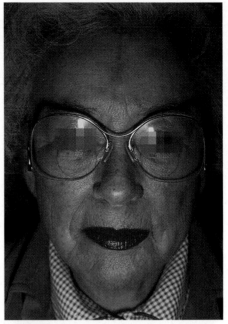

13-9B

CASE 2: Squamous Cell Carcinoma of Forehead

History (Figure 13-10, *A*)

This 64-year-old patient had a large squamous cell carcinoma of his right forehead. A diagnostic biopsy confirmed the clinical diagnosis. On referral the patient was informed of the surgical options, which included excision and primary closure, excision and coverage with a skin graft, or long-term expansion. An attempt at primary closure would elevate the right brow. Coverage with a local skin flap would result in larger scars and possible tissue distortion. Chronic expansion would necessitate two surgical procedures, with the first associated with a physical deformity.

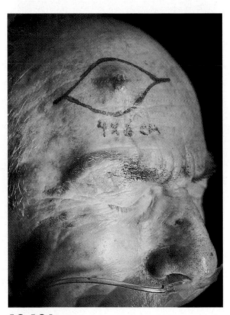

13-10A

Surgical Procedure (Figure 13-10, *B* and *C*)

After excision and frozen section demonstrated an absence of tumor cells at the periphery and deep margins of the specimen (4 × 6 cm), maximal undermining and releasing permitted a primary closure of the defect. When the approximation resulted in brow elevation 2 cm over its opposite side, intraoperative expansion was performed. A 50 cc round expander was positioned in the subgaleal plane of the adjacent upper forehead and scalp, and a 20 cc round expander was located in the subgaleal plane of the adjacent lower forehead. Three expansion periods stretched the tissues to permit a primary closure.

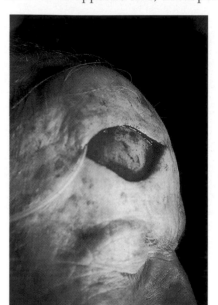

13-10B

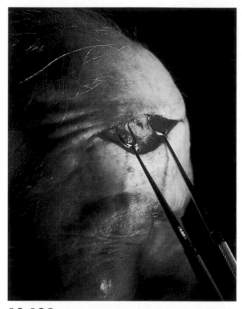

13-10C

Results (Figure 13-10, *D*)

Two years after surgery the patient has a fine horizontal scar resembling one of the upper forehead wrinkles. The patient remains free of tumor recurrence. In the resting state, both brows are at the same height. With movement, each brow elevates 1 cm in concert with the opposite side.

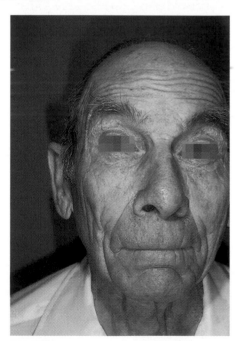

13-10D

CASE 3:   Large Basal Cell Carcinoma of Lateral Forehead

History (Figure 13-11, *A*)

This 51-year-old patient had a 1.5 × 1.5 cm basal cell cancer on his right forehead. A biopsy confirmed the clinical diagnosis. On referral, surgical options of excision and closure were discussed with the patient. With a skin graft the patient understood that hyperpigmentation could occur with graft maturation. On the other hand, distortion of the lateral tail of the brow could result from a tight primary closure. The use of any local flap would create larger scars. Chronic expansion would be too complex a procedure for reconstruction of this lesion. The patient favored intraoperative expansion as a means to close the defect with a primary closure, without brow distortion, and with minimal scarring.

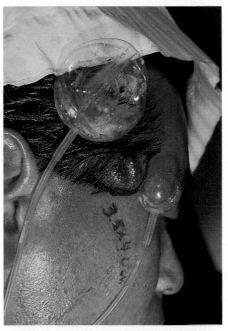

13-11A

Surgical Procedure (Figure 13-11, *B*)

After the basal cell cancer was excised through a 3.5 × 4 cm skin ellipse, tumor clearance of the deep and superficial margins was confirmed with a frozen section. A 50 cc round tissue expander was inserted under the adjacent scalp and a 10 cc round expander under normal skin lateral to the brow tail. Serial expansion three times provided an additional 1 to 2 cm of tissue. With each expansion the volume within the expanders increased as tissue stretching occurred. The balloons were removed, and a primary closure was possible.

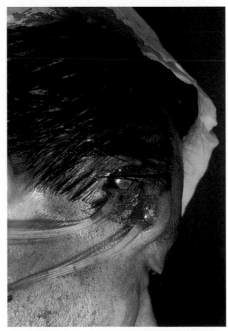

13-11B

Results (Figure 13-11, *C*)

Eight months after surgery the patient has no tumor persistence and no distortion of the brow position. The incision scar is maturing without scar hypertrophy.

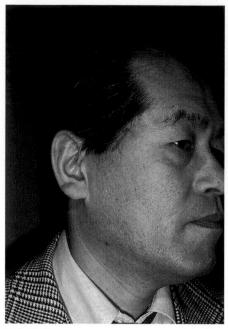

13-11C

CASE 4: Mohs' Surgical Defect Inferior and Lateral to Brow Tail

History (Figure 13-12, *A*)

This 53-year-old patient had a sclerosing basal cell cancer located lateral and inferior to the tail of her right brow. A Mohs' surgical procedure was performed 5 days before her reconstruction. Surgical options were discussed with the patient and included skin grafting, local flaps, or long-term expansion. The patient understood that a primary closure would result in a lateral displacement of her brow and eyelid commissure. The patient wanted the least amount of scars in this cosmetically apparent area.

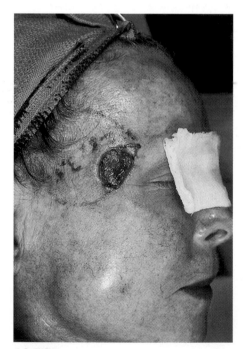

13-12A

Surgical Procedure (Figure 13-12, *B*)

A 50 cc round expander was inserted in the subcutaneous plane of skin lateral to the defect. A superficial dissection was made intentionally over the frontal branch of the facial nerve. Intraoperative expansion was performed through three expansion cycles. Sufficient tissue was gained to permit a primary closure.

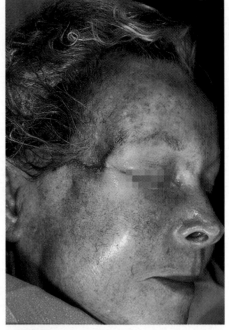

13-12B

Results (Figure 13-12, *C*)

One year after her surgery the patient has an acceptable scar. The position of the brow tail and lateral commissure is symmetric to the opposite side. The frontalis muscle is appropriately animated in concert with the contralateral side.

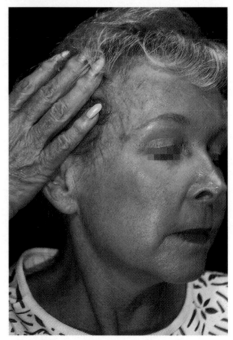

13-12C

CASE RESULTS: MIDFACE RECONSTRUCTION

Midface reconstruction by expansion is usually restricted to skin and fat replacement. The goals of surgery are to (1) provide similar facial tissue; (2) avoid transferring hair-bearing skin into hairless areas; (3) match color, texture, and sensation; (4) respect aesthetic lines of closure; and (5) prevent distortion of the lower eyelid and oral commissure.

Use of the intraoperative expansion technique to stretch local tissue has been most successful in achieving these goals in the midface and neck regions for coverage of small defects. Since the skin of the midface and neck is usually redundant and lined with wrinkles, aesthetic and functional closures are seen at long-term follow-ups. For nasomaxillary defects, expansion of the malar donor site has permitted a smaller rotation-advancement flap to be transferred without the need for skin grafts.

Selected defects of the upper and lower lip can be readily closed by rapid expansion of adjacent lip skin without distortion to the vermilion border and commissure. Local transposition flaps (e.g., nasolabial flaps) may be expanded to (1) increase the amount of tissue in select regions of the flap and (2) permit a donor site closure with minimal tension.

Intraoperative expansion has been used directly over facial muscles, branches of the facial nerve, the carotid artery, and the jugular veins without immediate or delayed complications. Expansion is generally performed in tissues above the facial muscles.

CASE REPORTS AND ANALYSES: Midface Reconstruction

CASE 1:   Port-wine Stain on Nasomaxillary Border

History (Figure 13-13, *A*)

This 33-year-old patient had a deep capillary hypertrophic vascular malformation that involved her lower lid margin, lateral nose, and cheek. The patient had undergone a laser procedure without significant reduction of the larger and deeper vessels. Surgical options included skin grafting, a local rotation-advancement flap, or chronic expansion. A primary closure would distort the lower lid. Intraoperative expansion was discussed as another option to close the defect while minimizing the subciliary-temporal skin release.

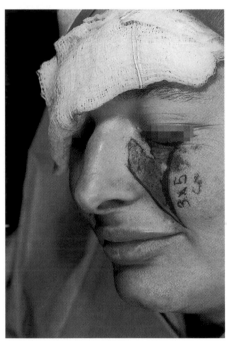

13-13A

Surgical Procedure (Figure 13-13, *B*)

A standard cervicofacial flap was designed along the subciliary border of the lower lid, curved upward and lateral from the lateral commissure, continued along the preauricular border, and proceeded to the post-auricular sulcus. This large exposure was required if intraoperative expansion did not provide sufficient tissue locally for advancement closure. A vertical incision was made along the lateral border of the vascular malformation.

A deep subcutaneous fat dissection under the mid-face skin to the ear's anterior border permitted placement of a 200 cc round expander. Serial expansions gained additional tissue so that a releasing subciliary incision terminated 2 cm lateral to the commissure along the previously described marking. Absorbable dermal-to-deep tissue sutures supported the flap advancement and minimized descent of the lower lid margin.

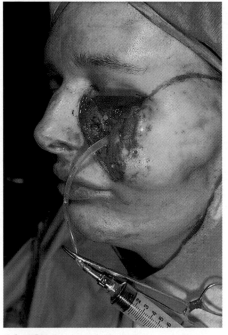

13-13B

Results (Figure 13-13, *C* and *D*)

Four years after surgery the vascular malformation has not recurred. The incisional scar has matured without hypertrophy or significant dyschromia. The lower lid is competent without bowing.

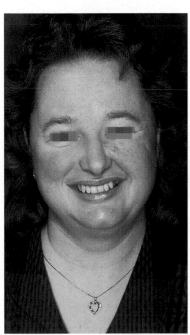

13-13C

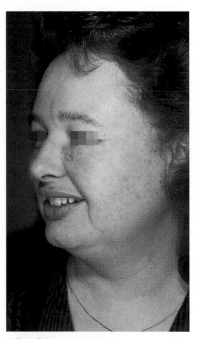

13-13D

CASE 2: Mohs' Surgical Defect on Right Chin Sulcus

History (Figure 13-14, *A, left*)

This 37-year-old patient underwent a Mohs' surgical excision of a sclerosing basal cell cancer within the sulcus of her right chin. After 3 weeks of healing the defect measured 3 × 4 cm. The surgical options included skin grafting, adjacent flaps, transposition flaps, or chronic expansion. Long-term expansion would be complicated by the insertion of a balloon adjacent to an open defect. A primary closure would result in a lower lip distortion.

Intraoperative expansion of the nasolabial flap, which would then be transposed to the chin defect, was offered to the patient as an alternative procedure. The rationale for rapidly expanding the nasolabial flap was to provide a sufficiently wide flap to close the defect without lip drooping. A 2 cc round expander would expand the distal end of a standard nasolabial flap before transfer. A 5 cc round expander would be inserted under the skin inferior to the chin defect to reduce downward forces on the lower lip.

First Surgical Procedure
(Figure 13-14, *A right* and *B left*)

Intraoperative expansion of the chin site was performed first with the 5 cc expander. After three expansion cycles, the skin from the lower chin was unable to be advanced superiorly without causing a deformation of the lower lip. The inferiorly based nasolabial flap was then elevated, de-epithelialized in its buried portion, and insetted into the released recipient chin site.

Results (Figure 13-14, *B right*)

One year after her procedure the patient has an acceptable nasolabial scar and a button knob from the flap within the sulcus. The patient wanted this "biscuit" flap removed and replaced with normal tissue.

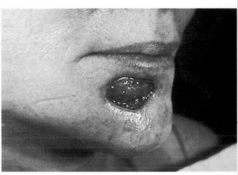

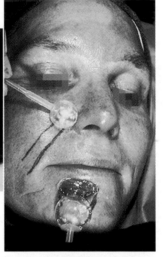

13-14A

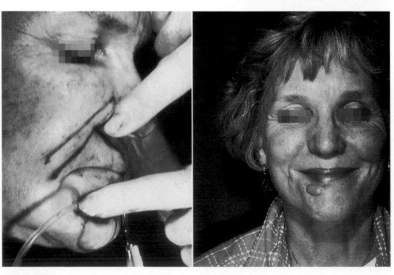

13-14B

Second Surgical Procedure

The tissue around the transposed flap remnant (1 × 1.5 cm) in the sulcus would be expanded to permit a primary closure. Intraoperative expansion with a 20 cc round expander under the ovoid-shaped flap remnant and adjacent tissue was performed in three cycles. The extra tissue obtained was sufficient to close the defect.

Results (Figure 13-14, *C* and *D*)

One year later the patient has minimal distortion of the lower lip.

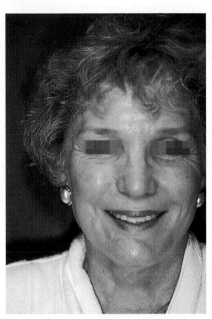

13-14C

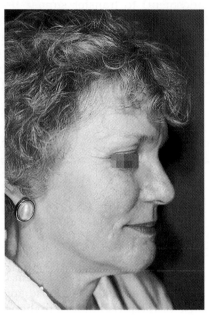

13-14D

CASE 2: Mohs' Surgical Defect on Central Nose

History (Figure 13-16, *A left*)
This 62-year-old patient had a 2.5 × 3 cm defect on the nasal dorsum at the supratip level after a Mohs' surgical resection for a nodular basal cell carcinoma. Surgical options included the use of a skin graft, local flaps, or transposition flaps. Chronic expansion would risk implant exposure or infection because of the open defect. The patient wanted minimal facial scars and like-skin coverage of her defect.

Surgical Procedure (Figure 13-16, *A right*)
The open area was permitted to close by secondary intention for 3 weeks, and the defect was reduced to a 2 × 2.5 cm defect. The patient was returned to surgery, where the skin edges were débrided sharply back to the defect's original size. After maximal undermining and trial closure, two 2.5 cc round expanders were inserted under the nasal skin and serially expanded. Sufficient tissue was generated to permit a primary horizontal closure.

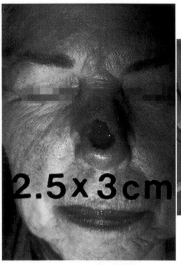
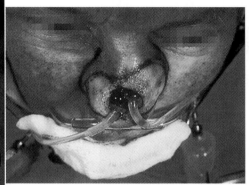

13-16A

Results (Figure 13-16, *B*)
One year after her surgical procedure the patient shows slight roughening of the closure line. The nasal profile on frontal and lateral views demonstrates a near-normal appearance without tip elevation or significant depression along the supratip. The patient has not requested further efforts at scar revision or resurfacing to smooth out the skin.

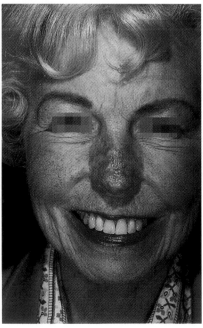

13-16B

CASE 3: Mohs' Surgical Defect on Left Nasal Tip and Alar Fold

History (Figure 13-17, *A*)
This 37-year-old patient underwent a Mohs' surgical procedure to excise a sclerosing basal cell carcinoma on the left nasal dome area. The resultant defect 2 days after surgery measured 2×2 cm. The area was permitted to heal by secondary intention for 3 weeks. At that time, surgical options included skin grafting, local and transposition flaps, or long-term expansion. Because the patient requested minimal scars and like-tissue coverage, intraoperative expansion was offered as an alternative procedure.

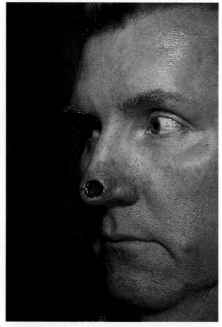

13-17A

Surgical Procedure (Figure 13-17, *B*)
A 10 cc round expander was inserted under the adjacent nasal skin that had been undermined from the nasomaxillary border to the opposite side. Serial expansions with up to 19 ml of saline produced sufficient tissue to attempt a primary closure. The cephalic flap was advanced to the opposite side as a straight advancement without a rotational component, resulting in a transverse closure.

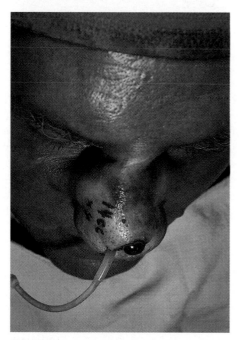

13-17B

Results (Figure 13-17, *C* and *D*)
Four years after his surgical procedure the patient's scar is barely noticeable even with no revisions. The nose has returned to symmetry without distortions to the alar rim, nasal dorsum, or tip.

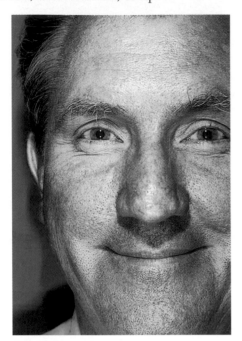

13-17C

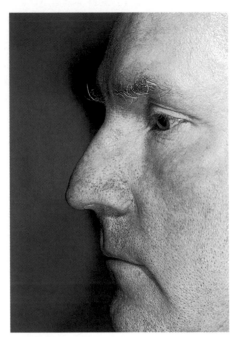

13-17D

CASE 4: Complex Middorsal Nasal Deformity

History (Figure 13-18, *A*)
This 42-year-old patient developed a nasal infection that required débridement of the medial aspects of his upper lateral cartilages, septum, and caudal portion of his nasal bone. A skin graft provided coverage over this area. The patient also was dissatisfied with the bifid nasal tip caused by loss of midline structures.

The patient sought consultation 5 years later to replace the skin graft and restore the normal contour of his nose. Surgical options included overgrafting, serial reduction procedures, local or transposed flap (nasolabial or glabellar) replacement, or chronic expansion. Since the defect measured 2.5 cm at its widest dimension, a primary closure would result in a nasal distortion. Intraoperative expansion was offered as a means to replace the defects with similar tissue that would support an underlying cartilaginous graft.

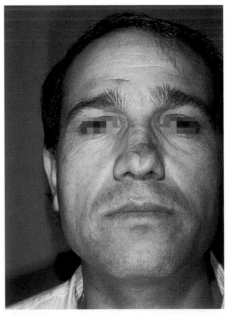

13-18A

Surgical Procedure (Figure 13-18, *B* and *C*)

A 1 × 3 cm conchal graft was harvested from the left ear and carved to replace the central bony and cartilaginous nasal deficiencies. An vertical incision was made through the center of the skin graft. The adjacent nasal skin from the nasomaxillary border to the opposite side was elevated. Two 10 cc expanders were inserted in this generous pocket. Serial expansions gained 2 cm of skin to provide normal skin cover. The structural defects of the septal, upper lateral, and bony architecture were exposed. The contoured cartilage graft was inserted and fixed with absorbing sutures. A vertical skin closure was performed.

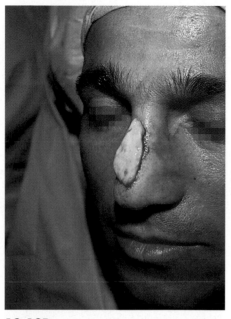

13-18B

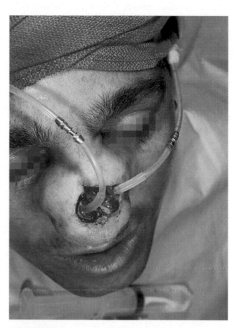

13-18C

Results (Figure 13-18, *D* and *E*)

Three years after his surgical procedure the patient's scar is acceptable with noticeable nasal tip support, a contoured dorsum, and correction of the bifid tip.

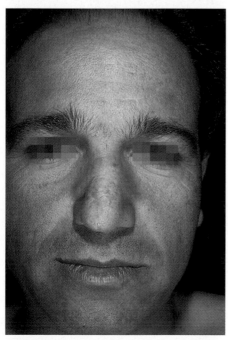

13-18D

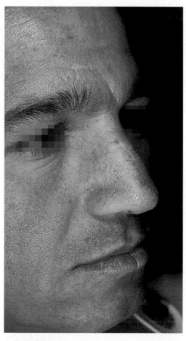

13-18E

CASE 5: Total Nasal Resurfacing for Multicentric Basal Cell Carcinomas

History

This 65-year-old patient has had multiple excisions of basal cell cancers to his nasal skin over the years. Recently, multicentric disease was determined from biopsies over most of his scarred nasal skin. The patient was advised to remove the entire nasal skin. Because of the 7 to 8 cm-wide skin loss, the suggested coverage was either a skin graft or a chronically expanded glabellar flap. The patient did not accept the skin graft coverage because of tissue discrepancy and a contour deficiency. Long-term expansion of his forehead skin was not an option because of the temporary deformation and the need for two surgical stages. Intraoperative expansion was offered as an alternative procedure.

Surgical Procedure (Figure 13-19, *A* and *B*)

A 7 cm–wide flap based on the left supraorbital vessels was designed on the midforehead. A 2.5 cm incision along each border of the forehead flap permitted dissection of generous subcutaneous pockets for each of the two 50 cc round expanders. Each expander was inserted above the frontalis muscle in a pocket that extended from the temporal hairline to the border of the designed flap. Three serial saline fillings up to volumes of 100 cc within each expander produced sufficient donor skin to close the midforehead defect.

The forehead skin flap was thinned at its distal end, infolded to create the columella, and transposed to the nose. The established nasal defect extended from one nasomaxillary border to the other (5 cm), across to the lateral aspects of each ala (7 cm), and down to the columella. No cartilage replacement was required.

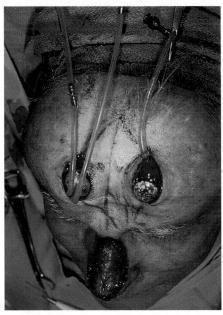

13-19A

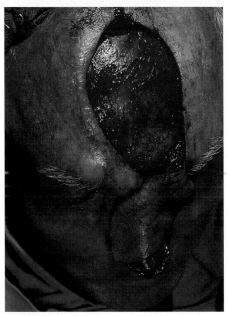

13-19B

Results (Figure 13-19, *C* and *D*)

The patient is shown 4 years after his subsequent reconstructive procedures, which included division and inset of the pedicle and two defattening procedures. The nasal contour has been reestablished without tumor recurrence within the transposed forehead skin. The forehead scar is acceptable to the patient. Each frontalis muscle elevates the brow by 1 cm. The medial aspect of each eyebrow has returned to its presurgical location.

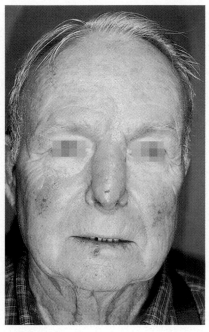

13-19C

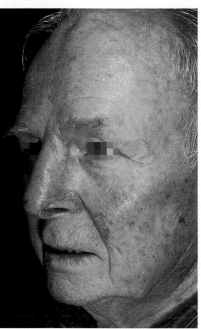

13-19D

CASE RESULTS: NECK RECONSTRUCTION

Small skin defects of the neck can usually be managed by undermining and primary skin closure in a vertical, transverse, or zigzag direction. For larger defects, skin grafting or local and regional flaps may provide adequate coverage but with additional scars. Chronic tissue expansion is ideal for larger defects because of similar tissue replacement and minimal scars. The drawbacks of long-term expansion are the temporary cosmetic deformities produced by the large balloon(s) and the need for two surgical procedures.

Intraoperative expansion of neck skin also provides like-skin coverage and minimal incisional scars. Its main advantages are no enlarging foreign body and only a single procedure. It is a useful technique for small and medium-sized defects.

CASE REPORT AND ANALYSIS: Breast Reconstruction

Contracted Breast Envelope

History (Figure 13-21, *A* and *B*)

This 49-year-old patient underwent bilateral modified radical mastectomies for breast cancers. Primary reconstructions were initiated by long-term tissue expansion technique. After 4 months of expansion, 500 cc gel implants were inserted with reconstruction of the inframammary folds. A postoperative infection of the left breast implant from a suture line exposure necessitated implant removal. A second attempt to insert another 500 cc implant was considered 6 months later. Since only a small amount of tissue contraction had occurred, intraoperative expansion was offered as an alternative procedure to the insertion of a conventional tissue expander.

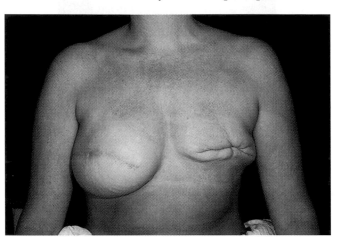

13-21A

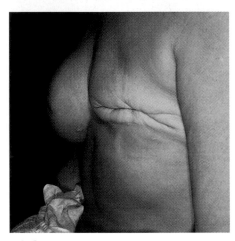

13-21B

Surgical Procedure (Figure 13-21, *C*)

An incision was made along the mastectomy scar to unfurl the contracted skin brassiere by removal of the anterior dome of the previous capsule and releasing any constricting bands of tissue. After a 600 cc round intraoperative expander was inserted in the submuscular plane, the expander was filled to 700 cc over three expansion cycles. Each expansion cycle lasted 5 minutes to stretch the tissue effectively to its maximal level. A 500 cc textured and profiled gel implant was exchanged for the intraoperative expander.

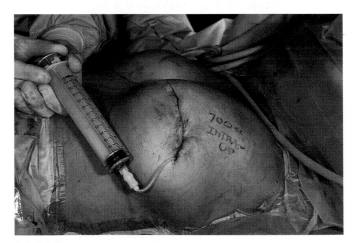

13-21C

Results (Figure 13-21, *D* and *E*)

Two years after the procedure the patient maintains a Baker II/III classification of capsule formation. The left breast mound is symmetric to the right. The patient did not want nipple-areolar reconstruction.

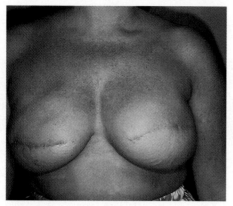

13-21D

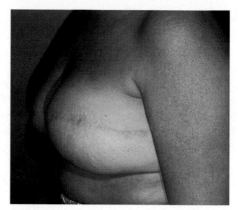

13-21E

CASE RESULTS: TRUNK AND EXTREMITY RECONSTRUCTION

The resurfacing of defects on the trunk and extremities employs skin grafts, local flaps, and regional and free tissue transfers. Chronic tissue expansion has also played a significant role in the reconstruction of these sites because of the inherent advantage of using local tissue with minimal donor site problems.

The intraoperative technique has been employed successfully to recruit local tissue rapidly for removal of small skin grafts, scars, tattoos, and benign and malignant tumors. The amount of tissue recruited may be as much as 2.5 cm for each expander, depending on the anatomic site and the patient's age. The expander(s) is placed under the subcutaneous tissue above the muscle fascia. Since exposure and infection may frequently occur in the distal sites of the upper and lower extremities, fingers, and sacral areas with placement of a chronic expander, intraoperative expansion has distinct advantages. Its obvious limitation is the amount of tissue that may be reliably stretched. Rapid expansion can result in flap margin ischemia (4% rate; see section on complications) in the lower third of the lower and upper extremities. Because the intrinsic blood supply to these areas is less reliable than in other areas, the observation of adequate dermal bleeding at the flap's leading margin is mandatory to reduce this complication.

In more than 100 clinical cases of intraoperative expansion reconstruction in the upper and lower extremities, no muscle wasting, neuropraxia, joint stiffness, or tendon adhesion has occurred. The expanded skin provided well-vascularized, innervated tissue with satisfactory color and contour match. Scar hypertrophy within the extremities and upper back and shoulder, however, has not been prevented with recruitment of adequate tissue by rapid expansion. Scar hypertrophy and keloid formation still appear to be related more directly to the site of reconstruction and amount of skin tension rather than to the type of procedure.

CASE REPORTS AND ANALYSES: Trunk and Extremity Reconstruction

CASE 1: Congenital Nevus on Lower Midabdomen

History (Figure 13-22, *A*)

This 16-year-old patient had a 5 × 12 cm congenital nevus on the midline of the lower abdomen. Because of the potential for malignant degeneration, surgical removal was indicated. The options for reconstruction included fractional reductions, skin grafting, local flaps, or chronic expansion. A primary closure of the defect was possible but could produce a secondary deformity at the pubis. Intraoperative expansion was selected as an alternative procedure.

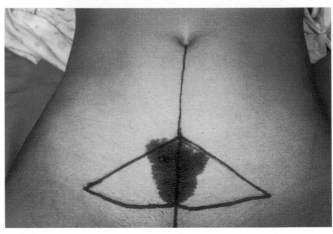

13-22A

Surgical Procedure (Figure 13-22, *B* and *C*)

A 300 cc round expander was inserted in the subcutaneous tissue above and below the nevus through an incision along its border. Serial expansions with up to 420 ml of saline produced sufficient tissue to close the defect in a horizontal direction after resection of the entire nevus.

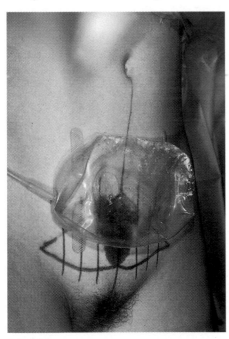

13-22B

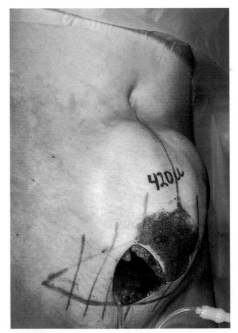

13-22C

Results (Figure 13-22, *D*)

Six months after surgery the patient demonstrates entire nevus removal with an extended suprapubic transverse scar. The pubic hairline was not elevated, and the distance between the umbilicus and pubis remained about 12 cm. Slight scar hypertrophy was controlled with one intralesional steroid injection.

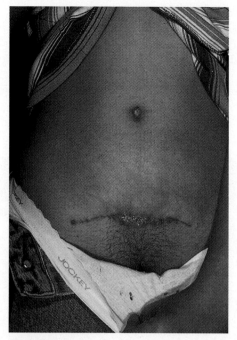

13-22D

CASE 2: Keloid Formation on Abdomen

History (Figure 13-23, *A*)

This 33-year-old patient had a cesarean section through a Pfannenstiel incision. Keloid formation along the scar line occurred 3 months later. Another cesarean section through the keloidal scar was performed for her second pregnancy. Tape was applied across the abdomen in various locations to hold the dressings in place. Four months later, keloid formation developed under areas of taping, involving almost the entire lower half of the abdomen. Keloidal patches occurred about 8 cm above the umbilical level on both sides of the anterior abdominal wall. Sinus tract infections were present above the pubic bone.

Options included fractional excisions, skin grafting, chronic expansion, radiotherapy, or intralesional steroid injections in the most symptomatic portions of the keloid. Intraoperative expansion was suggested as an alternative procedure. If the amount of tissue produced by rapid expansion did not satisfy the reconstructive requirements, a chronic tissue expander(s) could be left in place under the incompletely excised keloid skin. Serial expansion would proceed slowly until sufficient tissue was generated to complete the second stage.

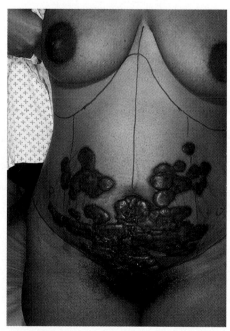

13-23A

Surgical Procedure (Figure 13-23, *B* and *C*)

Two 1000 cc rectangular expanders would be inserted under the skin of the upper half of the abdomen. The surgical procedure began as a conventional approach for an abdominoplasty. A 30 cm incision was made along each inguinal fold to elevate the abdominal wall from the deep fascial plane. Plication of the anterior rectus fascia corrected the diastasis recti abdominis deformity from the xiphoid process to the pubic sym-physis. All tissue below and including the umbilicus was excised.

After temporary closure of the skin edges, each expander was inserted and serially filled to 3000 cc. Sufficient tissue was generated to remove all the remaining patches except for a sentinel keloid spot in the upper left quadrant. Meticulous closure was performed with absorbable synthetic deep sutures and a permanent subcuticular suture.

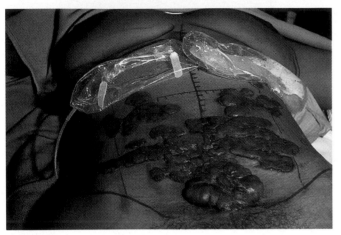

13-23B

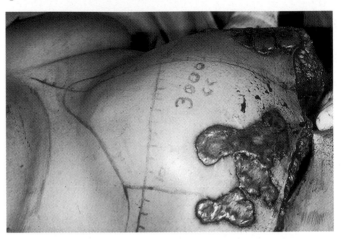

13-23C

Results (Figure 13-23, *D* and *E*)

Six months after surgery the patient shows a slight scar hypertrophy. The pubic hairline is not significantly elevated. Steroid taping, silicone sheeting, and intralesional steroids prevented keloid formation. Unfortunately, a year after surgery, keloid formation returned but was limited along the incision scar line.

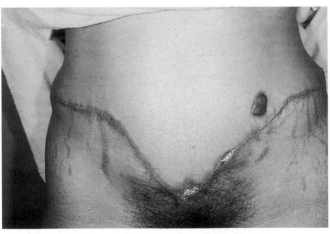

13-23D

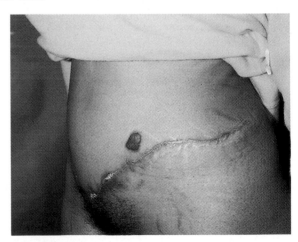

13-23E

CASE 3: Tattoo on Midback

History (Figure 13-24, *A*)

This 27-year-old patient had a 7 × 7 cm tattoo on her right midback done by a professional tattoo artist. The surgical options included laser removal, fractional excisions, skin grafting, local flaps, or chronic expansion. Intraoperative expansion was suggested as another method.

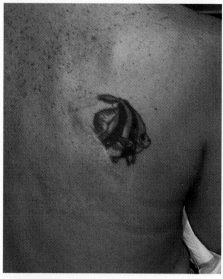

13-24A

Surgical Procedure (Figure 13-24, *B* and *C*)

Three 100 cc round intraoperative expanders would be inserted circumferentially under adjacent normal skin. The dissection in the subcutaneous plane was accomplished through a 3 cm incision along the tattoo's lower border. Generous pockets were created to maintain the expanders' positions during filling.

Serial expansions with 300 ml of saline within each balloon for three cycles created 9 cm hemispheric flaps. After the tattoo was removed, a closure in an oblique direction was possible. A series of advancing absorbable sutures from the dermis to the deep layer fixed the flaps under minimal tension at the incision line.

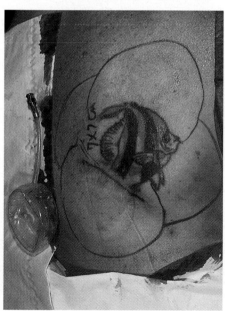

13-24B

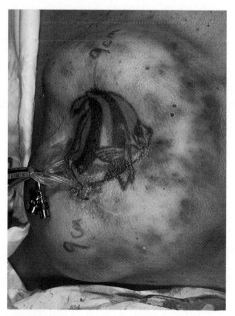

13-24C

Results (Figure 13-24, *D*)

The patient is shown 2 years after completion of her procedure. Scar maturation has occurred with a minimal degree of scar widening or thickening. Steroid tapes were used for 6 weeks after suture removal to reduce the opportunity for scar hypertrophy.

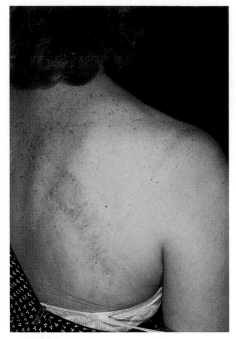

13-24D

CASE 4: Giant Congenital Nevus on Back

History (Figure 13-25, *A*)

This 3-year-old patient had an 11 × 12 cm congenital nevus on the lower back. Because of possible malignant degeneration, surgical removal was suggested. The options included fractional reductions, skin grafting, local flaps, or chronic expansion. Long-term expansion in a toddler's back risks a number of complications, including pressure skin necrosis and infection. These effects are likely to occur because of the thinness of toddlers' skin and their favored supine positioning. Intraoperative expansion was offered as an alternative method, which could be altered to a chronic expansion procedure if insufficient tissue was created.

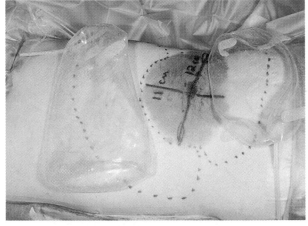

13-25A

First Surgical Procedure (Figure 13-25, *B*)

Two 100 cc intraoperative expanders were inserted through a 2.5 cm intralesional incision. The expander pockets were created around the defect in the subcutaneous plane. Serial expansions with saline up to volumes of 100 to 120 cc produced sufficient tissue that allowed removal of all but 2.5 cm of the nevus.

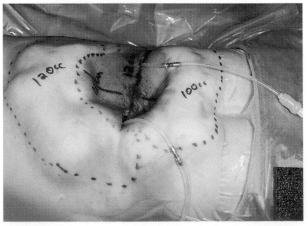

13-25B

Second Surgical Procedure (Figure 13-25, *C* and *D*)
After 6 months a second intraoperative procedure was performed with two 100 cc expanders. Serial expansions with 60 ml of saline in each expander for three cycles created enough tissue to remove the remnant completely.

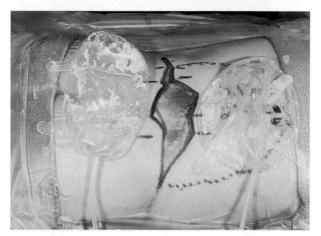

13-25C

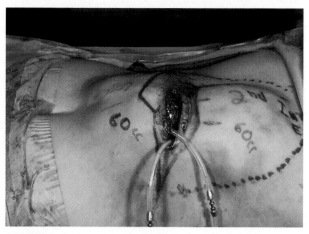

13-25D

Results (Figure 13-25, *E*)
Two years later the patient has an acceptable scar that has not hypertrophied or widened. Sensation has slowly returned to near-normal levels.

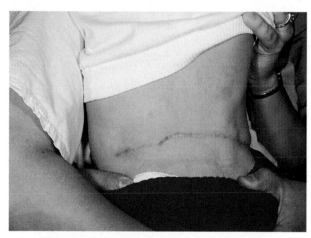

13-25E

CASE 5: Tattoo on Right Brachium

History (Figure 13-26, *A*)

This 26-year-old patient had a 4 × 6 cm tattoo on his right lateral brachium. Surgical options included skin grafting, fractional reductions, local flaps, and chronic expansion. Laser removal was not accepted by the patient because of the possible need to repeat the procedure up to six times. Intraoperative expansion was offered to the patient as an alternative procedure.

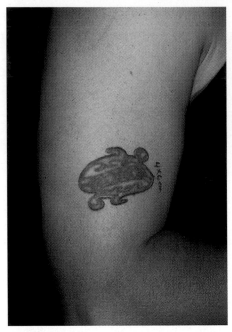

13-26A

Surgical Procedure (Figure 13-26, *B* and *C*)

Two 50 cc intraoperative expanders were inserted, one on each side of the tattoo, through a 2.5 cm intralesional incision. Because the tattoo's longest dimension was horizontal, the most effective skin closure was in an axial direction. This required that the expanders be placed cephalad and caudad to the tattoo. Serial expansions with 150 ml of saline in each balloon for three expansion phases created sufficient tissue to close the defect.

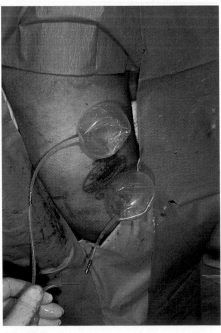

13-26B

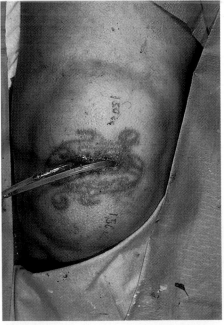

13-26C

Results (Figure 13-26, *D*)

Three years after his surgical procedure the patient shows slight scar widening. Scar hypertrophy was minimal after one injection of intralesional steroids.

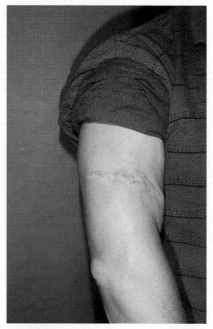

13-26D

CASE 6:   Congenital Nevus on Right Elbow

History (Figure 13-27, *A*)

This 3-year-old patient had a 4.5 × 5 cm congenital nevus on his right elbow. Because of possible malignant degeneration, surgical excision was recommended. The options included skin grafting, fractional reductions, local flaps, or chronic expansion. Intraoperative expansion was suggested as an alternative procedure.

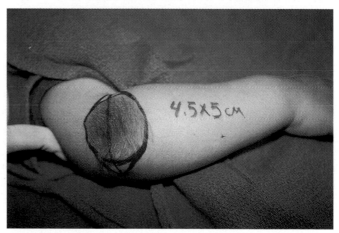

13-27A

Surgical Procedure (Figure 13-27, *B* and *C*)

Two 50 cc intraoperative expanders were inserted through a 2.5 cm intralesional incision in the subcuta-

neous level. Serial expansions with 100 ml of saline within each expander produced sufficient tissue to close the defect.

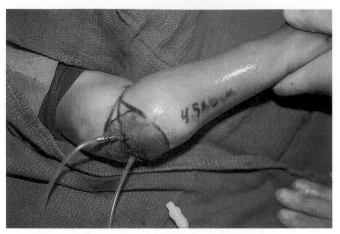

13-27B

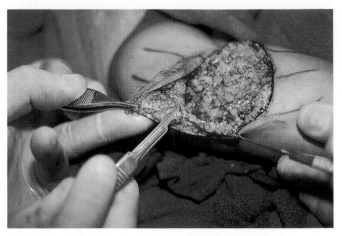

13-27C

Results (Figure 13-27, *D*)

One year after surgery the patient has minimal scar hypertrophy. Scar maturation has progressed with the use of steroid tapes without the need for steroid injections.

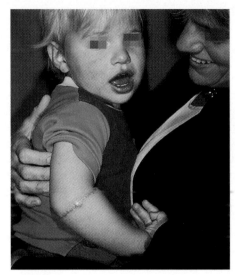

13-27D

CASE 7: Hypertrophic Skin Grafts to Lower Abdomen and Thighs

History (Figure 13-28, *A* and *B*)

This 13-year-old patient underwent hypertrophic skin grafting to her lower abdomen (5 × 20 cm), right upper and inner thigh (2 × 10 cm), and left upper and inner thigh (5 × 12 cm). The surgical options included serial reductions, local advancement flaps, or chronic expansion. Excision and primary closure would produce tissue distortions on the pubis and vulvae. Intraoperative expansion was offered to the patient as an alternative method. If only a partial excision resulted from the first procedure, a second intraoperative surgery could be performed later.

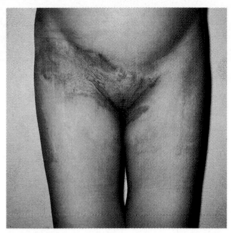

13-28A

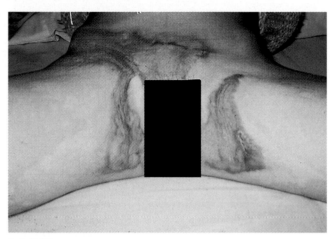

13-28B

Surgical Procedure (Figure 13-28, *C* and *D*)

A 400 cc rectangular expander was inserted in the subcutaneous plane of the lower abdomen through a 2.5 cm incision at the lateral aspect of the skin graft. A 200 cc rectangular expander was positioned in the subcutaneous plane below each thigh graft through a 2.5 cm intralesional incision. Serial expansions with 540 cc (ml) of saline stretched the lower abdominal skin and gained about 3 cm of tissue from a 12 cm hemispheric flap. Serial expansions with 240 cc of saline within each expander gained about 2.5 cm of tissue from 9 cm hemispheric thigh flaps. This extra tissue was sufficient to excise the entire skin graft scars and permit a primary closure by advancing the flaps.

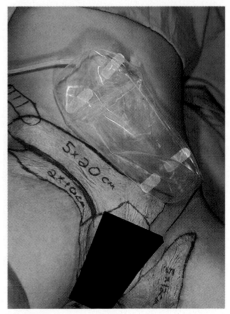

13-28C

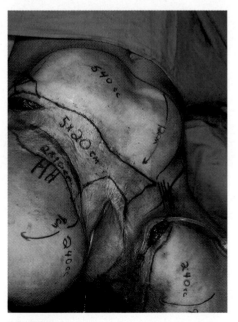

13-28D

Results (Figure 13-28, *E*)
Three years after her surgical procedure the patient's scars have matured and remain hidden within the groin creases and medial thighs. No hypertrophic scar formation developed. Prophylactic use of steroid tapes for 6 weeks may have prevented excessive scar formation.

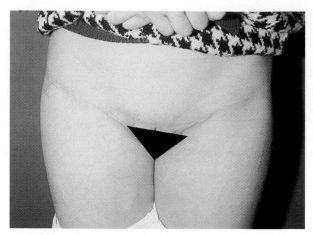

13-28E

CASE 8:   Type III Injury to Right Lower Extremity

History (Figure 13-29, *A* and *B*)
This 22-year-old patient was involved in a motorcycle accident and sustained a type III injury to his right lower extremity. The tibia and fibula were fractured and associated with arterial spasm to the posterior tibial and posterior interosseous vessels. Neurapraxia to the posterior tibial nerve was diagnosed at one of his surgical procedures. The patient required initial reduction and fixation of his fractures with an external fixation device and two-stage procedures of débridement (2.5 cm of skin loss) and tissue approximation. Plastic surgery consultation for closure of the soft tissue defect was initiated the night of the injury.

Six weeks after the injury the surgical options included skin grafting across the fracture site, skin-muscle flap coverage, chronic expansion, and free tissue transfer. The patient refused all options except skin grafting. Intraoperative stretching of adjacent skin was offered as an alternative to provide more stable coverage over the bony fracture line.

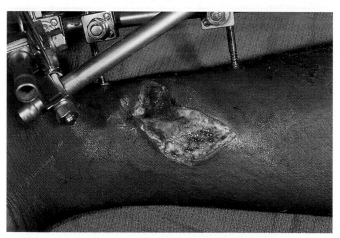

13-29A

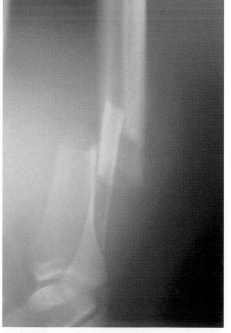

13-29B

Surgical Procedure (Figure 13-29, *C*)

A Suture Tension Adjustment Reel device (see Chapter 14) was positioned on both sides of the defect. Sutures were passed through the dermis of each skin edge and into both devices. Gradual tightening of the sutures by turning the rachet reels over 10 days stretched sufficient skin to permit a closure.

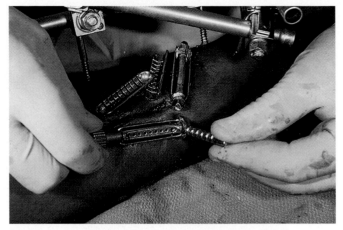

13-29C

Results (Figure 13-29, *D*)

Six months after his external fixation was removed, the patient is able to ambulate without assistance. Bone healing was progressive along fracture lines. The soft tissue approximation remained stable.

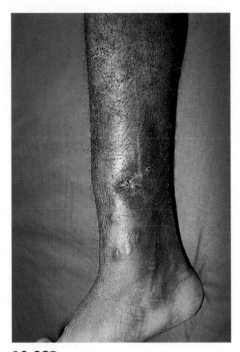

13-29D

REFERENCES

1. Neumann CG: The expansion of an area of skin by progressive distention of a subcutaneous balloon, *Plast Reconstr Surg* 19:124, 1957.
2. Gibson T: The physical properties of skin. In Converse JMS, editor: *Reconstructive plastic surgery,* vol 1, Philadelphia, 1977, Saunders.
3. Peng TJ, Landel RF, Brody GS: In vivo study of human skin rheology. In *Proceedings of the Sixth New England Biomedical Conference,* New York, 1978, Pergamon.
4. Gibson T, Kenedi RM: The structural components of the dermis and their mechanical characteristics. In Montagna W, Bentley JP, Dobson RL, editors: *The dermis,* New York, 1968, Appleton-Century-Crofts.
5. Landsman L, Mandy SH: Adjuncts to scalp reduction surgery, *J Dermatol Surg Oncol* 17:670-672, 1991.
6. Gibson T, Kenedi RM, Craik JE: The mobile microarchitecture dermal collagen: a bioengineering study, *Bio J Surg* 54:752-764, 1965.
7. Hirshowitz B, Kaufmann T, Ullman J: Reconstruction of the tip of the nose and ala by local cycling of the nasal skin and harnessing of extra skin, *Plast Reconstr Surg* 77:316, 1986.
8. Machida BK, Liu-Shindo M, Sasaki GH, Rice DH: Immediate versus chronic tissue expansion, *Ann Plast Surg* 26:227-231, 1991.
9. Siegert R, Weerda H, Hoffmann S, Mohadjer C: Clinical and experimental evaluation of intermittent intraoperative short-term expansion, *Plast Reconstr Surg* 92:248-254, 1993.
10. Sasaki GH: Intraoperative sustained limited expansion (ISLE) as an immediate reconstructive technique, *Clin Plast Surg* 14:563-573, 1987.

11. Sasaki GH: Intraoperative expansion as an immediate reconstructive (and aesthetic) technique, *Facial Plast Surg* 5:362-378, 1988.
12. Sugihara T, Ohura T, Kim C, et al: The extensibility in human skin. Paper presented at PSEF International Tissue Expansion Symposium, San Francisco, October 1987.
13. Ohura T, Sugihara T, Honda K: Post-operative evaluation in plastic surgery using the Bio-skin Tensiometer, *Ann Plast Surg* 5: 74-82, 1980.
14. Stark et al: Directional variations in the extensibility of human skin, *Br J Plast Surg* 30:105, 1977.
15. Chretien-Marquet B: Rapid intraoperative distension using isotonic saline solution, *Plast Reconstr Surg* 96:158-165, 1995.
16. van Rappard JHA, Sonneveld GJ, Borghouts JMHM: Geometric planning and the shape of the expander, *Facial Plast Surg* 5:287-290, 1988.
17. Mackay DR, Saggers GC, Kotwal N, Manders EK: Stretching skin: undermining is more important than intraoperative expansion, *Plast Reconstr Surg* 86:722, 1990.
18. Austad ED, Pasyk KA, McClatchey KD, Cherry GW: Histomorphic evaluation of guinea pigs skin and soft tissue after controlled tissue expansion, *Plast Reconstr Surg* 70:704-710, 1982.
19. Austad ED, Thomas SB, Pasyk KA: Tissue expansion: dividend or loan? *Plast Reconstr Surg* 78:63-67, 1986.
20. Nordstrom REA: "Stretch-back" in scalp reduction for male pattern baldness, *Plast Reconstr Surg* 73:422-426, 1984.
21. Lam AC, Nguyen QH, Tahery DP, et al: Decrease in skin-closing tension intraoperatively with Suture Tension Adjustment Reel, balloon expansion and undermining, *J Dermatol Surg Oncol* 20: 368-371, 1994.

CHAPTER

14 Intraoperative Expansion in Aesthetic Surgery

The management of skin in cosmetic surgeries may involve (1) removal of excess tissue (scalp reduction in male-pattern baldness, rhytidectomy, abdominoplasty), (2) skin recruitment and improvement of skin draping (facial, breast, and calf augmentation), and (3) contraction of redundant integument (suction-assisted lipectomy, endoscopic surgery). Intraoperative expansion, as a surgical technique, may be helpful in achieving these three management goals as follows:

1. Intraoperative expansion incrementally elongates skin to its limits of inherent extensibility. This "extra" tissue can then be excised without producing an overpulled appearance. The removal of prestretched skin may be beneficial in scalp reductions, face and neck lifts (cervicofacial rhytidoplasties), and abdominoplasties to minimize earlier onset of skin laxity in the postoperative period.
2. Intraoperative expansion recruits additional skin for improved draping over autogenous grafts or alloplastic implants. The retention of this prestretched skin over alloplastic implants may be important to the final outcome after nasal, cheek, chin, breast, and calf augmentation procedures.
3. Dermal injury after intraoperative expansion may produce delayed skin contraction months after the procedure. This secondary benefit of intraoperative expansion may be helpful in stimulating excess skin to shrink after minimally invasive surgical procedures, such as endoscopic forehead lifts, that are associated with small incisions and no skin resection.

The use of intraoperative expansion in aesthetic surgery has proceeded cautiously over the past 12 years (Table 14-1). It is still unclear whether the long-term results justify its use and whether immediate tissue stretching is required at surgery.

MALE-PATTERN BALDNESS

Chronic Versus Intraoperative Expansion

Long-term tissue expansion of flaps for correction of male-pattern baldness has achieved better results than those previously obtained with punch grafts, scalp reductions, and flaps. The goal of expansion procedures is to provide an even and dense coverage across the frontal hairline and occipital vertex, while minimizing scars and producing a natural direction of hair flow. Chronic expansion requires a two-stage approach: (1) insertion of the balloon(s) in the subgaleal pockets and (2) advancement of the skin flaps that have been expanded over time.

Long-term expansion is best indicated for the highly motivated patient who can cope with the physical deformity produced by the expanders. This temporary deformation slowly develops over a number of office visits throughout the 3- to 4-month expansion period and may result in social isolation and withdrawal from the workplace.

After expansion of the denser hair-bearing temporal and parietal scalp is completed, the stretched scalp is advanced toward the sagittal midline with maximum anterior advancement beyond the existing frontotemporal line. Since the face is divided into equal thirds, an optimal forehead height between 5 and 7 cm from the widow's peak to the brow is determined from the vertical heights of the lower two segments (brow to nasal sill and nasal sill to chin).

Chronic expansion for correction of male-pattern baldness may not achieve enough forward flap advancement to create a 5 to 7 cm forehead height after the first expansion period. Thus the same expanders may be reinserted as far forward as possible under the sagittal scalp after 4 months of healing, reexpanded for 6 to 10 weeks, and then removed. The additional tissue can be readvanced to create a symmetrically positioned precapillary line with a widow's peak and lateral recessions.

The presence of tissue expanders always increases the risk of infection because of exposure or contamination of the foreign body.

The introduction of intraoperative expansion techniques has simplified the surgical reduction of certain types of male-pattern baldness and made the procedure more accessible. Patients encounter neither the prospect of a physical deformity nor the risk of a foreign body infection. The results of this technique illustrate its limitations, however, because intraoperative expansion

■ **Table 14-1** Skin Removal and Retention Procedures in 356 Intraoperative Expansions in Aesthetic Surgery, 1986 to 1997

Procedure	Number
Removal of Prestretched Skin	
Male-pattern baldness	6
Cervicofacial rhytidectomy	137
Abdominoplasty	10
Retention of Prestretched Skin	
Nasal augmentation	30
Cheek augmentation	5
Chin augmentation	24
Breast augmentation	137
Calf augmentation	7

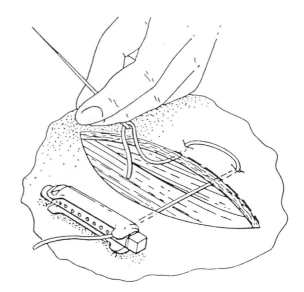

Figure 14-1 The Suture Tension Adjustment Reel (STAR) device consists of an active and a passive member. The active member is positioned adjacent to the defect, while the passive comb-shaped member is located on the opposite side. A double-stranded O, nonabsorbable suture is passed through the one of the lateral holes of the winder, located in the boat-shaped container of the active member. The suture is then passed into the skin, across the wound, and through the opposite skin. The suture is retraced back to the active member and tied. After the passive member is slipped under the exposed suture loop, gradual turning of the winder through a racheted bar forces the wound edges toward the midline. The STAR device may be either left in place for a short time to facilitate linear stretch or removed to permit closure. Since the components are of metal, the device may be autoclaved for repeat use. A number of STAR devices may be necessary to approximate larger wounds. (From Cohen BH, Cosmetto AJ: *J Dermatol Surg Oncol* 18:112-123, 1992.)

cannot produce the extra scalp tissue necessary for a greater degree of skin stretchback after closure.

Despite these limitations, this technique may provide an alternative for patients with a lax scalp who cannot tolerate enlarging scalp expanders over time. In these patients an S-shaped paramedian or sagittal midline incision permits adequate exposure for intraoperative expansion methods that can reduce extensive areas of alopecia. Expansion of the scalp's midline, however, involves areas where hair density is less than in the denser areas of the occiput and temporoparietal zones. The sagittal midline scar may also create an artificial part in the hair at the top of the head and produce an indentation in the midfrontal hairline.

In addition, significant forward advancement up to 5 cm anterior to the established temporofrontal hairline may be difficult to accomplish with intraoperative expansion techniques, let alone a single long-term expansion procedure. A short-term period of chronic expansion of the inadequately advanced frontal hairline may be necessary to achieve the final widow's peak position.

Regardless of these disadvantages, intraoperative expansion has gained acceptance as a staged procedure that obviates the presence of an enlarging foreign body and its attendant physical deformity and potential for infection.

Devices

Two devices have facilitated intraoperative expansion for reconstructive or aesthetic concerns. Both devices are reusable and may be autoclaved for subsequent surgeries.

Suture Tension Adjustment Reel[1,2]
The Suture Tension Adjustment Reel (STAR) device was developed to assist in conventional skin closure and to stretch skin (Figures 14-1 and 14-2). In contrast to the inflatable silicone tissue expander, the STAR device produces a linear tension vector instead of a spheric one.

Components of the device include an active member (winder in boat-shaped container), positioned on one side of the defect, and a passive member (comb-shaped edge) on the opposite side of the defect. Both elements are linked with a horizontal mattress suture (double-stranded O, nonabsorbable), which is passed through the members and the intervening tissues. The suture is tightened by rotating the winder, forcing the wound edges toward the midline.

Intraoperative Silicone Balloon
Silicone, smooth-wall, 800 to 1000 cc rectangular expanders with remote fast-fill valves are conventional expanders available from manufacturers (Figure 14-3). Smaller volume expanders may be used but offer no significant advantages over larger expanders. Rectangular expanders fit the donor sites more efficiently than other conventionally shaped balloons. Textured-surface implants do not provide any advantages over smooth-walled expanders during intraoperative expansion.

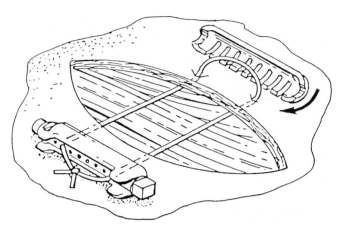

Figure 14-2 The passive comb-shaped member of the Suture Tension Adjustment Reel (STAR) device. (From Cohen BH, Cosmetto AJ: *J Dermatol Surg Oncol* 18:112-123, 1992.)

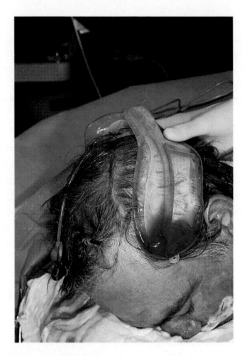

Figure 14-3 Rectangular expander for intraoperative scalp expansion.

Surgical Technique

Patients may receive a ring block of lidocaine (Xylocaine) 2% with 1:200,000 epinephrine alone or with general anesthesia. After skin preparation with Betadine paint, bitemporal incisions are made along the right and left frontotemporal recessions anteriorly and continued posteriorly along the border of fringe hair to the occipitoparietal junction. An alternative surgical approach is a sagittal midline incision within the bald area that extends from the predicted frontal hairline to the occiput. The bitemporal incisions are carried through the galea aponeurotica by angling the blade to parallel the direction of the hair follicles and minimizing damage of these adnexal structures along the incision line.

Each subgaleal pocket is widely undermined in the temporal area down to the ears and back to the nuchal line in the parieto-occipital area, but not under the central bald area. Galeotomies are performed in a crossing fashion to release this tough layer before application of the STAR device. Each component of the STAR device is positioned on each side of the bitemporoparietal incisions and linked by the double-stranded, O-strength suture. Since each STAR device spans about 5 cm along the wound edge, two separate devices may be positioned in line along a longer defect.

Lap pads (sterile gauze pads) may be placed under the bitemporal pockets to increase the efficiency of expansion. Linear stretch is begun by turning the drum and cranking the suture inward with maximum tension. After 3 minutes the drum is lifted from its carriage, releasing the suture and permitting reperfusion of the flaps for a short period. Suture tension is repeated for two series to obtain the most effective stretch of opposing flaps. The amount of sagittal advancement of flaps that have undergone linear stretch with the STAR device should be greater than that obtained with initial galeotomies.

Further recruitment of tissue can be expected when tissue expanders contribute spheric stretch in combination with the STAR devices. Two 800 cc smooth-wall rectangular expanders are inserted under the temporoparieto-occipital pockets with the STAR devices under suture tension. Intraoperative expansion is performed to tissue tolerance for 3 minutes, stretching the hair-bearing flaps. The volume introduced into each expander during the separate expansion phases is determined by tissue resistance, degree of blanching, and to some extent the awake patient's discomfort. In general a greater volume should be introduced into the expanders with each stretch period as the tissues become looser and thinner. After 3 minutes of deflation, reexpansion is done for 3 additional minutes. This sequence is repeated for a total of three expansion-deflation periods to gain maximal tissue.

The expanded flaps are mobilized toward the sagittal midline and as far anteriorly as possible after removal of the intraoperative expanders. Tailored resection of the central bald area is completed for an effective scalp reduction of 5 to 6 cm. The hair-bearing flaps are sutured to the central remnant of alopecia. Although the STAR devices may be left in place to reduce tension at closure, they are usually removed in turn from the flap edges as scalp approximation begins. Surgical drains may be positioned under the flaps to reduce hematoma collection.

The combination of linear (STAR) and spheric (expander balloon) intraoperative expansion may be repeated 4 to 6 months later when the scalp has relaxed and its blood supply has stabilized. This second advancement toward the midline should eliminate the central area of alopecia. However, scar spreading and alopecia may develop because of increased tension as the flaps heal over the next 6 months. In addition, the patient may request further anterior advancement of the widow's peak and frontal recessions.

If midline alopecia and a poorly positioned frontal hairline are to be corrected, a brief period of chronic expansion with one or two 800 cc smooth-wall rectangular expanders, located posterior to the frontal hairline to the scalp vertex, should provide additional tissue for an advanced widow's peak. The expansion period may vary from 4 to 6 weeks, depending on the final desired forehead height. Because of the short expansion period, the patient should not experience significant physical deformity that would restrict his work or social activities.

Alternative Surgical Approach

The surgeon may also plan a scalp reduction with a patient by suggesting the use of short-term chronic expansion first for 1 to 3 weeks (or until physical deformation develops) to reduce the physical embarrassment of enlarging balloons and to generate more available tissue than that obtained by only intraoperative stretching. At surgery, intraoperative expansion of the balloons along with linear stretching by the STAR devices, as just described, can remove a significant portion of the bald area. The amount of scalp excision varies but can be 6 to 10 cm in width.

Clinical experience has shown that the final amount of skin removal does not depend on whether one type of skin stretching (spheric) precedes the other (linear). The hair-bearing flaps are mobilized toward the sagittal line and sutured in a layered fashion to the central bald remnant. After 4 to 6 months of wound healing, either intraoperative stretching or short-term balloon expansion (with intraoperative stretching) may be repeated to complete the removal of the central bald spot and to advance the frontal hairline to its final position.

SUMMARY

Intraoperative expansion may provide an alternative method for reduction or removal of the bald areas in male-pattern baldness. The procedure may be best indicated for patients who present with the smaller areas of stable alopecia or who may not be able to accommodate the visible scalp deformity produced by chronic expansion. Of course, chronic expansion may be terminated whenever cosmetic or functional deformity of expansion becomes a patient's concern. Intraoperative expansion technique can then be employed at that time to increase tissue recruitment.

When intraoperative expansion is the only method used, either spherical stretching (balloon) or linear stretching (STAR) techniques are available to the surgeon.

CASE REPORTS AND ANALYSES: Male-Pattern Baldness

CASE 1: Serial Intraoperative Expansions

History (Figure 14-4, *A* to *C*)
This 48-year-old patient selected surgical correction of his male-pattern baldness by serial intraoperative stretching techniques rather than long-term balloon expansion because of his business schedule during reconstruction. Four years earlier the patient underwent a bicoronal forehead lift that left a 35 cm linear scar. Two years later, hair-plug transplantation was successfully performed to fill in the anterior frontal bald areas.

On preoperative examination the anterior area of progressive alopecia measured 12 cm across behind the reconstructed anterior tuft filled with hair plugs, 10 cm across at the midscalp, and 8 cm across at the vertex (Figure 14-4, *C*). The sagittal length of the bald spot measured about 16 cm. The forehead height from the central brow to the transplanted frontal hairline was 10 cm on each side.

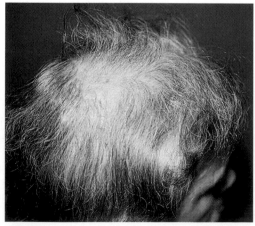

14-4A

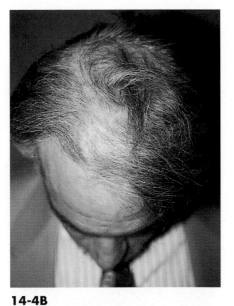

14-4B

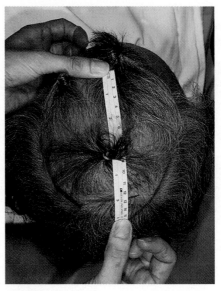

14-4C

First Surgical Procedure (Figure 14-4, *D* to *F*)

A bitemporal incision was made along the edges of the central bald spot. Crossing galeotomies released to some extent the elevated temporoparieto-occipital flaps. STAR stretching with two devices permitted about 2 cm of advancement from each side toward the midline. Intraoperative expansion with two 800 cc rectangular balloons in combination with the STAR devices resulted in a 5 to 6 cm reduction of the central area of alopecia.

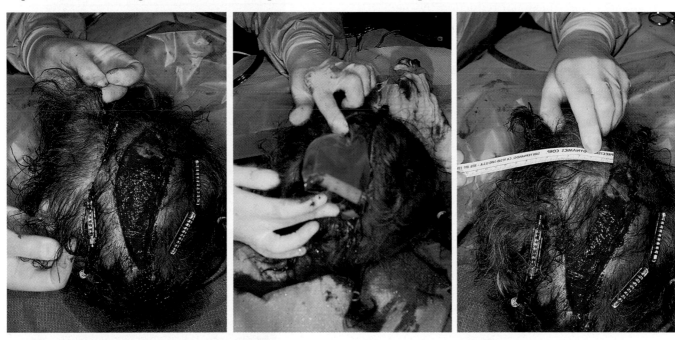

14-4D   **14-4E**   **14-4F**

Second Surgical Procedure (Figure 14-4, *G* and *H*)
Nine months later, intraoperative stretching by both techniques was repeated on the soft, pliable donor

flaps. About 4 cm of additional alopecia was removed, leaving a central 1 to 2 cm remnant of stretch-back scar.

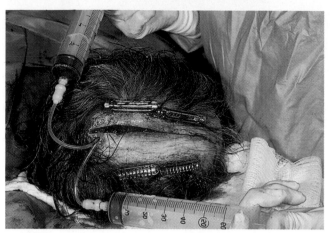

14-4G

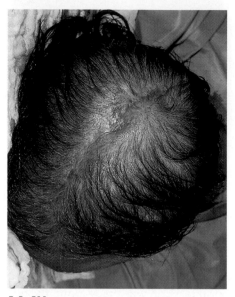

14-4H

Third Surgical Procedure (Figure 14-4, *I*)
Four months later, fractional reduction by the STAR technique removed the remaining area of scar alopecia.

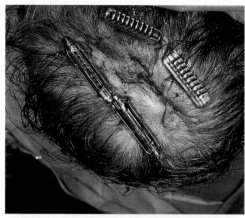

14-4I

Results (Figure 14-4, *J*)
Although the scar widened 1 cm postoperatively, the patient is satisfied with the results.

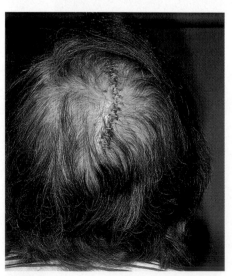

14-4J

CASE 2: Short-term Chronic Expansion and Intraoperative Expansion

History (Figure 14-5, *A* to *C*)

A 56-year-old patient developed the first stages of male-pattern baldness at age 25. He had never sought consultation for correction of his baldness before his initial introduction to the benefits of expansion technique.

On preoperative examination the central area of alopecia measured 12 cm across the anterior temporal hairline, 8 cm across the midscalp, and 5 cm across the vertex (Figure 14-5, *C*). The sagittal length of the bald spot was 18 cm. The forehead height from the brow to the anterior temporal junction was 10 cm on each side.

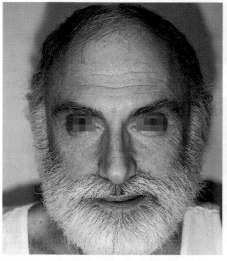

14-5A

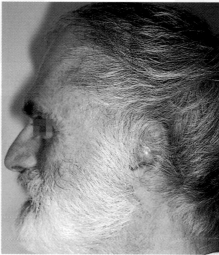

14-5B

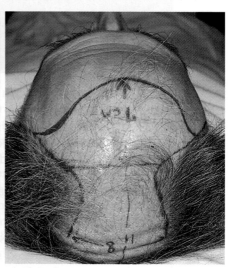

14-5C

First Surgical Procedure (Figure 14-5, *D* to *H*)

Two 800 cc smooth-wall rectangular long-term expanders with buried valves were positioned under the hair-bearing temporoparieto-occipital scalp on each side through a 3 cm horizontal incision at the scalp vertex. Short-term chronic expansion over 2 to 3 weeks resulted in a 100 cc volume in each balloon. The patient tolerated the minimal scalp deformity during this short duration. A month later, galeotomies along with STAR stretching and intraoperative expansion of the balloons permitted the removal of 5 to 6 cm of central alopecia (Figure 14-5, *H*).

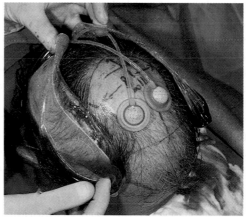

14-5D

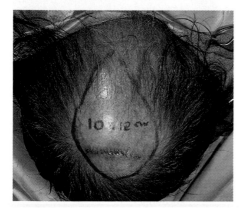

14-5E

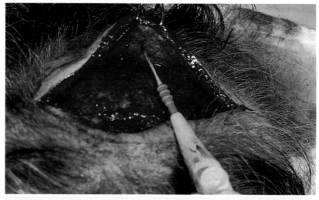

14-5F

Continued

about 3 cm in a medial direction to the parotid gland's anterior border. The fascia is pulled in a posterior direction, resected, and fixed with interrupted absorbable sutures (4-0). The attachment of the platysma muscle along the sternocleidomastoid muscle is also incised, with elevation of the platysma muscle anteriorly to the facial vessels. The platysma muscle is tightened in a posterosuperior direction, resected, and sutured (4-0) to the sternocleidomastoid fascia.

Surgical Technique

A temporary skin closure sets the tension across the midface and neck before intraoperative expansion. A 1 to 1.5 cm first incision is made into the midface flap at the level of the helical root (Figure 14-6, *D*). The midface flap is pulled upward and in a posterior direction. At the level of the previously made dart, the flap is sutured to the ear's superior aspect. A second incision is made into the postauricular curve of the neck flap. The flap is sutured to the apex of the postau-

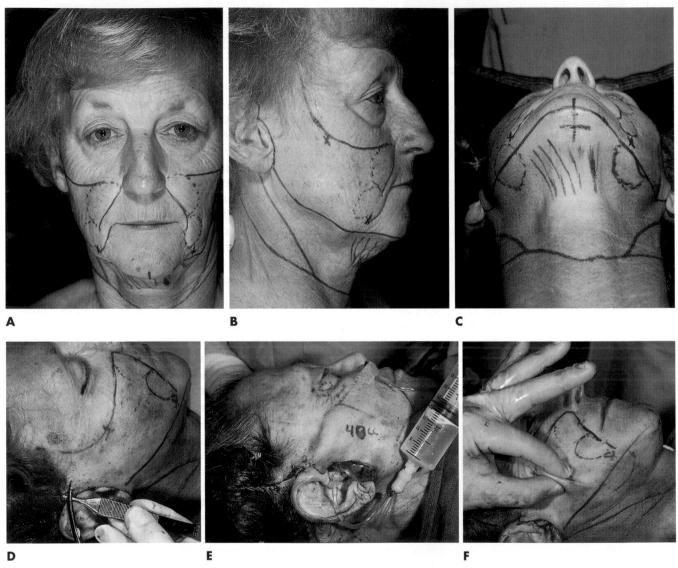

A   B   C

D   E   F

Figure 14-6 **A** to **C,** This 53-year-old patient demonstrates the preoperative markings of an expansion-assisted cervicofacial rhytidoplasty for ptosis of the cheek fat along the nasolabial line, laxity of the platysma muscles with production of marionette folds, jowls, anterior submental fullness, and creeping (crinkling) of the lateral neck. In addition, skin laxity accentuates drooping of the deeper structures. The nasolabial lines, marionette lines, mandibular borders, anterior border of the sternocleidomastoid muscles, and zygomatic and mandibular ligaments are outlined with the patient in the sitting position. The temporal, preauricular and postauricular, and submental incision lines are marked. The inferior extent of the neck dissection is designated along with the locations of the ptotic submandibular glands. **D,** After SMAS resection and tightening, the ptotic submandibular glands were repositioned by imbrication technique. Minimal fat suctioning was performed lateral to the marionette and nasolabial lines instead of fat repositioning with suture fixation. The facial and neck skin was draped in a cephalad and posterior direction. After key incisional darts in the redraped skin were made at the level of the helix, postauricle, and lobule, temporary suture fixations secured the skin flap at optimal tension. *Continued*

ricular skin. A third incision into the overlapping flap at the ear lobe level insets the flap without tension.

Round expanders of various volumes (50 to 200 cc) may be inserted under each facial flap and serially expanded and deflated three times for 1- to 3-minute cycles (Figure 14-6, *E* and *F*). The amount of saline fill is determined by the clinical appearance of flap viability and perfusion characteristics. Intraoperative expansion of the flap permits additional skin removal at the preauricular edge, the pull of which

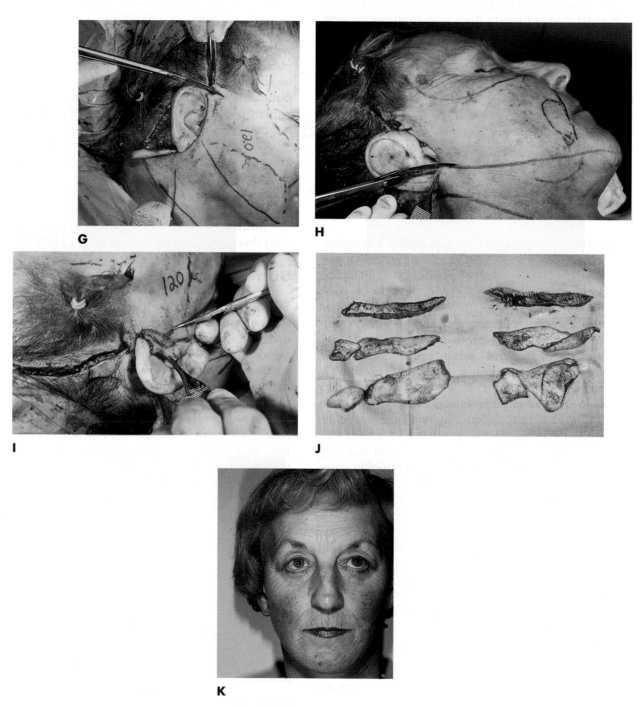

Figure 14-6 cont'd E to H, Round 40 cc expander was inserted under each midface skin flap. Both expanders were simultaneously filled with 120 cc (ml) of saline for 1 to 3 minutes and then deflated for 1 to 3 minutes to permit flap reperfusion. Usually, three cycles of intraoperative expansion "gained" 1 to 3 cm of tissue from each midfacial flap. The key incisional darts were extended to resect a greater amount of skin without producing an overpulled appearance with tension lines. **I** and **J,** An additional 1 cm of preauricular skin, beyond the original skin markings for resection, preempted to some degree the postoperative skin laxity. Additional temporal and postauricular skin resection was possible because of the effects of intraoperative expansion. **K,** Two years after her surgical procedure the patient has excellent contouring of her mandibular angle and margin without a significant return of nasolabial and marionette folds.

Results (Figure 14-7, *E* and *F*)
The patient is shown 2 years after his surgery. The nasolabial and marionette folds, as well as the jowls, have not significantly recurred to require additional corrective surgery. The neck architecture has maintained its contour, with no significant skin ptosis.

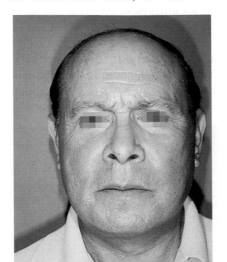

14-7E

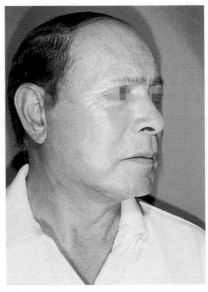

14-7F

CASE 2:   Flaccid Skin and Moderate Fat

History (Figure 14-8, *A* and *B*)
This 54-year-old patient had ptosis of her cheek fat pads, nasolabial and marionette folds, jowls, and neck. An SMAS rhytidectomy with intraoperative expansion was offered as an alternative for her cosmetic corrections.

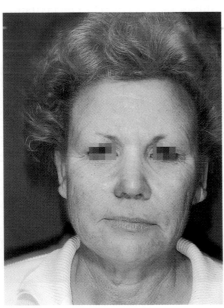

14-8A

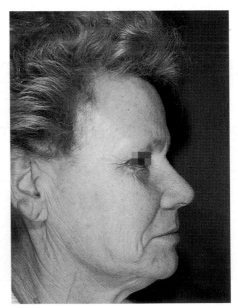

14-8B

Surgical Procedure (Figure 14-8, *C* and *D*)

After SMAS resection and tightening was completed, 100 cc midface expanders and a 100 cc round anterior neck expander were inserted under the elevated skin flaps. Serial expansion of both midface expanders up to 120 cc was repeated for three cycles. The anterior neck expander was inflated up to 100 cc and deflated for three cycles. An additional 2 cm of preauricular and postauricular skin beyond the initial estimate was able to be removed.

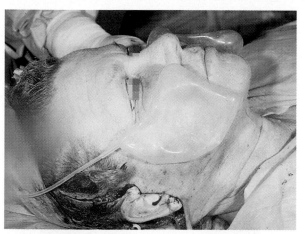

14-8C

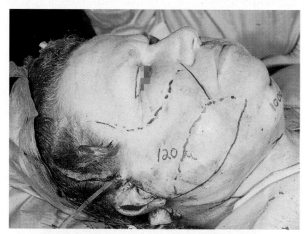

14-8D

Results (Figure 14-8, *E* and *F*)

The patient is shown 2 years after her expansion-rhytidectomy. Correction of her midface and neck ptosis has been maintained without an overpulled appearance.

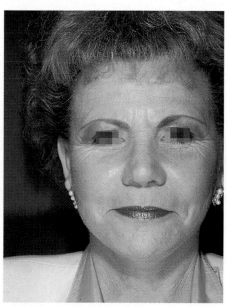

14-8E

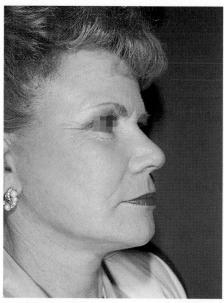

14-8F

CASE 3: Flaccid Skin and Minimal Fat

History (Figure 14-9, *A* and *B*)
This 49-year-old patient had early midface ptosis associated with nasolabial and marionette folds, jowls, and neck bands. An SMAS rhytidectomy with expansion was offered to correct these findings.

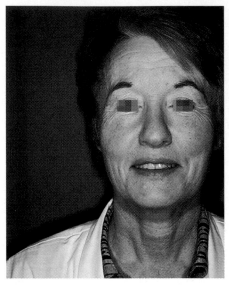

14-9A

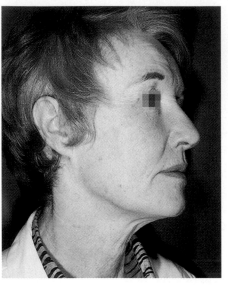

14-9B

Surgical Procedure (Figure 14-9, *C* and *D*)
At surgery, two 150 cc expanders were inserted under the elevated skin after SMAS resection and tightening. The skin was adjusted to an appropriate tension by temporarily tacking the key points of fixation. Serial expansions with saline up to 185 cc stretched the tissue for three cycles. After the balloons were removed, an additional 2 to 3 cm of preauricular and postauricular skin was resected.

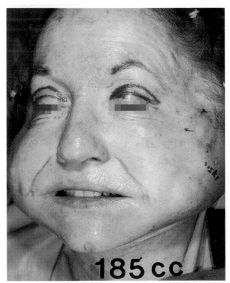

14-9C

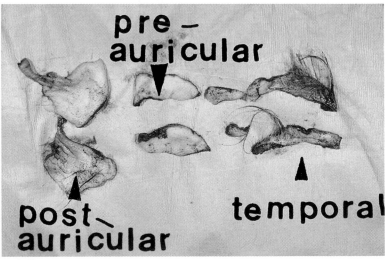

14-9D

Results (Figure 14-9, *E* and *F*)

The patient is shown 2 years after her surgical procedures. The nasolabial folds and marionette lines are corrected without an overpulled appearance to the midface or neck.

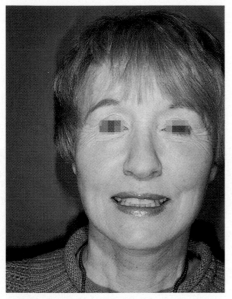

14-9E

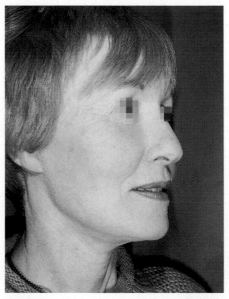

14-9F

ABDOMINOPLASTY

The goals of abdominoplasty are to remove the pannus of skin and fat, repair the diastasis recti abdominis deformity, and contour the anterior torso. The final transverse suprapubic scar should be kept low without an exaggerated upward displacement of the pubic hairline. Occasionally a patient has a significant distance (greater than 12 cm) between the umbilicus and pubis. After a conventional lower abdominal resection, this distance may result in a high transverse scar and pubic hairline. In these patients, intraoperative expansion of the tissue above the umbilicus may permit an acceptable closure.

The use of intraoperative expansion of the abdominal skin can generate additional tissue to aid in the closure of a wide defect. In the following case, intraoperative expansion permitted a low skin closure after abdominoplasty to camouflage the scar and maintain the optimal position of the pubis.

CASE REPORT AND ANALYSIS: Abdominoplasty

Wide Distance (15 cm) Between Umbilicus and Pubis

History (Figure 14-10, *A* and *B*)

This 48-year-old mother of three children had a moderate pannus, diastasis recti abdominis deformity of 3 cm, and a wide lower half of the abdomen. The patient wanted an abdominoplasty but was concerned about an elevated transverse scar and pubic hairline. Intraoperative expansion of the upper abdominal skin was offered as a possible solution to prevent these postoperative sequelae.

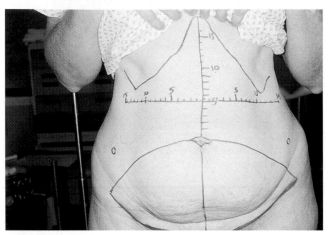

14-10A

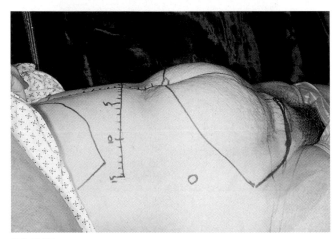

14-10B

Surgical Procedure (Figure 14-10, *C* and *D*)

At surgery the lower half of the abdominal skin and fat were excised from the suprapubic line to the umbilicus, extending 24 cm on each side from the midline of the abdomen (Figure 14-10, *C*). The cephalic flap was elevated from side wall to side wall and above the subcostal margin. The anterior rectus fascia was plicated from the xiphoid process to the pubic symphysis. Minimal liposuction was performed under the flap and hips. A temporary closure of the cephalic skin flap to the midline of the suprapubic flap raised the pubis to a higher-than-acceptable level.

Two 900 cc rectangular expanders (9 × 20 cm) were inserted under the cephalic flap and filled for three cycles with up to 1300 ml of saline within each expander (Figure 14-10, *D*). About 2 cm of "extra" skin was obtained after three cycles. The excess amount of distal flap was trimmed. The umbilical button was brought through a 2.5 cm horizontal skin incision and sutured for closure.

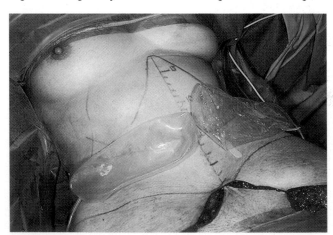

14-10C

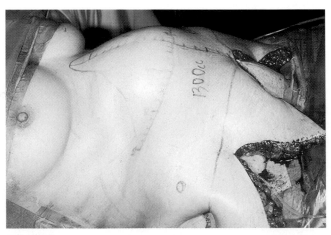

14-10D

Results (Figure 14-10, *E* and *F*)

One year after her abdominoplasty the patient has a contoured figure. The pubis is not elevated from the closure. Minimal scar hypertrophy developed.

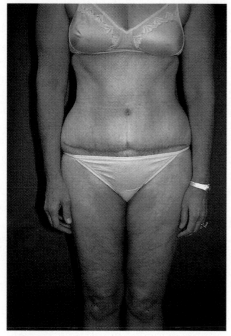

14-10E

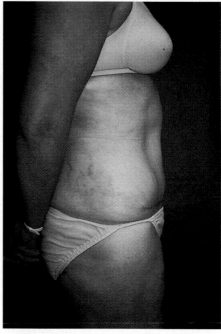

14-10F

AUGMENTATION MAMMOPLASTY

The goals of augmentation mammoplasty are to increase the volume, define the shape, and improve the symmetry of a small breast to create a larger one. Intraoperative expansion can benefit augmentation mammoplasty by providing extra tissue for improved draping over a larger implant. Soft tissue limitations, however, often prevent the insertion of a larger prosthesis, which, if positioned in the subglandular or subpectoral pocket, produces an ectopic implant position, fullness of the superior breast mound, and a downward- positioned nipple. The expansion of an intraoperative balloon under the glandular tissue or pectoralis muscle stretches the overlying restrictive tissues and helps to correct these anomalies produced by a sizable implant.

Surgical Protocol

Ranging in age from 18 to 57 years (median age about 32), 135 patients were indicated for breast enhancement between 1986 and 1997 in the author's series. Only 55 patients could be evaluated 2 years or more after surgery. Three patients had undergone previous augmentation mammoplasties but were indicated for implant exchanges because of capsular contracture.

Each candidate underwent extensive consultation on the benefits and side effects of the procedure, especially in regard to the potential unique problems that have been associated with the use of an alloplastic silicone implant. Standard photographs, including Polaroid views, were taken during the initial visit and subsequent postoperative appointments. All patients were required to obtain a mammogram at least 3 months before surgery.

Patients underwent mammoplasties under general anesthesia in an outpatient setting and received systemic antibiotics at the start of surgery. The surgical approach, location of the pocket dissection, and type of implant were discussed in detail. Preoperative markings of the hypoplastic breasts were outlined on the patient in the upright position before surgery.

Definition of Breast Hypoplasia

The hypoplastic breast possesses at least the following three inadequate dimensions (see Chapter 12):

1. The inframammary fold line (DCE) extends for a short distance from its medial point (E) to the lateral splay point (D). In patients with an A-cup size the length of the inframammary line is about 13.1 ± 1 cm

(Table 14-5), shorter compared with similar lines in B-cups (15.1 ± 2 cm) and C-cups (17.4 ± 3 cm). Clinically these patients do not possess significant cleavages because the breasts are distant from the midsternal line (FG).

2. The nipple to inframammary line (BC) is short in patients with A-cups (5.7 ± 0.2 cm) compared with such lines in B-cups (7.7 ± 0.1 cm) and C-cups (9.8 ± 0.1 cm). A short nipple-inframammary distance produces a small undercupping that is absent in the fuller ptotic breasts.

3. The transverse breast line (DBE) is small in A-cups (17.3 ± 0.2 cm) compared with similar lines in B-cups (20.1 ± 0.2 cm) and C-cups (22.5 ± 0.2 cm). A short transverse line usually translates into a flattened breast mound.

Thus, to enlarge a hypoplastic breast, all three dimensions should be increased to form a fuller, but symmetric mound. Other features of the hypoplastic breast, such as nipple-areolar deficiencies, should be noted when a breast enlargement procedure is considered.

Measurements of these anatomic breast landmarks were recorded in 100 consecutive patients, who were evaluated on the basis of their stated cup size and clinical examination. The length of every landmark was noted, averaged for each cup size, and tabulated (Table 14-5).

Surgical Technique

Before anesthetic induction the patient sits upright for surgical markings (Figure 14-11, *A*). First, the midsternal line is drawn from the sternal notch to the umbilicus. The inframammary line is outlined from the observed medial point of cleavage to the lateral splay point, which divides into the posteriorly directed brassiere line and the upwardly curved line of the later breast mound. A plumb line is dropped from the midclavicle through the nipple to intersect with the inframammary line. The superior breast is palpated and outlined from the lateral splay point across the superior border of the breast to the medial point of the cleavage.

In addition to these basic anatomic landmarks, reference lines are drawn to define the larger dimensions of the anticipated augmented breast.

Additional Reference Lines (Figure 14-11, *B*)

Cleavage.   The new medial point of the inframammary line is marked 1 to 2 cm from the midsternal line, shifting the original medial end of the cleavage fold higher and closer to the midline.

Undercup fullness.   The new inframammary fold is lowered 1 to 2 cm below and parallel to the original line. This design effectively adds 1 to 2 cm to the vertical meridian line, raises the nipple, and produces a more generous undercup.

Projection.   The new transverse breast line is drawn from the lateral splay point, parallel to but about 3 cm above the superior aspect of the breast mound, to meet the new medial point of the inframammary line. This increases the breast's transverse dimension, producing added projection after expansion and implant exchange.

Access Sites

After induction of general anesthesia the patient's arms are comfortably extended and padded. The wrists and elbows particularly are stabilized to prevent nerve compression. Local anesthesia of 0.5% lidocaine (Xylocaine) with epinephrine (1 : 200,000) is injected as a field block to diminish bleeding after surgery and minimize postoperative pain. The final amount of injected anesthetic agent varies from 50 to 100 ml.

Surgical accesses include the transaxillary, periareolar, and inframammary approaches. The surgeon will have discussed the benefits and drawbacks of each incision with the patient. The author prefers a subpectoral positioning of a textured implant through an inframammary approach to (1) reduce the incidence and deformities of capsular contracture, (2) reduce the visible and palpable presence of implant folds, (3) permit a more reliable interpretation of a mammogram by effective breast displacement, and (4) perhaps retard the

■ **Table 14-5**   Profiles of Breast Dimensions* (in cm) in 100 Consecutive Augmentations

Patients	Cup size	Age (years)	Height (inches)	Weight (pounds)	AC	DCE	ABC	AB	BC	DBE
67	A	24.9	65.6	121.2	19.7	13.1	24.3	18.4	5.7	17.3
		±6	±3	±5	±0.3	±1	±0.1	±0.1	±0.2	±0.2
25	B	38.6	66.3	125.0	19.6	15.1	27.0	19.3	7.7	20.1
		±3	±4	±4	±0.2	±2	±0.2	±0.2	±0.1	±0.2
8	C	34.0	65.5	131.5	21.0	17.4	31.0	22.0	9.8	22.5
		±5	±5	±6	±0.3	±3	±0.1	±0.1	±0.1	±0.2

*AC, Breast position; DCE, inframammary line; ABC, vertical meridian line; AB, clavicle-nipple line; BC, nipple-inframammary line; DBE, transverse line. (See Chapter 12.)

"bottoming out" of the implant from elongation of the undercup length with time.

An incision is made just above and parallel to the new inframammary line by beginning from the vertical meridian line and extending laterally for 3.5 to 5 cm. A dissection plane is developed down to the extended pectoralis fascia, lifting up the parenchymal breast tissue, to gain exposure to the lower lateral border of the pectoralis muscle. The pectoralis major muscle is dissected off the sixth rib, allowing a subpectoral pocket to be developed by transecting the muscle slips from their parasternal origins between the fourth to sixth ribs (Figure 14-11, C).

Parasternal dissection begins at the new medial point of the inframammary line and then continues upward past the thickened portion of the pectoralis major muscle that intrudes on the fourth rib from the sternum. This muscle bundle consistently contains one of the large perforating branches of the internal mammary artery. This tongue of muscle must be transected to expand the pectoralis muscle effectively later from the thorax. The lateral portion of the subpectoral pocket is developed by following the external skin markings along the midaxillary line, freeing the lateral border of the pectoralis major muscle from its connections along this border. The subpectoral dissection continues cephalad to about 5 cm above the superior border of the breast tissue, leaving intact the pectoralis minor muscle below.

Expansion and Implant Exchange

A fast-fill tissue expander (about 300 to 600 cc) is filled to the "best-fit" volume to assess the breast profile in the upright position (Figure 14-11, D). The most appropriate expander volume is recorded on the basis of adequate pocket fill. Further areas of dissection, usually along the inframammary and lateral axillary lines, may be required to create a more symmetric pocket. The expander is overexpanded slowly by 100 to 200 ml of saline for 10 to 15 minutes while dissection is begun on the opposite breast.

After expansion is completed, the balloon is removed. The pocket is irrigated with an antibacterial solution. Although the expansion process controls

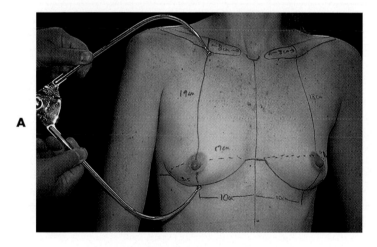

A

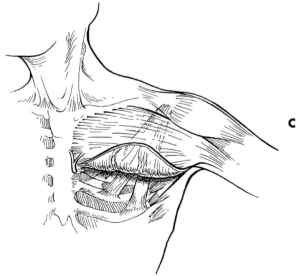

Figure 14-11 **A,** Before anesthetic induction, surgical markings are outlined with the patient in an upright position (see text). **B,** Additional reference lines indicate anticipated cleavage, undercup fullness, and projection of the augmented breast. **C,** Dissection of the pectoralis major muscle off the sixth rib permits development of subpectoral pocket by transecting the muscle slips from their parasternal origins between the fourth to sixth ribs. *Continued*

PRE-OPERATIVE EXTENDED
MARKINGS

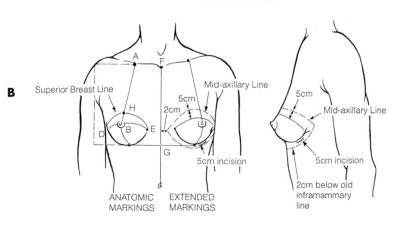

B

C

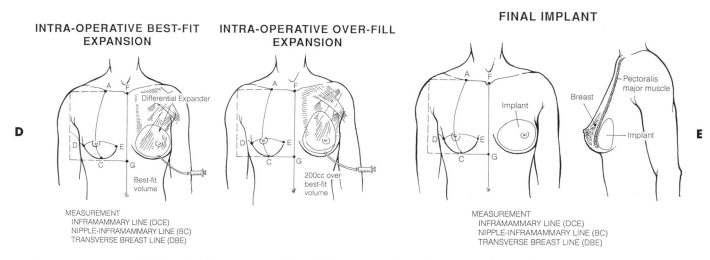

INTRA-OPERATIVE BEST-FIT EXPANSION

INTRA-OPERATIVE OVER-FILL EXPANSION

FINAL IMPLANT

Figure 14-11 cont'd   D, *Left,* Intraoperative "best-fit" expansion. *Right,* Intraoperative overfill expansion. Fast-fill skin expander (300 to 600 cc) is filled to the estimated optimal volume to assess the breast profile with the patient in an upright position. **E,** Larger saline or gel textured implant, usually 50 to 100 cc greater than the original "best-fit" volume, is inserted and evaluated for breast projection and symmetry with the patient upright.

■ **Table 14-6**   Profile Measurements (in cm) of Augmented Breasts Before and After Intraoperative Expansion in 55 Patients

| Preoperative cup size | Patients | Measurement* | Preoperative | Intraoperative | | Postoperative (2 or more years) | Implant volume (cc) | |
				Extended pocket	After expansion		Extended pocket	After expansion
A	22	DCE	13 ± 1	14 ± 2	15 ± 1	16 ± 2	200 ± 50	275 ± 50
		BC	4.5 ± 3	5.5 ± 1	6 ± 2	6 ± 1		
		DBE	15 ± 2	16 ± 1	18 ± 2	17 ± 2		
B	26	DCE	15 ± 2	16 ± 2	17 ± 2	18 ± 1	250 ± 50	325 ± 25
		BC	6 ± 1	7 ± 1	8 ± 1	8 ± 1		
		DBE	18 ± 2	19 ± 2	21 ± 1	20 ± 2		
C	7	DCE	17 ± 2	18 ± 2	20 ± 1	20 ± 1	325 ± 50	400 ± 25
		BC	10 ± 1	11 ± 1	12 ± 2	12 ± 2		
		DBE	20 ± 2	21 ± 2	22 ± 2	21 ± 2		

*DCE, Inframammary line; BC, nipple-inframammary line; DBE, transverse line.

most of the oozing smaller vessels, absolute hemostasis must be obtained before closure.

A larger saline or gel textured implant, usually 50 to 100 cc more than the original "best-fit" volume, is inserted and evaluated for projection and symmetry in the upright position (Figure 14-11, *E*). Since 1993 the author has favored the use of the adjustable saline implant with a buried remote valve and tubing to (1) size the final implant volume and shape, (2) minimize implant irregularities, and (3) adjust implant softness postoperatively. Final measurements of the new pocket are made after closure to confirm the previous measurements. In general the lengths of the inframammary line, nipple to inframammary line, and transverse breast line have increased by 1 to 2 cm.

A meticulous approximation of Scarpa's fascia and the subdermis is done with 4-0 Vicryl (polyglactin 910) sutures with a 3-0 proline subcuticular skin closure. A support dressing consisting of a soft roll and elastic bandage is applied. Drainage is usually not required. A sports brassiere is useful after surgery for continued support for an additional 3 weeks. No postoperative massages are routinely recommended.

Case Results

Intraoperative expansion in augmentation mammoplasty is indicated in patients who want a natural-looking but larger breast profile than could be obtained by simply increasing the pocket dimensions. Relative contraindications to expansion apply to patients with severely atrophic skin and glandular tissue, which require a breast lift with augmentation.

Fifty-five patients who underwent expansion surgery from 1986 to 1990 were evaluated at a 1992 follow-up (Table 14-6). The extended dimensions of the enlarged breasts were measured postoperatively and the data compared with the preoperative measurements. A 3-year assessment of the incidence of capsular contracture and return of nipple sensation were also evaluated in some patients.

Twenty-two patients were designated before surgery to be an A-cup size by brassiere cup and measurements of their inframammary line (DCE), nipple-inframammary line (BC), and transverse breast line (DBE). After expansion surgery these measurements increased by 1.5 to 3 cm. Two years or more later, measurements remained about the same (DCE, 16 ± 2 cm; BC, 6 ± 1 cm; DBE, 17 ± 2 cm) as those after expansion surgery. Patients reported that their size increased from an A-cup to a regular B-cup. Final implant volume was 275 ± 50 cc, about 75 cc larger than the postexpansion volume of the "best-fit" implant in Table 14-6.

Twenty-six patients were determined to be a B-cup size. Measurements after expansion surgery were 2 to 3 cm larger than those obtained before surgery. Two or more years later, measurements reflected a change in cup size from a small C to a regular C (DCE, 18 ± 1 cm; BC, 8 ± 1 cm; DBE, 20 ± 2 cm). The final implant size was 350 ± 50 cc, compared with the 325 ± 25 cc volume of the "best-fit" implant in the extended pocket.

Seven patients were determined to be a C-cup size before surgery. Measurements after expansion were 2 to 3 cm greater than those obtained before surgery. Two or more years later, measurements indicated a change in cup size to a full C, or small D (DCE, 20 ± 1 cm; BC, 12 ± 2 cm; DCE, 21 ± 2 cm). Patients noted an increase in cup size. Final implant size (425 ± 50 cc) was larger than preexpansion volume of the "best-fit" implant (400 ± 25 cc).

Complications

Capsular contracture (Baker III/IV) developed in four of 62 patients followed 3 years or more after expansion surgery. Sensation to the nipple-areolar complex returned to near-normal levels in most patients 3 years later. None of the patients developed complications such as bleeding, infection, or skin loss.

Summary

Tissue expansion represents an adjunctive procedure that offers advantages during augmentation mammoplasty. A permanent increase in the profile measurements of a hypoplastic breast produces a more natural shape from a larger prosthesis than the original "best-fit" implant. The incidence of capsular contracture with textured-wall implants did not favorably change with the addition of tissue expansion, but nipple-areolar sensation did return to "normal."

CASE REPORTS AND ANALYSES: Augmentation Mammoplasty

CASE 1:   A-Cup to B-Cup

History (Figure 14-12, *A* and *B*)
This nulliparous 28-year-old patient had 32-A-cup breasts. She wanted to increase her breast volume and

size to a full-B-cup. Intraoperative expansion was offered to accomplish these goals.

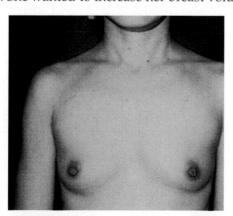

14-12A

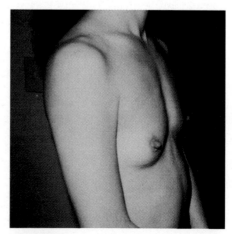

14-12B

Surgical Procedure (Figure 14-12, *C*)

At surgery a subpectoral pocket was dissected through a transaxillary approach to accommodate a 350 cc intraoperative expander. Serial expansions up to 410 cc for 10 to 15 minutes were repeated over three cycles to stretch the overlying tissues. A textured 325 cc saline adjustable implant was inserted and filled to an operative volume to 275 cc.

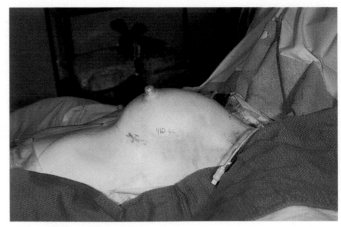

14-12C

Results (Figure 14-12, *D* and *E*)

The patient is shown 5 years after her augmentation mammoplasty. Her final volume adjustment was 315 to 325 cc (ml) of saline. The remote fill valve and tubing were removed 4 months after surgery. Her breasts were classified as a Baker II encapsulation.

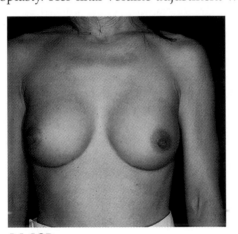

14-12D

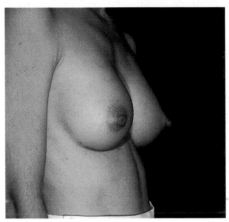

14-12E

CASE 2: A-Cup to C-Cup

History (Figure 14-13, *A* and *B*)

This 32-year-old nulliparous patient had A-cup-size breasts and wanted to augment them to a C-cup volume. Intraoperative expansion was offered as an alternative to accomplish this goal.

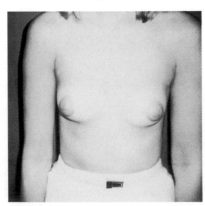

14-13A

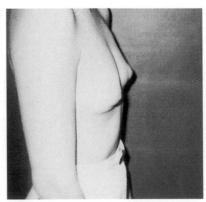

14-13B

Surgical Procedure (Figure 14-13, *C* and *D*)

At surgery a subpectoral pocket was dissected through a transaxillary approach for the insertion of a 600 cc intraoperative expander. Serial expansions up to 600 cc

for 3 to 10 minutes stretched the overlying soft tissue to permit the insertion of a textured 350 cc saline adjustable implant. The intraoperative fill volume was 300 cc.

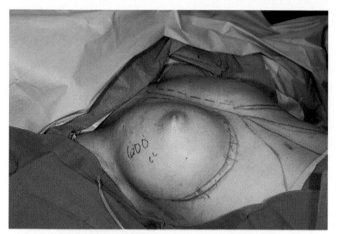

14-13C

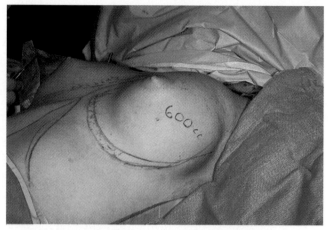

14-13D

Results (Figure 14-13, *E* and *F*)

The patient is shown 4 years after her surgical procedure. The final volume adjustment was about 350 to

360 cc of saline. The remote valve and tubing system were removed about 1 year after her augmentation mammoplasty. Her breasts remain a Baker II classification.

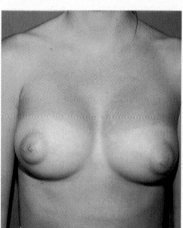

14-13E

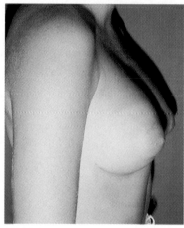

14-13F

CASE 3:   Small B-Cup to C-Cup

History (Figure 14-14, *A* and *B*)
This gravida I patient presented with small B-cup-size breasts and desired to increase their volumes to regu-lar C-cups. The patient chose intraoperative expansion to accomplish this goal.

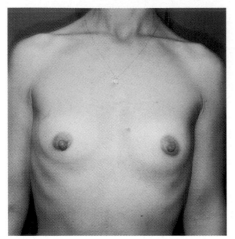

14-14A

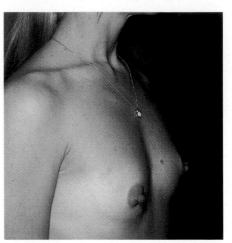

14-14B

Surgical Procedure (Figure 14-14, *C*)
At surgery a 350 cc intraoperative expander was in-serted in the subpectoral pocket dissected through an inframammary approach. Serial expansions up to 420 cc stretched the tissues for three cycles. A 375 cc silicone textured gel implant was positioned under the muscle layer.

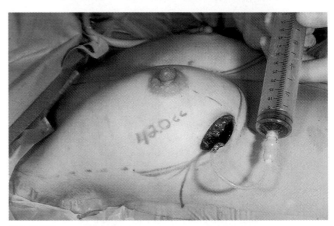

14-14C

Results (Figure 14-14, *D* and *E*)
The patient is shown 5 years after her surgery. Her breasts were classified as Baker II, with regular C-cup volume.

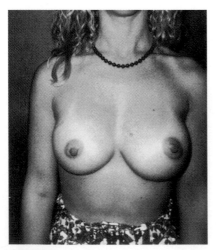

14-14D

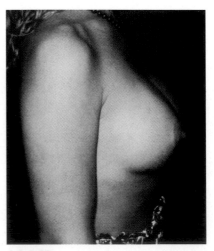

14-14E

AUGMENTATION RHINOPLASTY AND MENTOPLASTY

Intraoperative expansion may favorably alter the characteristics of soft tissue draping over an alloplastic implant during an augmentation rhinoplasty or mentoplasty (nose or chin reconstruction). Rapid stretching of the periosteum creates a pocket in which the contoured implant fits snugly without compression. This technique permits the insertion of the larger volume implants that may be required to achieve an optimal result.

CASE REPORTS AND ANALYSES: Augmentation Rhinoplasty and Mentoplasty

CASE 1: Poorly Defined Nasal Dorsum

History (Figure 14-15, *A* and *B*)

This 48-year-old patient had excess skin and fat on the upper eyelids and a flattened nasal dorsum. The patient requested an upper lid blepharoplasty, which also would define her supratarsal crease lines. An augmentation rhinoplasty with an L-shaped silicone implant was recommended to enhance her midface features.

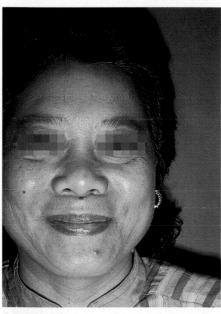

14-15A

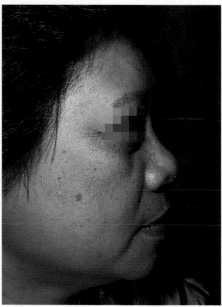

14-15B

Surgical Procedure (Figure 14-15, *C* and *D*)

After the upper lid blepharoplasties were completed, intercartilaginous nasal approaches were used to create a midline subperiosteal pocket slightly above the nasofrontal angle. A 2 cc rectangular expander (2 × 5 cm) was inserted in the subperiosteal cavity. Intraoperative expansions over three cycles stretched the overlying tissues so that a trimmed implant with a columellar strut was lodged in its pocket without exposure of the implant at the incisional sites. A Steri-Strip dressing maintained the optimal position of the implant for 7 days.

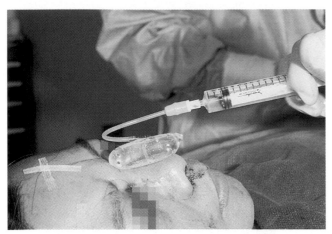

14-15C

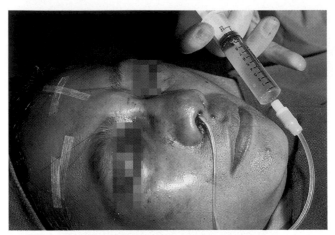

14-15D

Results (Figure 14-15, *E* and *F*)

The patient is shown 3 years after her surgical procedures. Nasal projection at the tip and dorsum added a dimensional appearance to the midface that was complemented by the results of the upper lid blepharoplasties.

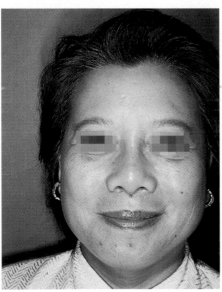

14-15E

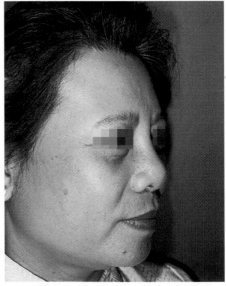

14-15F

CASE 2: Chin Recession

History (Figure 14-16, *A* and *B*)

This 47-year-old patient had a recessed chin that produced an imbalance to facial symmetry. The patient did not want changes to his nasal profile or anterior neck.

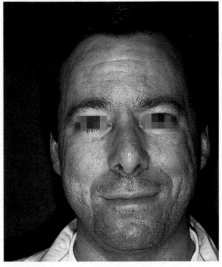

14-16A

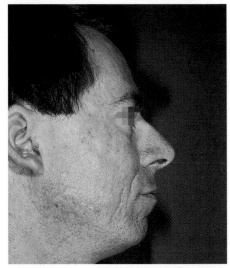

14-16B

Surgical Procedure (Figure 14-16, *C* to *E*)

A silicone elastomer chin implant (7 × 42 mm) was inserted under the mental periosteum through a labial-alveolar approach. After pocket dissection a 1 × 3 cm expander was inserted in this subperiosteal space and serially inflated three times to stretch the overlying structures. The chin implant was exchanged for the balloon.

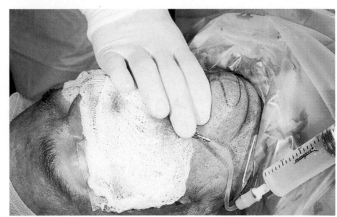

14-16C

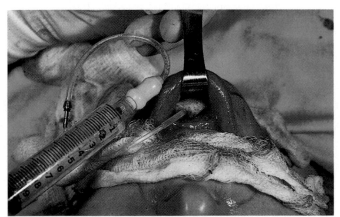

14-16D

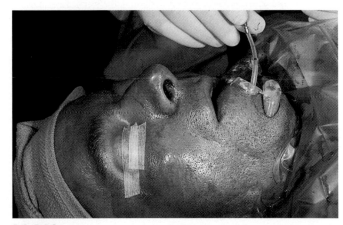

14-16E

Results (Figure 14-16, *F* and *G*)

The patient is shown 2 years after his chin augmentation. Facial balance is improved on lateral gaze, with the nasal tip in better alignment with the chin projection.

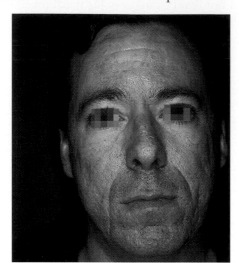

14-16F

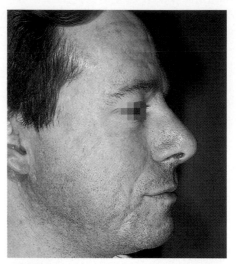

14-16G

REFERENCES

1. Cohen BH, Cosmetto AJ: Suture Tension Adjustment Reel: a new device for the management of skin closure, *J Dermatol Surg Oncol* 18:112-123, 1992.
2. Ersek RA, Vazquez-Salisbury A: Wound closure using a skin stretching device, *Contemp Orthop* 28:495-500, 1994.

CHAPTER 15

Intraoperative Expansion for Correction of Aesthetic Complications

The technique of intraoperative expansion has been most useful in providing tissue for revision of hypertrophic scars that result after surgery for male-pattern baldness. The creation of additional tissue by intraoperative expansion may also be used to reverse the detrimental effects of tissue deficiency that may occur after forehead lifts, blepharoplasties, and rhytidoplasties. In the following anecdotal cases, intraoperative expansion corrected adverse results after aesthetic surgery (Table 15-1).

Intraoperative expansion may represent another technique to manage difficult skin deficiency problems that result from conventional aesthetic surgeries. This innovative technique provides specific appealing benefits to correct such complications. The method represents a single-stage procedure that releases and stretches tethered, identical skin for tissue replacement. Often, skin grafts may create additional problems when used in facial areas of the aesthetic surgical patient. Intraoperative expansion, however, can supply only a limited amount of tissue, which may be insufficient to correct significant tissue shortage complications.

■ **Table 15-1** Intraoperative Expansion for Complications After 15 Aesthetic Surgeries

Aesthetic surgery/complication	Number
Male-pattern baldness	
Scar alopecia	7
Postoperative hair loss	1
Coronal forehead lift	
Elevated eyebrows	2
Lower lid blepharoplasty	
Bowing	2
Xantholasma (cholesterol collections)	1
Abdominoplasty	
Elevated pubis	2

CASE REPORTS AND ANALYSES

CASE 1: Scar Alopecia and Hair Loss After Forehead Lift

History (Figure 15-1, *A*)

This 55-year-old patient underwent a coronal forehead lift for male-pattern baldness that resulted in an area of traumatic alopecia behind the right forehead recession line. The triangular area measured 3.5 × 6 cm anterior to the bicoronal scar line. The patient was offered long-term expansion or intraoperative expansion to provide hair-bearing tissue to replace the defect.

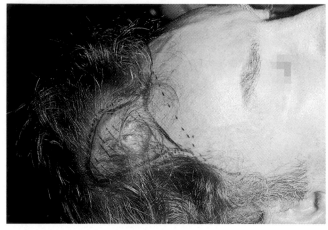

15-1A

Surgical Procedure (Figure 15-1, *B* and *C*)

A 100 cc round expander was inserted through a 2 cm incision under the galea aponeurotica of surrounding hair-bearing scalp. After saline serial expansions up to 150 cc volume, the entire area of alopecia was excised and covered with adjacent normal scalp.

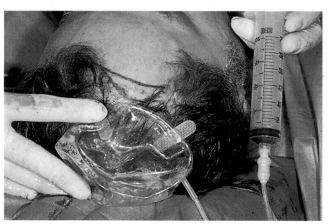

15-1B

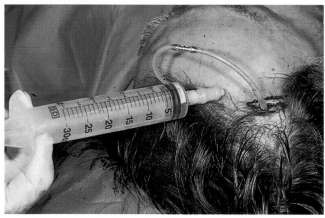

15-1C

Results (Figure 15-1, *D*)

Three years after surgery, the patient has a symmetric anterior hairline. The expanded scalp has retained its hair density, eliminating the area of alopecia.

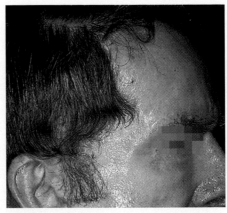

15-1D

CASE 2:   Excessive Brow Elevation After Forehead Lift

History (Figure 15-2, *A*)

The patient in Case 1 underwent a precapillary forehead lift 3 years before his consultation. The patient complained of a "surprised" appearance with excessive brow elevation. The midportion and tail of the eyebrows were arched and produced an angry look. The patient wanted to lower the lateral half of the eyebrows to create a more masculine appearance.

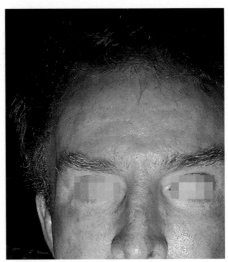

15-2A

Surgical Procedure (Figure 15-2, *B* and *C*).
A 200 cc rectangular intraoperative expander was inserted in the subgaleal plane through a 4 cm incision in a portion of the original scar line. Serial expansions up to 300 cc over three cycles stretched the tissues.

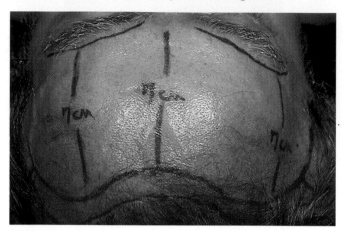

15-2B

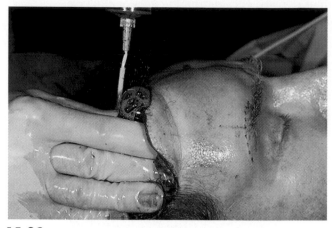

15-2C

Results (Figure 15-2, *D*)
Three years later the patient has a more masculine and natural appearance after intraoperative expansion lowered the lateral half of each brow by 1 cm. The frontalis muscles function appropriately after rapid stretching.

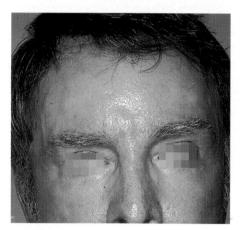

15-2D

CASE 3: Bowing of Lower Lids After Subciliary Blepharoplasty

History (Figure 15-3, *A*)

The patient in Cases 1 and 2 also complained of tearing from his weakened lower lids 2 years after a subciliary blepharoplasty. The patient exhibited lateral bowing of the lids, primarily from skin shortness rather than ptosis of the orbicularis oculi muscle sling. The contribution of orbital septum fibrosis to bowing could not be accurately determined from the physical examination. The pinch test did not elicit any degree of horizontal laxity to the lower lids. Because the patient did not accept full-thickness skin grafting, intraoperative expansion of the tight skin was offered as a means to elevate the lids.

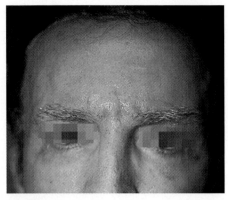

15-3A

Surgical Procedure (Figure 15-3, *B* and *C*)

A 5×35 mm rectangular expander was inserted through a 1 cm incision at the lateral canthus under the lower lid skin. Serial expansion up to 2 cc (ml) of saline for three cycles created additional skin. After the balloon was removed, the lower lid was supported for 3 weeks with taping. A lateral canthopexy or tarsal strip procedure was not performed.

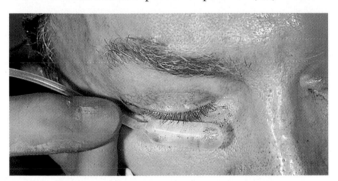

15-3B

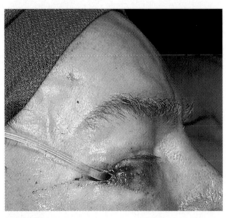

15-3C

Results (Figure 15-3, *D* and *E*)
The patient is shown 1 year after intraoperative expansion of the skin to the lower lids. Lateral bowing

was improved to the degree that tearing did not occur postoperatively.

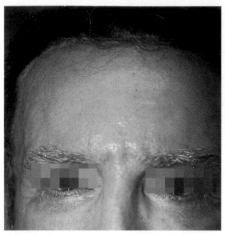

15-3D

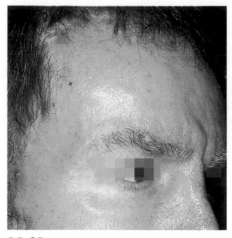

15-3E

CASE 4: Xantholasma to Lower Lids

History (Figure 15-4, *A* and *B*)
This 38-year-old patient had large cholesterol plaques under both lower lids. She requested removal of the plaques with minimal scarring. Intraoperative expan-

sion was suggested to stretch sufficient lower lid skin to excise the involved skin through a subciliary incision and reduce the incidence of lower lid bowing or ectropion.

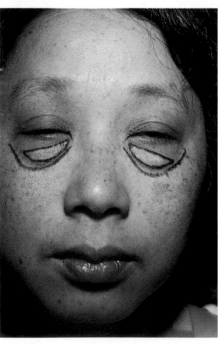

15-4A

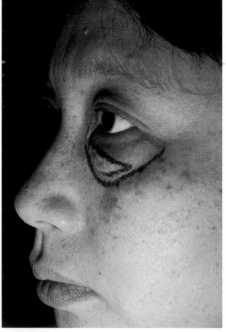

15-4B

Surgical Procedure (Figure 15-4, *C* and *D*)

A 1 cm subciliary incision permitted dissection of a skin pocket 2 cm below the lowest level of the cholesterol plaques. A rectangular intraoperative balloon (1 × 3.5 cm) was inserted and serially expanded through three cycles to gain as much tissue as possible. After the expander was removed, the involved skin was excised through an extended subciliary incision across the entire distance of the lower lid and canthus.

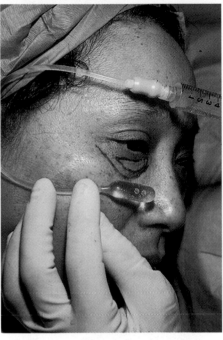

15-4C

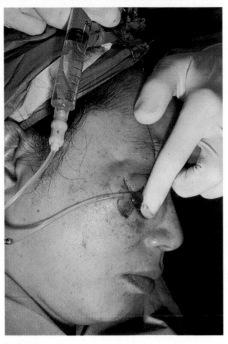

15-4D

Results (Figure 15-4, *E* and *F*)

Two years after her surgery the patient shows complete removal of the cholesterol plaques. The lesions have not recurred. The patient exhibits an acceptable subciliary scar without bowing or ectropion.

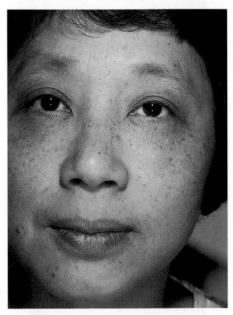

15-4E

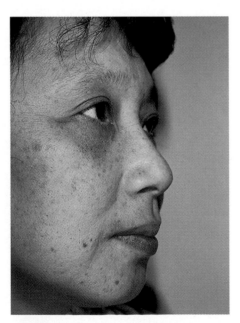

15-4F

CASE 5: Absence of Temporal Hair
After Rhytidectomies

History (Figure 15-5, *A*)

This 65-year-old patient had undergone two previous rhytidectomies that resulted in an absence of temporal hair. The patient would not accept hair transplantations, transposition flaps, or chronic expansion as a means to recreate the original hairline. During a "skin tuck" procedure for the midface and neck, intraoperative expansion of the receded temporal hair was attempted to obtain a small amount of hair-bearing skin that would be advanced downward to recreate temporal hair.

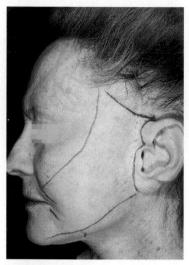

15-5A

Surgical Procedure (Figure 15-5, *B*)

A 50 cc round expander was inserted in the subgaleal space under the frontotemporal hair. After intraoperative expansion up to 120 cc volume for three cycles, the balloon was removed. The extra amount of scalp was advanced downward to create a semblance of the normal hairline.

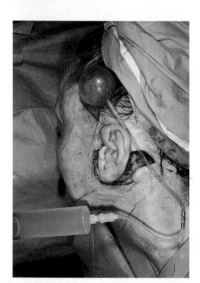

15-5B

Results (Figure 15-5, *C*)

The patient is shown 2 years after temporal hair reconstruction. The scars have healed without hypertrophy, and hair density remains unchanged.

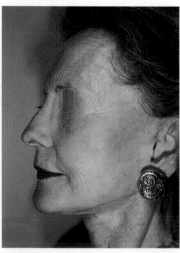

15-5C

PART

Four SPECIALIZED AREAS

Results (Figure 16-1, *C*)
Three months after the third procedure the width of the remaining back nevus ranges from 6 to 14 cm. Scar widening was 4.5 to 5 cm.

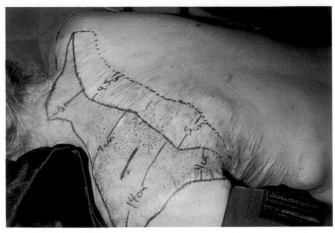

16-1C

Fourth Surgical Procedure (Figure 16-1, *D* and *E*)
Two 800 cc round expanders with remote valves were inserted through a 2.5 cm incision at the posterior axillary fold under the previously expanded back tissue.

Serial expansions for 3 months created 28 cm hemispheric flaps. After capsulectomies the flaps were advanced as far cephalad as possible.

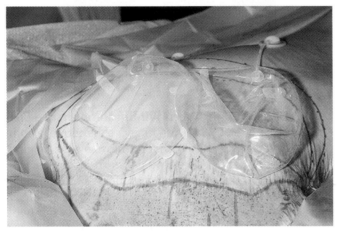

16-1D

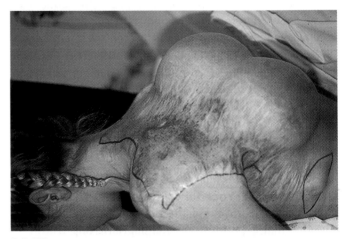

16-1E

Results (Figure 16-1, *F*)
The patient is shown 3 weeks after surgery with almost all the back nevus removed. The flap could be advanced to the nape of the neck and across the left crest of the posterior shoulder.

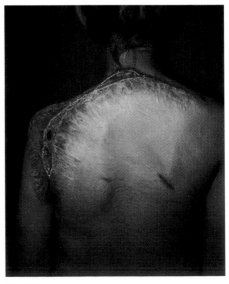

16-1F

Fifth Surgical Procedure (Figure 16-1, *G* to *I*)

An 800 cc rectangular expander was inserted under the skin of the left groin. Serial expansions over 3 months created a hemispheric flap 15 cm across and 21 cm long. The entire expanded flap was thinned over a wire strainer, creating a full-thickness skin graft. The skin graft covered the supraclavicular fossa, anterior chest wall, and shoulder tip.

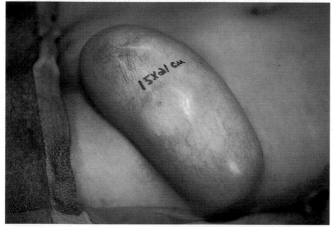

16-1G

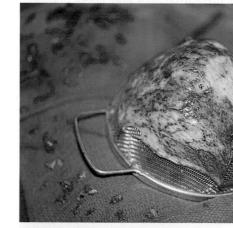

16-1H

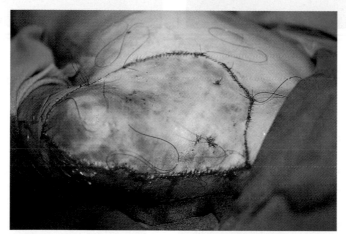

16-1I

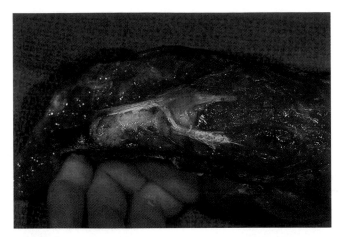

16-2C

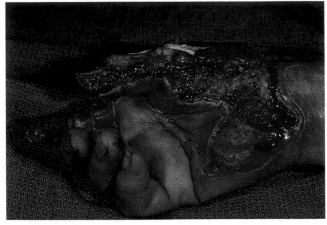

16-2D

Surgical Procedure (Figure 16-2, *E* to *I*)

A 500 cc round expander was inserted under the skin of the deltoid aspect of the shoulder through a 3 cm incision within the supraclavicular fossa. Serial expansions continued for 6 weeks to create a 12 × 15 cm expanded hemispheric dome within the extended portion of the deltopectoral flap.

After the expander was removed, the deltopectoral flap was elevated, based on the axial vessels from the thoracic perforators (Figure 16-2, *H*). Capsulectomy unfurled the domed flap, which was thinned to provide supple coverage around the reconstructed thumb. A cortical bone graft from the iliac crest was fashioned to resemble the distal phalanx of the thumb. The graft was positioned on the distal end of the proximal phalanx by Kirschner-wire fixation (Figure 16-2, *I*). The flap was wrapped around the thumb and applied to the radial aspect of the hand.

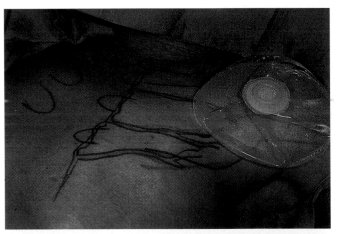

16-2E

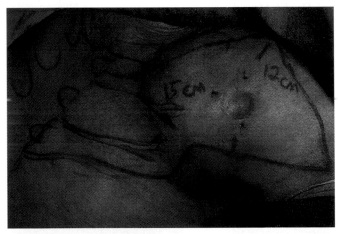

16-2F

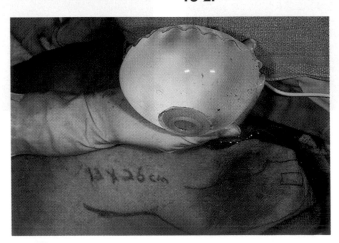

16-2G

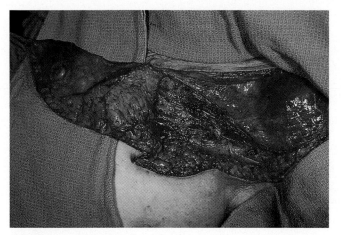

16-2H

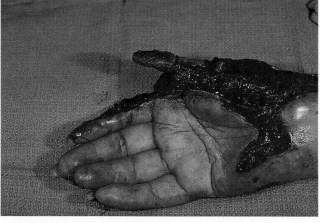

16-2I

Results (Figure 16-2, *J* and *K*)
The flap, divided and insetted 8 weeks later, provided stable and aesthetic coverage to the thumb, radial aspect of the hand, and a portion of the palm. Thumb length was preserved for approximation and prehension functions with the other phalanges. A full-thickness skin graft successfully covered the radial aspect of the index finger.

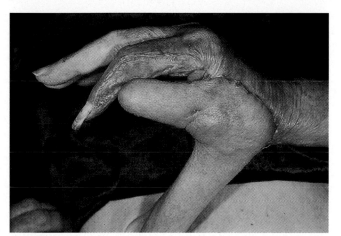

16-2J

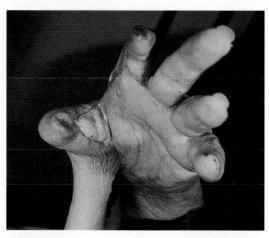

16-2K

EXPANDED MYOCUTANEOUS FLAPS

A defined area of skin and subcutaneous tissue may be transferred with a specific muscle unit. Occasionally the planned myocutaneous flap with its established width and length may not be sufficient to cover a defect. Expansion of the muscle-skin unit serves to increase the transferable surface area and encourage more blood flow, ensuring the safety of the reconstructive procedure.[15] Experimentally, Forte and colleagues[19] and Leighton and associates[20] demonstrated an increase in the microvascularity of expanded myocutaneous flaps over that found in controls.

Table 16-3 lists the author's experience with expanded myocutaneous flaps since 1986 for a variety of reconstructive problems.

■ **Table 16-3** Expansion of Myocutaneous Flaps in Five Patients

Flap	Expander (cc)	Duration (mo)	Transferred end (cm)	Defect (cm)
1. Latissimus dorsi	800	3	20 × 20	Radiated tumor, chest wall (15 × 17)
2. Latissimus dorsi (see Case 1)	800	3	15 × 24	Radio-osteonecrosis, chest wall (15 × 24)
3. Latissimus dorsi (see Case 2)	1000	3	18 × 22	Radiated tumor, chest wall (22 × 22)
4. Pectoralis major	600	3	9 × 15	Radionecrosis, midface (10 × 15)
5. Pectoralis major	600	3	15 × 15	Ear reconstruction

CASE REPORTS AND ANALYSES: Expanded Myocutaneous Flaps

CASE 1: Necrosis and Infection After Chest Wall Radiotherapy

History (Figure 16-3, *A* and *B*)
This 76-year-old patient underwent a left modified radical mastectomy with postoperative radiotherapy. Radio-osteonecrosis and infection were observed about 6 months after chest wall radiation. Serial biopsies of the exposed area and metastatic workup did not demonstrate tumor recurrence. Because the amount of débridement was expected to be significant, a large latissimus dorsi flap was required for coverage of the defect. An 800 cc round expander was inserted under the fascial extension of the ipsilateral latissimus dorsi flap. Serial expansions for 3 months produced a 24 × 24 cm domed flap over the random blood flow portion of the myocutaneous flap.

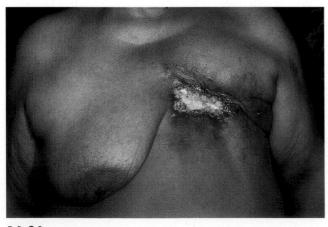

16-3A

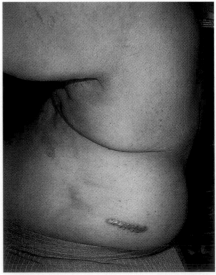

16-3B

Surgical Procedure (Figure 16-3, *C* to *E*)
At surgery the chest wall was débrided widely back to clinically noninfected tissue. A 15 × 22 cm chest wall defect resulted after removal of the infected fourth to sixth ribs. After the expander was removed from its pocket, the delayed preexpanded random skin paddle was raised continuous with the muscle unit and insetted into the chest wall defect.

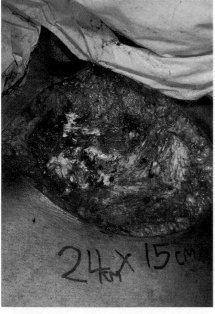

16-3C

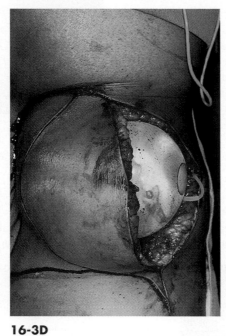

16-3D

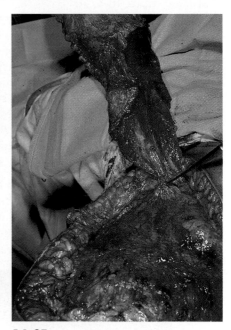

16-3E

Results (Figure 16-3, *F* and *G*)
The insetted flap, shown at completion of the surgical procedure, provided full coverage of the radiated recipient site. Wound healing proceeded without complications. The donor site was able to be approximated with a primary closure.

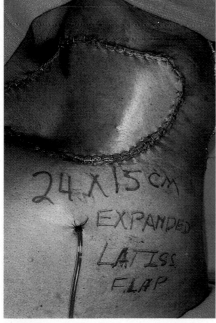

16-3F

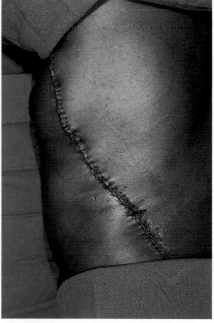

16-3G

CASE 2: Tumor Recurrence after Radiotherapy

History (Figure 16-4, A)
This 67-year-old patient underwent a right modified radical mastectomy and radiation therapy for advanced breast cancer. Two years later an area of ulceration appeared at the anterior axillary fold. Biopsy of the ulcerated site demonstrated tumor recurrence. Workup did not reveal any obvious systemic involvement. An expanded latissimus dorsi myocutaneous flap was required to cover the expected size of the resection that was planned to control local disease.

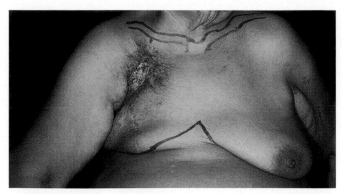

16-4A

Surgical Procedure (Figure 16-4, B and C)
A 1000 cc round expander was inserted under the fascial extension of the latissimus dorsi muscle-skin unit. Serial expansion over 8 weeks created a 24 × 24 cm domed flap. The chest wall was resected, including portions of the sixth to eighth ribs. A large skin paddle, measuring about 18 × 22 cm, was transposed anteriorly to cover the composite tissue defect. The donor site, approximated under moderate tension, progressed to primary healing.

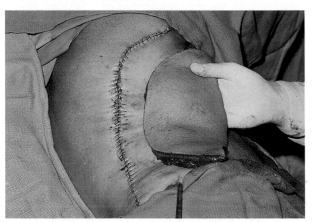

16-4C

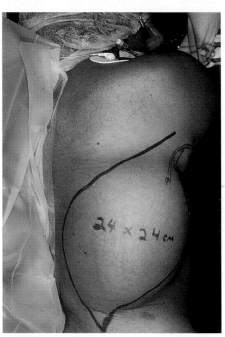

16-4B

Results (Figure 16-4, D)
Six months after her procedure the patient has a stable transposed flap. No evidence of tumor spread has been seen. The expanded flap did not demonstrate problems of delayed healing along its interface with radiated tissue.

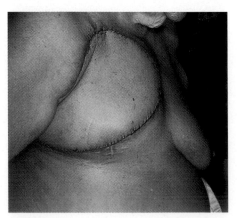

16-4D

EXPANDED FREE FLAPS

With their fixed axial length and width, available flaps sometimes are not adequate to satisfy a particular reconstruction. Although the use of free tissue transfers obviates this concern, the use of preexpanded free flaps permits coverage of large defects with a single flap and closure of the donor site. Almost any established free flap (fascial, cutaneous, myocutaneous, osseomyocutaneous) may be expanded before microvascular transfer.

Table 16-4 summarizes the author's limited experience with preexpanded free tissue transfer. Postexpansion of free flaps may be considered the same as for any tissue subjected to long-term expansion.

■ **Table 16-4** Preexpansion of Free Tissue Transfers in Three Patients

Flap	Expander (cc)	Duration (mo)	Transferred end (cm)	Defect (cm)
1. Latissimus dorsi (see Case 1)	1000	3	20 × 20	Pressure sores, hip sacrum (20 × 20)
2. Latissimus dorsi	1000	3	17 × 17	Tibial fracture (15 × 15)
3. Latissimus dorsi	800	3	15 × 18	Trimalleolar fracture (11 × 12)

CASE REPORT AND ANALYSIS: Expanded Free Flaps

Large Pressure Sores

History (Figure 16-5, *A* and *B*)
This 32-year-old paraplegic had pressure sores from his hips to the ankles. Hospital admission was necessary because of a subfascial infection to his right lower extremity.

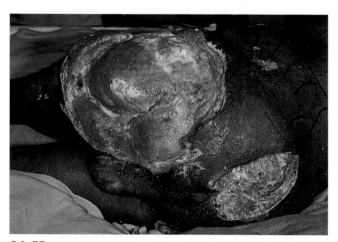

16-5A   **16-5B**

First Surgical Procedure (Figure 16-5, *C* and *D*)
The patient required multiple débridements, regular visits to the whirlpool, and nutritional support to manage most of his ulcers. Despite the addition of systemic antibiotics, suppuration and wet gangrene continued to progress in his right leg. The patient accepted a hip disarticulation, with coverage provided by a buttock flap.

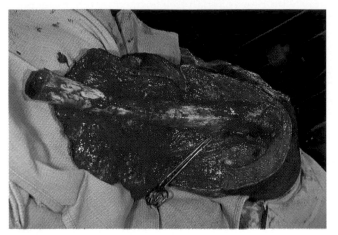

16-5C

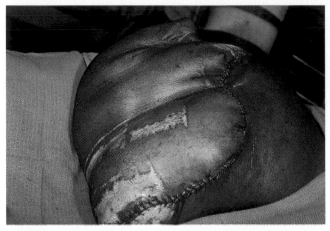

16-5D

Second Surgical Procedure (Figure 16-5, *E*)
To provide stable coverage for the large decubitus ulcer over his left hip and sacrum, a 1000 cc round tissue expander was inserted under the fascial extension of the left latissimus dorsi muscle. The patient had refused a second hip disarticulation procedure for coverage of the remaining open wound. Serial expansion over 8 weeks created a 20 × 20 cm skin paddle over the distal portions of the muscle-fascia complex.

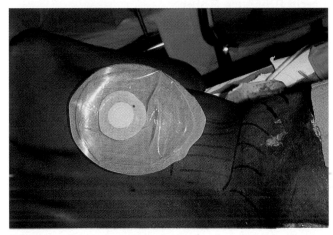

16-5E

Third Surgical Procedure (Figure 16-5, *F* to *H*)
At surgery the expander was removed from its pocket. The dissection elevated the latissimus dorsi muscle with isolation of the thoracodorsal pedicle. The expanded skin paddle contracted on creation of the distal flap but was able to be reexpanded to its original size during flap inset. The microvascular transfer was performed with a primary anastomosis of the flap's artery to the superior gluteal artery. Venous drainage was facilitated by approximating both venae comitantes of the thoracodorsal pedicle to the superior gluteal veins. Neural anastomosis was not performed.

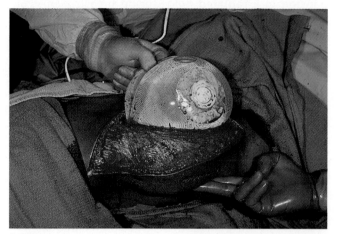

16-5F

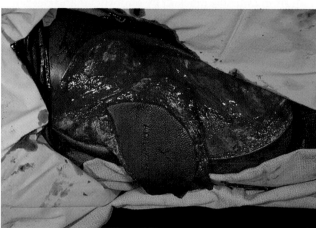

16-5G

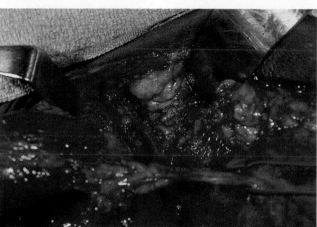

16-5H

Results (Figure 16-5, *I* and *J*)
The patient is shown 1 year after his numerous surgical procedures. Stable coverage was provided by the right buttock flap and the free latissimus dorsi myocutaneous flap to the problem sites. Cutaneous sensation to both reconstructed areas is still absent.

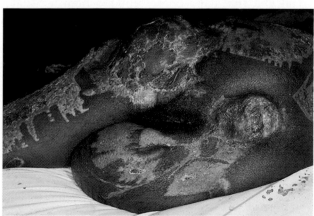

16-5I

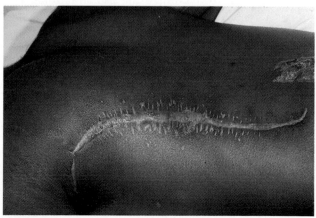

16-5J

EXPANDED RADIATED FLAPS AND SPECIAL PATIENT CONDITIONS

Radiated Tissue Considerations

Radiation injury is marked by superficial and deep tissue changes that can delay wound healing and contribute to necrosis and tissue sloughing beyond the original surgical field. Severely damaged skin is characterized by a dry, parchment appearance with telangiectasias, pigmentations, and nodules of hyperkeratosis. Histologic changes mirror these external findings and consist of endarteritis obliterans, lymphatic pooling, and massive fibrosis.[21,22] Delayed effects may result in radiation-induced carcinomas, recurrent carcinomas, and infections.[23,24] These characteristics contribute directly to the complications encountered with surgical intervention in an irradiated field.

The use of tissue expansion in altered environments must be circumspect because of the high potential for complications in this two-stage procedure. During the first stage of expander insertion, incisions should be small and placed distant from the expander unit to minimize injury to the vascular and lymphatic supply. The dissected pocket should be deep and limited to the expander size to reduce the chances for infection, bleeding, and skin blisters or loss. The remote valve system should be positioned deeply under "stable" tissue to decrease the opportunity for infections or exposure. Parenteral antibiotics should be given at surgery, with continuation of oral antibiotics in the immediate postoperative period.

In the filling phase, adherence to sterile technique must be observed during antibacterial preparation of the skin over the valve; handling of needles, syringes, and saline solutions; and application of antibacterial ointment over the puncture site. The amount of saline fill should not elicit ischemic blanching of the skin in order to prevent skin necrosis with exposure of the implant system. Consequently, expansion proceeds slowly over a longer period, with smaller increments of saline filling to maximize the ischemic margin of safety.

During the reconstructive phase, incisions and elevation of flaps should be minimized to maintain maximal lymphatic and blood supply. Since delayed healing often occurs at the interface of suture lines,[25] short incision lines should result in less postoperative morbidity. The concerns and implementation of tissue expansion in a radiated field during breast reconstruction are similar to those addressed in these clinical cases (see Chapter 12).

Special Patient Considerations

Similar precautions and strategic planning as those just discussed should be exercised in patients who have a history of diabetes, collagen disorders, and smoking. Tissue expansion in these patients is accompanied by higher complication rates, and these clinical problems should be considered relative contraindications for expansion. However, the use of judgment and caution in these risky clinical situations may result in a "successful" effort with the expansion technique.

Case Results

Table 16-5 summarizes the author's experience with tissue expansion in compromised tissue. Although significant increased morbidity was not observed, the number of cases is too small to generalize on the choice of using expansion in these specific cases. Other methods of reconstruction (e.g., free tissue transfer) would be preferable to tissue expansion in radiated fields that results in compromised tissue coverage. In addition, the expanded tissue often is inadequate because of the intrinsic tissue deficiencies from fibrosis and ischemia.

Expanded Skin Grafts

Tissue expansion may successfully provide larger areas of full-thickness skin grafts to cover significant defects when skin deficiencies cannot be resurfaced by alternative methods. Some patients cannot provide regional and free flaps or present too high a risk for reconstruction.

■ **Table 16-5** Expansion of Compromised Tissue in Five Patients

Etiology	Defect area (cm)	Expander (cc)	Duration (mo)	Average fill (cc)	Morbidity
1. Radiation ulcer (see Case 1)	Face (3 × 5)	200	4	10-15	Inadequate tissue
2. Radiation dermatitis	Cheek (5 × 5)	200	4	10-15	Inadequate tissue
3. Radiation ulcer	Scalp (4 × 4)	400	5	10-15	Inadequate tissue, hair loss
4. Radiation dermatitis	Knee (2 × 3)	200	5	10-15	Delayed healing
5. Radiation dermatitis, in situ squamous cell carcinoma (see Case 2)	Nose	200 (radiated forehead)	4	10-15	Delayed healing

In the author's limited experience, expanded full-thickness grafts maintain the characteristics of nonexpanded grafts, which include durability, ability to adapt to normal growth patterns, and aesthetics. Expanded supraclavicular donor skin produces optimal match for facial defects, and expanded groin donor skin provides functional qualities for deficiencies in other areas. Donor sites for expanded skin grafts may be approximated by primary closure.

Summary

Tissue expansion of vascularly compromised skin, as found in radiated tissue and in the diabetic or collagen-diseased patient, can provide useful coverage in these special circumstances. During the expansion procedure, skin is subject to delayed healing, infections, and resistance to expansion forces. The surgeon must exercise caution and judgment during the entire expansion procedure to prevent serious complications.

CASE REPORTS AND ANALYSES: Expanded Radiated Flaps

CASE 1:   Radiation Dermatitis of Cheek

History (Figure 16-6, *A*)
This 55-year-old patient had invasive squamous cell carcinoma of her right lower lid and infraorbital skin. A 5 × 5 cm split-thickness skin graft was successfully applied to the defect. The patient received 6 weeks of radiation therapy (2500 R) to the graft site and adjacent cheek skin. Because of severe radiation dermatitis with cellulitis and skin breakdowns, the patient requested more stable coverage. Tissue expansion was offered as a means to resurface the area with an expanded cheek flap. The patient refused free tissue transfers to import stable and nonradiated tissue.

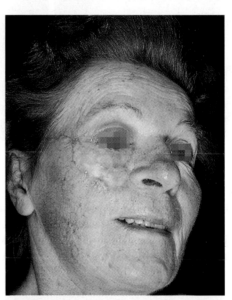

16-6A

First Surgical Procedure (Figure 16-6, *B*)
A 200 cc round expander with a remote valve system was inserted under the radiation-exposed cheek skin through a 2 cm retrolobular incision. The small incision away from the radiated field would be expected to heal without complications. The pocket dissection was in the deep subcutaneous plane and limited to the expander's size. Serial expansions with 10 to 15 ml of saline per week over 4 months created a domed flap about 16 cm across. Overexpansion with tissue ischemia was avoided during filling.

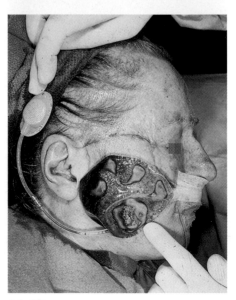

16-6B

Second Surgical Procedure (Figure 16-7, *D*)

At surgery an 8 cm-wide glabellar flap, based on the right supraorbital vascular pedicle, was elevated and cautiously defatted to produce a "thinned-out" flap. The entire skin of the nasal complex was excised, sparing the skin of the columella and alar rims. The flap was insetted over the entire nasal dorsum. The donor site was able to be closed primarily with minimal tension.

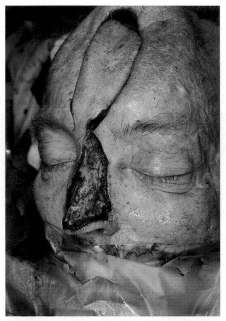

16-7D

Results (Figure 16-7, *E* and *F*)

One year after flap division and inset the patient's radiation-exposed forehead tissue provides coverage over the nasal defect. Inspection of the transposed skin has not revealed malignant changes on follow-up visits. Although delayed healing occurred along the suture seam lines, no widened scars, infection, or fibrous skin contraction have developed in this dimensional reconstruction. The forehead midline incision healed primarily without tissue loss.

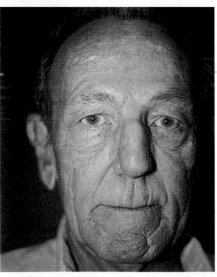

16-7E

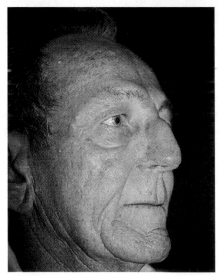

16-7F

REFERENCES

1. Gemperli R: The use of tissue expanders for induction of facial skeletal growth. Paper presented at The Third International Tissue Expansion Symposium, Sapporo, Japan, 1991.
2. Van Damme PA, Heidbuchel KL, Kuijpers-Jagtman AM, et al: Tissue expansion in aesthetic cranio-maxillo-facial surgery: experimental rationalism or clinical empiricism? Paper presented at The Third International Tissue Expansion Symposium, Sapporo, Japan, 1991.
3. Furrey JA, Manders EK, Rossi J, et al: Elongation of human peripheral nerve. Paper presented at the Soft Tissue Expansion Symposium, Hershey, Penn, March 1984.
4. Mackinnon SE: Surgical management of the peripheral nerve gap, *Clin Plast Surg* 16:587-603, 1989.
5. Mander EK, Saggers GC, Diaz-Aloneso P, et al: Elongation of peripheral nerve and viscera containing smooth muscle, *Clin Plast Surg* 14:551-562, 1987.
6. Hwang KH, Kojima T, Hirakawa M, et al: Elongation of sciatic nerve with tissue expander: report of two cases. Paper presented at The Third International Tissue Expansion Symposium, Sapporo, Japan, 1991.
7. Romo T, Jablonski RD, Shapiro AL, et al: Long-term nasal mucosal tissue expansion use in repair of large nasoseptal perforations, *Arch Otolaryngol Head Neck Surg* 121:327-331, 1995.
8. Ruiz-Razura A, Layton EG, Williams JL, et al: Clinical applications of acute intraoperative arterial elongation, *J Reconstr Microsurg* 4:6, 1993.
9. Ruiz-Razura A, Sozer SO, Layton EG, et al: Comparative study between acute intraoperative arterial elongation and the use of the interpositional vein graft for arterial reconstruction. Paper presented at 9th Annual Meeting of the American Society for Reconstructive Microsurgery, Kansas City, Mo, September 1993.
10. Argenta LC, Marks MW, Iacobucci JJ, et al: Expanded full-thickness skin grafts, *Plast Surg Forum* 11:176, 1988.
11. Bauer BS, Vicari FA, Richard ME: The role of tissue expansion in pediatric plastic surgery, *Clin Plast Surg* 17:101, 1990.
12. Felman JJ: Reconstruction of the burned face in children. In Serafin D, Georgiade NG, editors: *Pediatric plastic surgery,* St Louis, 1984, Mosby.
13. Baur BS, Vicari FA, Richard ME, et al: Expanded full-thickness skin grafts in children: case selection, planning, and management, *Plast Reconstr Surg* 92:59-69, 1993.
14. Middleton WG, Ellis DA, Trimas SJ: Expanded pectoralis major myocutaneous flaps in head and neck surgery, *J Otolaryngol* 24: 42, 1995.
15. Thornton JW, Marks MW, Izenberg PH, et al: Expanded myocutaneous flaps: their clinical use, *Clin Plast Surg* 14:529-534, 1987.
16. Hallock GG: Refinement of the radial forearm flap donor site using skin expansion, *Plast Reconstr Surg* 81:21-25, 1988.
17. Hallock GG: Free flap donor site refinement using tissue expansion, *Ann Plast Surg* 20:566, 1988.
18. Kenney JG, DiMercurio S, Angel M: Tissue expanded radial forearm free flap in neck burn contracture, *J Burn Care Rehabil* 11:443-445, 1990.
19. Forte V, Middleton WG, Briant TD: Expansion of myocutaneous flaps, *Arch Otolaryngol* 111:371, 1985.
20. Leighton WD, Russell RC, Marcus DE, et al: Experimental expansion of cutaneous and myocutaneous free flap donor sites: anatomical, physiological, and histological changes, *Plast Surg Forum* 9:262, 1986.
21. Hayward RH: Arteriosclerosis induced by radiation, *Surg Clin North Am* 52:359-366, 1972.
22. Wells FR: The lymphatic vessels in radiodermatitis: a clinical and experimental study, *Br J Plast Surg* 16:253-256, 1969.
23. Malbec EF, Quaife JV, Viegra Urquiz HA: Carcinoma complications in radiodermatitis, *Plast Reconstr Surg* 32:447-450, 1963.
24. Neuman Z, Ben-Hur N, Shulman J: The relationship between radiation injury to skin and subsequent malignant change, *Surg Gynecol Obstet* 117:559-562, 1969.
25. Robinson DW: Surgical problems in the excision and repair of radiated tissue, *Plast Reconstr Surg* 55:41-49, 1975.

17 Endoscopic Expansion Surgery

Endoscopy facilitates expansion surgery's goal of creating more tissue for reconstructive purposes.[1] Advantages include the use of mini-incisions, which may be placed away from the expansion pocket; precise endovisualization and dissection of the pocket; and minimal trauma during endoinsertion. During the interval stage of slow expansion, endodiagnosis of implant and capsule problems permits early corrective intervention so that minimal disruption occurs during the expansion process. At the final stage, endoscopic capsulotomy releases the initial expander pocket and allows more effective intraoperative expansion to gain more tissue.

Disadvantages of endoscopy include indirect contact with the tissue, reduced depth perception, restricted visual field, injury to the expander system, and additional training and equipment. Further experience is needed to weigh the benefits and complications of this new technique against those of conventional expansion techniques.[2]

INSTRUMENTS AND EQUIPMENT

Endoscopy employs the standard equipment used in tissue expansion surgery. The endoscopic system itself consists of the endotube and camera with an incorporated reliable and bright light source, the monitor, and the recording unit. An extension sheath or hood, secured on the front of the endoscope, elevates the tissues away from the lens and assists in dissection (Figure 17-1).

Different instrumentation may be required with soft tissue endoscopy to create and maintain the optical window. Expander insertion under endoscopic control is frequently hampered by soft tissue collapse around the lens and bleeding and staining within the operative field.

The use of an endosheath, umbrella, button, or small intraoperative balloon artificially opens the optical cavity to permit safe, effective dissection in the subcutaneous or submuscular plane (Figure 17-2). The use of endodissectors, scissors, graspers, and suction and irrigation systems facilitates this portion of the procedure.

INDICATIONS

The primary indication for endoscopy in expansion surgery is to aid in elevation of the soft tissue envelope so that the expander lies comfortably flat within its pocket. The port incisions are usually smaller (1 to 1.5 cm) than those made during conventional insertion of expanders. The mini-incisions are usually located away from the planned pocket to reduce implant exposure or infection. Certain anatomic circumstances favor endoscopic-assisted insertion procedures. Dissection under the periosteum or galea aponeurotica of the forehead and scalp creates an advantageous situation for endoscopy because of the glistening white, bloodless ceiling and nonencroaching calvaria. Similarly, development of a submuscular or fascial pocket is effectively performed by endoscopy because of an unobstructed visual cavity.

A second indication for endoscopy is to diagnose and correct any situation that prevents a safe, effective expansion period, including expander exposure, infection, malposition, and system failure. Endoscopy may assist in diagnosing the site of implant malfunction (e.g., valve turnover, implant leak) and can more precisely replace the defective part. Endoscopic capsulotomy may also reposition an expander that has withdrawn from its most effective area for expansion.

A third indication is to address problems at the final stage of expansion with endoscopic assistance. This may involve a more effective intraoperative expansion process using endoscopic capsulotomy.

SURGICAL TECHNIQUE

Endoinsertion

After skin preparation with Betadine paint the area is infiltrated with 0.5% lidocaine (Xylocaine) with epi-

---

Parts of this chapter were modified from Sasaki GH: Endoscopic Tissue Expansion, In Sasaki GH: Endoscopic, Aesthetic, and Reconstructive Surgery, Lippincott-Raven, 1996.

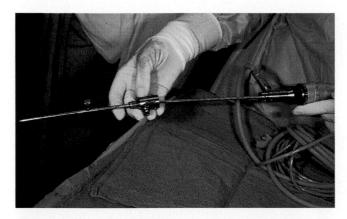

Figure 17-1 Endoscopic sheath is placed over the 4 mm endoscope to elevate the soft tissue during creation of an optical cavity.

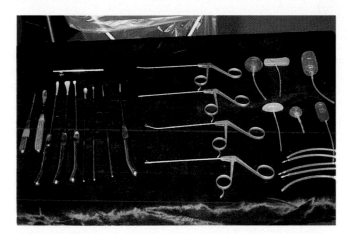

Figure 17-2 Endodissectors, scissors, and graspers are longer and narrower than conventional instruments to permit dissection through 1 to 2 mm port sites. *Upper right,* Small intraoperative expanders may be inserted through the access sites to facilitate soft tissue dissection, open the optical window, and control venous bleeding.

nephrine (1:200,000). The patient receives 1 g of cefazolin (Ancef) and 1.5 mg/kg body weight of gentamicin (Garamycin) before surgery. Two 5 to 10 mm access ports are strategically placed 3 to 5 cm apart (Figure 17-3, *A* and *B*). One port admits the 4 mm, 30-degree angle endoscope, and the other port receives any manipulator, such as a dissector or scissors. Initial dissection begins to open the optical window with elevation and release of tissues using dissectors and scissors (Figure 17-3, *C*).

The outline of the expander is marked on the skin to determine the dimensions of the pocket dissection. The pocket should be about 1 cm larger than the expander's "shoulders." If significant collapse of soft tissue occurs around the lens of the endoscope, the optical window must be kept open with an umbrella, button, intraoperative expander, or marionette sutures. Pocket irrigation with saline containing Betadine or bacitracin may be done to evacuate the pocket of blood or debris. The expander system is pretested before insertion to ensure no leakage or valve malfunction.

After balloon deflation the implant is rolled on itself and insinuated gently through one of the access ports. If this maneuver is unsuccessful, a leading edge of the deflated expander is introduced into the access port with the tip of a cotton swab. Once the balloon is inserted, the microvalve is inserted into its own pocket from one of the incision ports. The incisions are closed in layers (Figure 17-3, *D*).

Management of Defective Expander System

During serial expansion a defective expander system may not allow effective inflation to continue.

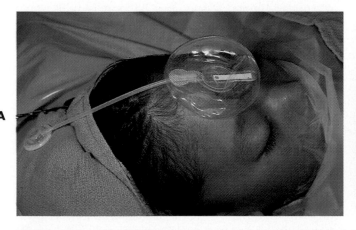

A

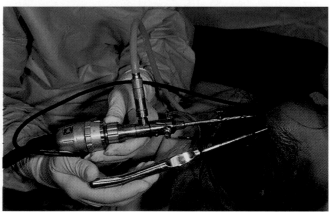

B

Figure 17-3 **A,** This 7-year-old patient received 3 × 5 cm hyperpigmented skin graft to her glabella after excision of a hemangioma. Long-term expansion was planned with insertion of a 100 cc round expander under the defect. **B,** Two 1 cm incisions were made behind the frontal hairline to permit insertion of a 4 mm scope in one port and an endodissector in the other.

Continued

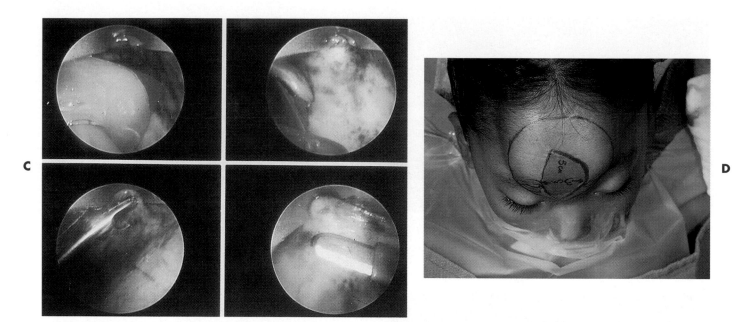

Figure 17-3, cont'd C, Endodissection was facilitated by the hood on the end of the expander. A larger optical window was created by inserting a small intraoperative expander, which was inflated and adjusted within the elevated superiosteal pocket as exposure was needed. Dissection was done with an endodissector and scissors. **D,** At completion of the procedure the deflated expander was inserted through one of the ports and intraoperatively filled to tissue tolerance with 50 ml of saline. The distant, closed small incisions permitted early postoperative expansion within a week of surgery.

Problems may involve malposition of the balloon, tubing, or valve or a balloon inappropriately positioned to stretch the donor tissue. The expander may have shifted from its original position, thus, negating any effective expansion of tissue adjacent to the defect. The tubing may be too close to the skin surface or curled on itself, partially obstructing flow. The valve may be too near the expanding balloon or overturned. All these defects may be accurately diagnosed by endoscopy and managed by capsulotomy or repositioning of the balloon, tubing, or valve. An overturned valve may be uprighted by endomanipulation with a grasper.

A defective expander system may also involve leakage from the balloon, tubing, or valve. An endoscope can confirm the leakage site, identifying which portion of the expander unit needs replacement. A leak within the balloon proper or tubing necessitates replacement with a new unit. However, an isolated valve leakage problem may require only valve replacement with an in-line connector to a new valve and its tubing.

The development of a septum between expanders prevents effective expansion. Endoscopic capsulotomy or capsulectomy removes this barrier and allows expansion to continue. The balloons are first deflated and removed from the pocket to prevent inadvertent injury to them during this corrective procedure.

Advancement of Expanded Flap

When expansion is completed, endoscopy can still help to maximize tissue recruitment during the final stage. At surgery the balloon(s) is deflated and temporarily removed from its pocket through one of the incision ports. The endoscope is inserted through this port to visualize the capsular cavity. The endoknife or dissector is inserted through the other port to perform the distal capsulotomy. After adequate flap release the balloon is reinserted. Intraoperative expansion is performed on the modified pocket to recruit additional tissue. The balloon is withdrawn from the pocket and the defect covered with the unfurled flap.

CASE RESULTS

In the author's series, 80 tissue expanders were endoscopically inserted in 50 patients. Thirty-nine patients had only one expander inserted, 13 patients received two expanders, and five had three expanders inserted at the same surgery. The expanders were positioned in most areas of the body (Table 17-1). Scalp and forehead expanders were placed under the galea aponeurotica or periosteum. The breast tissue expanders were positioned under the pectoralis muscle in delayed reconstructions. All other expanders were dissected in the subcutaneous planes.

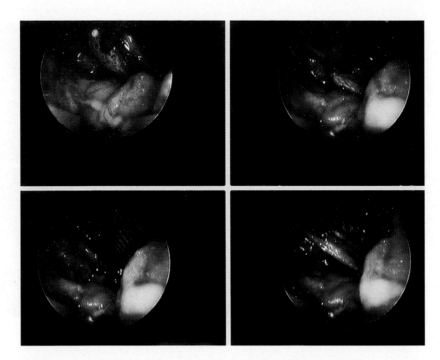

Figure 17-4 Tissue expander and its remote valve system were endoinserted in the lower extremity. An overturned valve could not be righted after insertion. Through the 1.5 cm access scar between the expander and its valve, a tract was endodissected toward the valve. The valve was grasped and overturned to its correct position.

■ **Table 17-1** Areas of Endoinsertion of 80 Expanders

Area of insertion	Number	Defect
Scalp	15	Baldness, scar, nevus
Forehead	5	Scar, nevus
Face	10	Scar, nevus, hemangioma
Neck	2	Scar
Breast	17	Postmastectomy
Trunk	17	Scar, nevus
Upper extremity	11	Scar, nevus
Lower extremity	3	Scar

■ **Table 17-2** Eight Complications After Diagnosis by Endoscopy Expander Endoinsertion

Complication	Number
Balloon malposition	2
Valve malposition	1
Balloon leakage	1
Tubing leakage	1
Valve leakage	1
Septum between expanders	2

COMPLICATIONS

Complications during endoscopic-assisted tissue expansion were negligible. Only one balloon puncture by the endoscopic dissector occurred during a capsulotomy. Skin flap injuries, hematomas, seromas, or infections were not observed after use of the endoscope.

During the expansion period, eight complications occurred with the 80 expanders, including balloon or valve malposition; leakage from the balloon, tubing, or valve; and development of a restricting septum between expanders (Table 17-2). These complications were noted and confirmed by endoscopic examination and corrected at the same time with endoscopic assistance.

The displaced balloons were repositioned closer to the defect's edge by endoscopic capsulotomy. The overturned valve was repositioned with a grasper instrument to its upright state (Figure 17-4). A major leak from the envelope required endoscopic verification and replacement of the unit (Figure 17-5, *top left*). A leak defect was noted in the tubing as it entered the valve from a needle entry (Figure 17-5, *top right*). A new valve and tubing replaced the perforated tubing. A transected tubing was identified by endoscopy as the source of deflation (Figure 17-5, *bottom left*). The tubing was shortened and attached to the metal in-line connector. Persistent leakage from the soft spot on a valve was remedied by insertion of a new valve (Figure 17-5, *bottom right*). A restricting septum was removed with an endoscopic scissors, which released the capsule for more effective expansion by the two balloons.

Figure 17-5 *Top left,* Tear in the envelope resulted in unsuccessful saline filling. A new balloon replaced the defective expander using endoinsertion through a 1.5 cm distant incision. *Top right,* Puncture of the tubing adjacent to the valve. A new valve unit replaced the original unit through an extended incision. *Bottom left,* Site of deflation from transected tubing. After endodiagnosis the tubing was shortened and attached to the metal in-line connector through an extended incision. *Bottom right,* Slow valve leak from a needle perforation of the dome produced gradual balloon decompression after each filling. After endodiagnosis a new valve replaced the damaged unit through an extended incision.

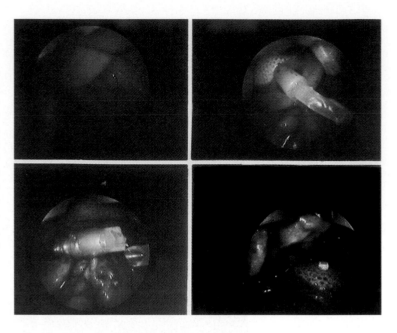

CASE REPORT AND ANALYSIS

Congenital Nevus on Left Cheek, Forehead, and Scalp

History (Figure 17-6, *A* and *B*)

This 3-year-old patient had a 16 × 20 cm congenital giant nevus on her left cheek, forehead, and frontoparietal and occipital scalp areas. The patient is shown before the insertion of expanders to remove the residual giant nevus. The forehead nevus measured 5 × 5 cm and the temporoparietal strip 4 × 7 cm. An intervening curvilinear 3 × 14 cm scar extended the area to be resurfaced by the expanded flap.

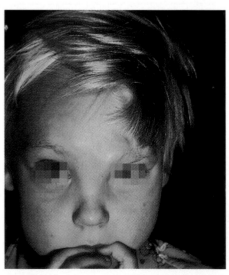

17-6A

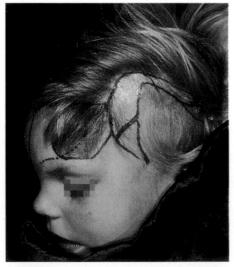

17-6B

First and Second Surgical Procedures

Initial surgical management began with the insertion of two scalp expanders through a generous paralesional incision in the frontoparietal and occipital scalp. The anterior expander became exposed and was removed about 4 weeks after insertion.

The patient was referred for further expansion management. She returned to surgery for insertion of a 640 cc rectangular expander to the forehead and frontoparietal area, a 400 cc expander to the occiput, and a 100 cc round expander to the cheek. After 4 months of serial expansion the nevus was partially removed. The remaining nevus involved the left forehead and a segment along the left temporoparietal scalp.

Third Surgical Procedure: Endoinsertion
(Figure 17-6, *C* and *D*)

Endoinsertion of a 640 cc expander under the forehead and scalp skin and a 100 cc rectangular expander under the occiput was accomplished 6 months later through two 1.5 cm incisions in the contralateral scalp (Figure 17-6, *C*). The deflated expanders were insinuated through the small incisions with a blunt plastic suction cannula and positioned in their subperiosteal pockets. The expanders were filled with saline to tissue tolerance. Endoscopic elevation of the scalp was performed in the subperiosteal plane to create pockets for each expander.

Serial expansion began 1 week after endoinsertion of the expanders (Figure 17-6, *D*). After 3 months of weekly expansions, sufficient tissue was generated to resurface the excised nevus and scar. The anterior dome flap measured 12 cm in diameter and the occipital flap 10 cm. The expanders were removed, with complete excision of the remaining nevus after 4 months of expansion. The position of the left brow was also adjusted at surgery.

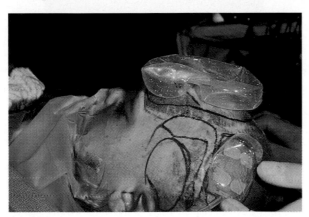

17-6C

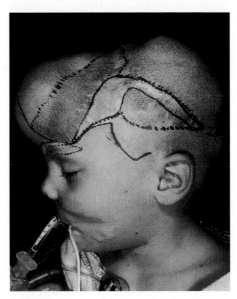

17-6D

Results (Figure 17-6, *E* and *F*)

Six months after her surgery the patient shows complete removal of the nevus. Her left brow will be adjusted later to achieve symmetry with the opposite side.

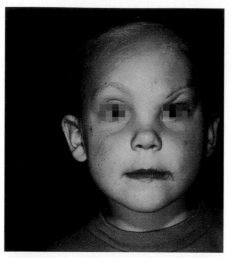

17-6E

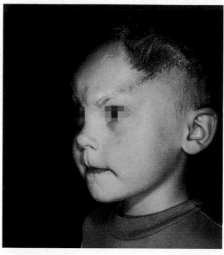

17-6F

SUMMARY

The advantages of using endoscopy during expansion surgery include the use of small incisions for insertion of expanders, diagnosis and correction of defective systems, and release of capsules before flap advancement. Small, distant access incisions permit earlier, safer expansions. Complications from endoscopy usually are minor during the expansion process.

REFERENCES

1. Anger J, Szego T: Use of videoscopy as an aid in the placement of tissue expanders, *Rev Paul Med* 111:363, 1993.
2. Sasaki GS: Tissue expansion. In Jurkiewicz MJ, Krizek TJ, Mathes SJ, Ariyan S, editors: *Plastic surgery: principles and practice,* St Louis, 1990, Mosby.

Bibliography

GENERAL REFERENCES

Argenta LC: Controlled tissue expansion in reconstructive surgery, *Br J Plast Surg* 37:520, 1984.

Argenta LC, Marks MW, Pasyk KA: Advances in tissue expansion, *Clin Plast Surg* 12:305, 1984.

Argenta LC: Controlled tissue expansion, *Surgical Rounds*, 65, 1986.

Argenta LC, Adson MH, Iacobucci JJ: Tissue expansion revisited, *Adv Plast Reconstr Surg* 4:113, 1988.

Aubert JP: *Etude clinique et experimentale de l'expansion tissulaire*, Marseille, 1987, These Medecine.

Aubert JP, Magalon G: Skin expansion. A new weapon in the therapeutic arsenal of plastic surgeons, *J Chir* 129(2):107, 1992.

Aubert JP, Magalon G: Treatment of skin lesions. Contribution of tissue expansion, *Presse Med* 22(9):417, 1993.

Bricout N: Chirurgie du sein: l'expansion cutanee. In *Medecine Sciences,* 1987, Flammarion.

Bricout N, Le Danvic D, De Roquancourt M, Banzet P: Protheses et accidents des silicones, *Ann Chir Plast Esthet* 31:268, 1986.

Clodius L: Temporary expander, *Plast Reconstr Surg* 71:279, 1983.

Davis-Boutte W, Taherpour SR, Moy RL, Kaplan B, Cohen B, Sasaki GH: Tissue expansion, *Prin Tech Cutan Surg* 44:605, 1996.

Fenton O: Expanding possibilities, *Br Med J* 295:684, 1987.

Greff A De: Tissue expansion in reconstructive surgery, *S Afr Med J* 69:705, 1986.

Hallock GG: Tissue expansion, *Contemp Surg* 29:34, 1986.

Kolkcraig A, Mc Cann JJ, Knight KR, O'Brien B: Some further characteristics of expanded tissue, *Clin Plast Surg* 14:447, 1987.

Malata CM, Williams NW, Sharpe DT: Tissue expansion: an overview, *J Wound Care* 4(1):37, 1995.

Malata CM, Williams NW, Sharpe DT: Tissue expansion: clinical applications, *J Wound Care* 4(1):37, 1995.

Malata CM, Williams NW, Sharpe DT: Tissue expansion: clinical applications, *J Wound Care* 4(2):88, 1995.

Manders EK, Mottaleb MA, Hetzler PT: Soft tissue expansion. In *Current therapy in plastic and reconstructive surgery,* vol 1, St. Louis, 1988, Mosby.

Mottaleb M, Wong RKM, Manders EK, Sasaki GH: Tissue expansion. In Riley WB, editor: *Instructional courses, vol 1: Plastic Surgery Educational Foundation,* St. Louis, 1988, CV Mosby Company.

Nordstrom REA: On tissue expansion. In *Proceedings of the 35 Cong. Nationale della Societa Italiana di Chirurgia Plastica,* Milan, 1986, Monduzzi Ed.

Nordstrom RE: Tissue expansion, *Tidsskr Nor Laegeforen* 112(14):1832, 1992.

Nosaki M, et al: Soft tissue expansion: procedures and complications, *Jap J Plast Reconstr Surg* 31:641, 1988.

Radovan C: Tissue expansion in soft tissue reconstruction, *Plast Reconstr Surg* 74:482, 1984.

Ramaswamy CN: Tissue expander for developing countries, *Plast Reconstr Surg* 82:553, 1988.

Robinson JK: Tissue expansion. A new way to achieve an old goal in dermatologic surgery, *J Dermatol Surg Oncol* 19:1063, 1993.

Sasaki GH, Berg J: Tissue expansion of the head and neck. In Krause C, editor: *Otolaryngology—head and neck surgery,* St. Louis, 1998, Mosby-Yearbook.

Sasaki GH: Tissue expansion, In Jurkiewicz MJ, Krizek TJ, Mathes SJ, Ariyan S, editors: *Plastic surgery. Principles and practice,* vol 2, St. Louis, 1990, CV Mosby Company.

Sellers DS, Miller SH, Demuth RJ: Tissue expansion as an adjunctive technique for the management of difficult wounds, *Am J Surg* 151:603, 1986.

Van Rappard JHA: Controlled tissue expansion in reconstructive surgery, *Thesis Groningen,* 1988.

Versaci AD, Balkovitch ME: Tissue expansion, In Hatal M, editor: *Advances in plastic and reconstructive surgery,* Chicago, 1984, Year Book Medical Publishers.

HISTORICAL REFERENCES

Burnett W: Yank melts native, *Nat Geogr* 88:124, 1945.

Caputo R: Ethiopia: revolution in ancient empire, *Nat Geogr* 165:614, 1983.

Chippaux C: Mutilations et deformations chroniques dans les races humaines, *Hist Med* 11:43, 1961.

Craig GT: Obituary: Radovan Ch, M.D., 1932–1984, *Plast Reconstr Surg* 77:356, 1986.

Neumann CG: The expansion of an area of skin by progressive distension of a subcutaneous balloon, *Plast Reconstr Surg* 19:121, 1957.

Weeks GS: Into the heart of Africa, *Nat Geogr* 100:257, 1956.

EXPERIMENTAL REFERENCES

Austad ED, Pasyk KA, Mc Latchey KD, Cherry GW: Histomorphologic evaluation of guinea pig skin and soft tissue after controlled tissue expansion, *Plast Reconstr Surg* 70:704, 1982.

Austad ED: The origin of expanded tissue, *Clin Plast Surg* 14:431, 1987.

Bartell TH, Mustoe TA: Animal models of human tissue expansion, *Plast Reconstr Surg* 83:681, 1989.

Belkoff SM, Naylor EC, Walshaw R, Lanigan E, Colony L, Haut RC: Effects of subcutaneous expansion on the mechanical properties of porcine skin, *J Surg Res* 58:117, 1995.

Chretien-Marquet B: Rapid intraoperative distension using isotonic saline solution, *Plast Reconstr Surg* 96:158, 1995.

Codvilla A: On the means of lengthening in the lower limbs, the muscle and tissues which are shortened through deformity, *Am J Orthop Surg* 2:353, 1905.

Codvilla A: On the means of lengthening in the lower limbs, the muscle and tissues which are shortened through deformity, *Am J Orthop Surg* 2:405, 1905.

Cohen BH, Cosmetto AJ: The suture tension adjustment reel. A new device for the management of skin closure, *J Dermatol Surg Oncol* 18:112, 1992.

Goni Moreno I: Le pneumoperitoine dans la preparation preoperatoire des grandes eventrations, *Mem Acade Chir* 96:1970.

Hirshowitz B, Kaufman T, Ulman J: Reconstruction of the tip of the nose and ala by load cycling of the nasal skin and harnessing of extra skin, *Plast Reconstr Surg* 77:716, 1986.

Hirshowitz B, Jackson IT: An attempt to harness the viscoelastic properties of skin in face lift operations. A preliminary report, *Ann Plast Surg* 18:188, 1987.

Hirshowitz B, Lindenbaum E, Har-Shai Y: A skin-stretching device for the harnessing of the viscoelastic properties of skin, Comment in: *Plast Reconstr Surg* 96(3):747, 1996, *Plast Reconstr Surg* 92(2):260, 1993.

Liang MD, Briggs P, Heckler FR, Futrell JW: Presuturing: a new technique for closing large skin defects: clinical and experimental studies, *Plast Reconstr Surg* 81:694, 1988.

Mac Guire MF: Studies of the excisional wound: biomechanical effects of undermining and wound orientation on closing tension and work, *Plast Reconstr Surg* 66:419, 1980.

Magnuson PS: Lengthening shortened bones on the leg by operation, *Univ Penn Med Bull* 103, 1908.

Matev I: Thumb reconstruction after amputation at the metacarpophalangeal joint of bone lengthening, *J Bone Joint Surg [Am]* 52A:957, 1970.

Pierard GE: Investigating the rheological properties of skin by applying a vertical pull, *Bioeng Skin* 2:31, 1980.

Putti V: The operative lengthening of the femur, *JAMA* 77:934, 1921.

Stough DB, Spencer DM, Schauder CS: New devices for scalp reduction. Intraoperative and prolonged scalp extension, *Dermatol Surg* 21(9):777, 1995.

EXPANDER SYSTEMS AND MATERIALS

Austad ED, Rose GL: A self-inflating tissue expander, *Plast Reconstr Surg* 70:107, 1982.

Clauss LC: *Biomateriaux et biocompatibilite: les silicones medicales,* Paris, 1985, These.

Cohen IK: Silicone expander with self-contained valve, *Plast Reconstr Surg* 75:279, 1985.

Dickson WA, Sharpe DT, Jackson IT: Experience with an external valve in small volume tissue expanded, *Br J Plast Surg* 41:373, 1988.

Duits HA, Molenaar J, Van Rappard JHA: The modeling of skin expander, *Plast Reconstr Surg* 83:362, 1989.

Elliott MP, Dubrul BP: Magne site tissue expander: an innovation for injection site location, *Plast Reconstr Surg* 81:605, 1988.

Frisch CE: *Biomaterials in reconstructive surgery,* Rubin L, editor: St. Louis, 1983, Mosby.

Hallock GG: Puncture threshold prior to leakage from tissue expanders reservoirs, *Plast Reconstr Surg* 82:666, 1988.

Manders EK: Used tissue expanders for developing nation: you can help, *Plast Reconstr Surg* 80:643, 1987.

Nordstrom REA: The Nordstrom system: a specially devised tissue expander. The Nordstrom flap: excision and advancement flaps. In Unger JNWP, Nordstrom REA, editors: *Hair transplantation,* ed 24, New York, 1987, Marcel Dekker.

Victor WH, Hurwitz M, Gruss JL: The development of a new tissue expander for the use in ophthalmic plastic surgery, *Ophthalmic Surg* 17:661, 1986.

PHARMACOLOGY

Liang MD, Dick GO, Narayana K: Enhancement of tissue expansion using DMSO, *Am Coll Surg Surg Forum* 38:593, 1987.

Lee P, Squier CA, Bardach J: Enhancement of tissue expansion by anticontractile agents, *Plast Reconstr Surg* 76:604, 1985.

TECHNIQUE

Argenta LC, Austad ED: Principles and techniques of tissue expansion. In McCarthy JG, editor: *Plastic surgery,* Philadelphia, 1990, WB Saunders.

Aubert JP, Paulhe P, Bardot J, Magalon G: L'apport des valves externes dans l'expansion cutanee, *Ann Chir Plast Esthet* 36:218, 1991.

Baker SR, Johnson TM, Nelson BR: Technical aspects of prolonged scalp expansion, *Arch Otolaryngol Head Neck Surg* 120:431, 1994.

Cohen IK: Lidocaine to relieve pain with tissue expansion of the breast, *Plast Reconstr Surg* 79:489, 1987.

Cuono CB: Caulking gun for tissue expansion, *Plast Reconstr Surg* 83:923, 1989.

Ditmars DM Jr: The caulking gun, an aid to inflate tissue expander prosthesis, *Plast Reconstr Surg* 72:672, 1987.

Guero SJ, Lacroix PA: An experimental model of scalp expansion: a method of optimizing flap size and shape, *Plast Reconstr Surg* 87:766, 1991.

Hallock GG, Rice DC: Objective monitoring for safe tissue expansion, *Plast Reconstr Surg* 77:416, 1986.

Hallock GG: Maximum overinflation of tissue expanders, *Plast Reconstr Surg* 80:567, 1987.

Iwahira Y, et al: An investigation of tissue expansion techniques, centering around sub-acute rapid tissue expansion, *Jpn J Plast Reconstr Surg* 31:632, 1988.

Iwahira Y, Maruyama Y: Combined tissue expansion: clinical attempt to decrease pain and shorten placement time, *Plast Reconstr Surg* 91(3):408, 1993.

Jackson J: Use of external reservoirs in tissue expansion, *Plast Reconstr Surg* 80:266, 1987.

Lawrence WT: Huber needles for tissue expander inflation, *Plast Reconstr Surg* 78:541, 1986.

Logan SE, Hayden JJ: A control unit for maximal-rate continuous tissue expansion (CTE), *Biomed Sci Instrum* 25:27, 1989.

Marks MW, Argenta LC, Thornton JW: Rapid expansion. Experimental and clinical experience, *Clin Plast Surg* 14:3, 1987.

Mustoe TA, Bartell TH, Garner WL: Physical, biomechanical, histologic and biochemical effects of rapid versus conventional tissue expansion, *Plast Reconstr Surg* 83:687, 1989.

Nahai F, McCain L: A method for the exteriorization of tissue expander tubing, *Plast Reconstr Surg* 82:723, 1988.

O'Connel HB, Chalfamian T: Use of transillumination in tissue expansion, *Plast Reconstr Surg* 83:574, 1989.

Patel PK: Estimating the tissue expander volume: a poor man's recipe, *Plast Reconstr Surg* 78:426, 1986.

Pennisi VR: Making a definitive inframammary fold under a reconstructed breast, *Plast Reconstr Surg* 60:523, 1977.

Pietila JP, Nordstrom REA, et al: Accelerated tissue-expansion with the "overfilling" technique, *Plast Reconstr Surg* 81:204, 1988.

Saouma S, Bricout N, Servant JM, Banzet P: Technique de l' expansion tissulaire, *J Chir* 126:34, 1989.

Sasaki GH: *Tissue expansion: guidelines and case analysis,* Arlington, TN, 1985, Dow Corning Wright.

Schmidt SC, Logan SE, Hayden JM, Ahn ST, Mustoe TA: Continuous versus conventional tissue expansion: experimental verification of a new technique, *Plast Reconstr Surg* 87:10, 1991.

Schneider M: Comparison of rapid versus slow tissue expansion on skin-flap viability, *Plast Reconstr Surg* 92:1126, 1993.

Sharpe DT, Palmer JH: Tissue expander tube exteriorization using a stylet, *Plast Reconstr Surg* 84:363, 1989.

Shively RE: Skin expander volume estimator, *Plast Reconstr Surg* 77:482, 1986.

Wickman M: Rapid versus slow tissue expansion for breast reconstruction: a three-year follow-up, *Plast Reconstr Surg* 95:712, 1995.

Yang CC: Pitfalls in percutaneous filling of the tissue expander, *Plast Reconstr Surg* 77:339, 1986.

HEAD AND NECK

Argenta LC, Watanabe MJ, Grabb WC, et al: Soft tissue expanders in head and neck surgery: a new method of reconstruction, *Plast Surg Forum* 4:55, 1981.

Argenta LC, Watanabe MJ, Grabb WC: Use of tissue expansion in head and neck reconstruction, *Ann Plast Surg* 11:31, 1983.

Argenta LC: Tissue expansion: tissue expansion in head and neck reconstruction. In Versacia AD, Balkowitch EM, editors: *Advances in plastic surgery,* Chicago, 1984, Year Book Publishers.

Azzolini A, Riberti C, Cavalca D: Skin expansion in head and neck reconstructive surgery, *Plast Reconstr Surg* 90:799, 1992.

Baker SR, Neil AS: Tissue expansion of the head and neck, *Arch Otolaryngol Head Neck Surg* 116:1990.

Carruthers A: Tissue expansion and Mohs micrographic surgery, *J Dermatol Surg Oncol* 19:1106, 1993.

Jackson IT, Grothaus P, Ryan: Treatment options in hemifacial atrophy, *Eur J Plast Surg* 9:22, 1986.

Magalon G, Auber JP: Apport de l'expansion dans le traitement des tumeurs malignes cutaness, *Cancer Commun* 2:413, 1988.

Manders EK: Soft tissue expansion for reconstruction in the head and neck. In: Stark RB, editor: *Plastic surgery of the head and neck,* New York, Churchill.

Marcus J, Esterly NB, Bauer BS: Tissue expansion in a patient with extensive nevus comedonicus, *Ann Plast Surg* 29(4): 362, 1992.

Morselli PG, Marconi F, Pistorale T, Cavina C: Tissue expansion in head and neck regions, *Acta Otorhinolaryngol Ital* 14:575, 1994.

Niranjan NS: Webbing of the neck: correction by tissue expansion, *Plast Reconstr Surg* 84:985, 1989.

Nordstrom REA, Pietila JP, Rintala AC: On clinical experience of tissue expansion, *Facial Plast Surg* 5:317, 1988.

Pestalardo CM, Cordero A, Jr, Ansorena JM, Bestue M, Martinho A: Acne keloidalis nuchae. Tissue expansion treatment, *Dermatol Surg* 21(8):723, 1995.

Pitanguy L: Tissue expansion and multiple partial resection. Boletin de cirurgia plastica, *Rev Bras Cir* 87:41, 1987.

Romo T 3d, Goldberg J: Versatile use of skin expanders in facial plastic surgery, *Arch Otolaryngol Head Neck Surg* 118: 333, 1992.

Shively RE, Bermant MA, Bucholz RD: Separation of craniopagus twins utilizing tissue expanders, *Plast Reconstr Surg* 76:765, 1985.

Snyder CC: Discussion about "separation of craniopagus twins utilizing tissue expanders" by Shively RE, *Plast Reconstr Surg* 76:765, 1985.

Spitz L, Stringer MD, Kiely EM, Ransley PG, Smith P: Separation of brachio-thoraco-omphalo-ischiopagus bipus conjoined twins, *J Pediatr Surg* 29:477, 1994.

Tse DT, McCafferty LR: Controlled tissue expansion in periocular reconstructive surgery, *Ophthalmology* 100(2):260, 1993.

Wieslander JB: Repeated tissue expansion in reconstruction of a huge combined scalp-forehead avulsion injury, *Ann Plast Surg* 20:1988.

SCALP

Argenta LC, Dingman RD: Total reconstruction of aplasia cutis congenita involving scalp, skull and dura, *Plast Reconstr Surg* 77:650, 1986.

Chang TS, Jin YT: Applications of tissue expansion to the treatment of post burn skin contracture and alopecia, *Eur J Plast Surg* 9:7, 1986.

Chassagne JF, Brice M, Maxant P, Flot R, Dinh-Doan G, Sticker M: Evolution des idees dans les techniques de reparation du scalp, *Ann Chir Plast Esthet* 31:325, 1986.

Dingman RO, Argenta LC: The surgical repair of traumatic defects of the scalp, *Clin Plast Surg* 9:131, 1982.

Edmond JA, Padilla JF 3rd: Preexpansion galeal scoring, *Plast Reconstr Surg* 93:5, 1087, 1994.

Laitung JKG, Brough MD, Orton CI: Scalp expansion flaps, *Br J Plast Surg* 39:542, 1986.

Leighton WD, Johnson ML, Friedland JA: Use of the temporary soft tissue expander in post traumatic alopecia, *Plast Reconstr Surg* 77:737, 1986.

Leonard AG, Small JO: Tissue expansion in the treatment of alopecia, *Br J Plast Surg* 39:42, 1986.

Manders EK, Graham WP: Alopecia reconstruction by scalp expansion, *J Dermatol Surg Oncol* 10:967, 1984.

Manders EK, Graham WP, Schenden MJ, Davis TS: Skin expansion to eliminate large scalp defects, *Ann Plast Surg* 12:305, 1984.

Nordstrom REA: Tissue expansion and flaps surgical correction of male pattern baldness, *Br J Plast Surg* 41:154, 1988.

Olshansky K: Tissue expansion in conjunction with rhytidectomy, *Plast Reconstr Surg* 85:828, 1990.

Persoff MM: Expansion-augmentation of the breast, *Plast Reconstr Surg* 91:393, 1993.

FUTURE OF EXPANSION

Cherskov M: Tissue expansion "Future of plastic surgery, for next 20 years," *JAMA* 247:3039, 1982.

Le Winn LR, Ruetschi MS: Tissue expansion: a fascinating frontier of reconstructive surgery, *Postgrad Med* 79:189, 1986.

Kojima T: Recent advance and future of plastic and reconstructive surgery, *Nippon Geka Gakkai Zasshi* 96:355, 1995.

TEXTBOOKS AND TREATISES

Magalon G, Aubert JP, Bardot J, Paulhe P: Tissue expansion, *Diffusion generale de librairie,* Marseille, 1992,

Olenius M: *The expanded skin in breast reconstruction: an experimental and clinical study,* Stockholm, 1995, Repro Print.

Index

Key: Entries followed by t refer to tables; entries in italic print refer to figures.